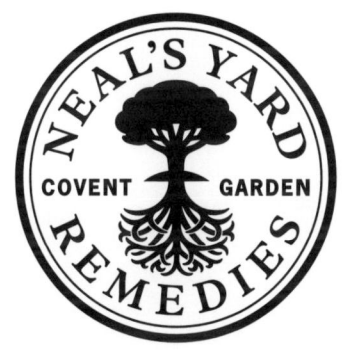

ESSENTIAL
HERBS

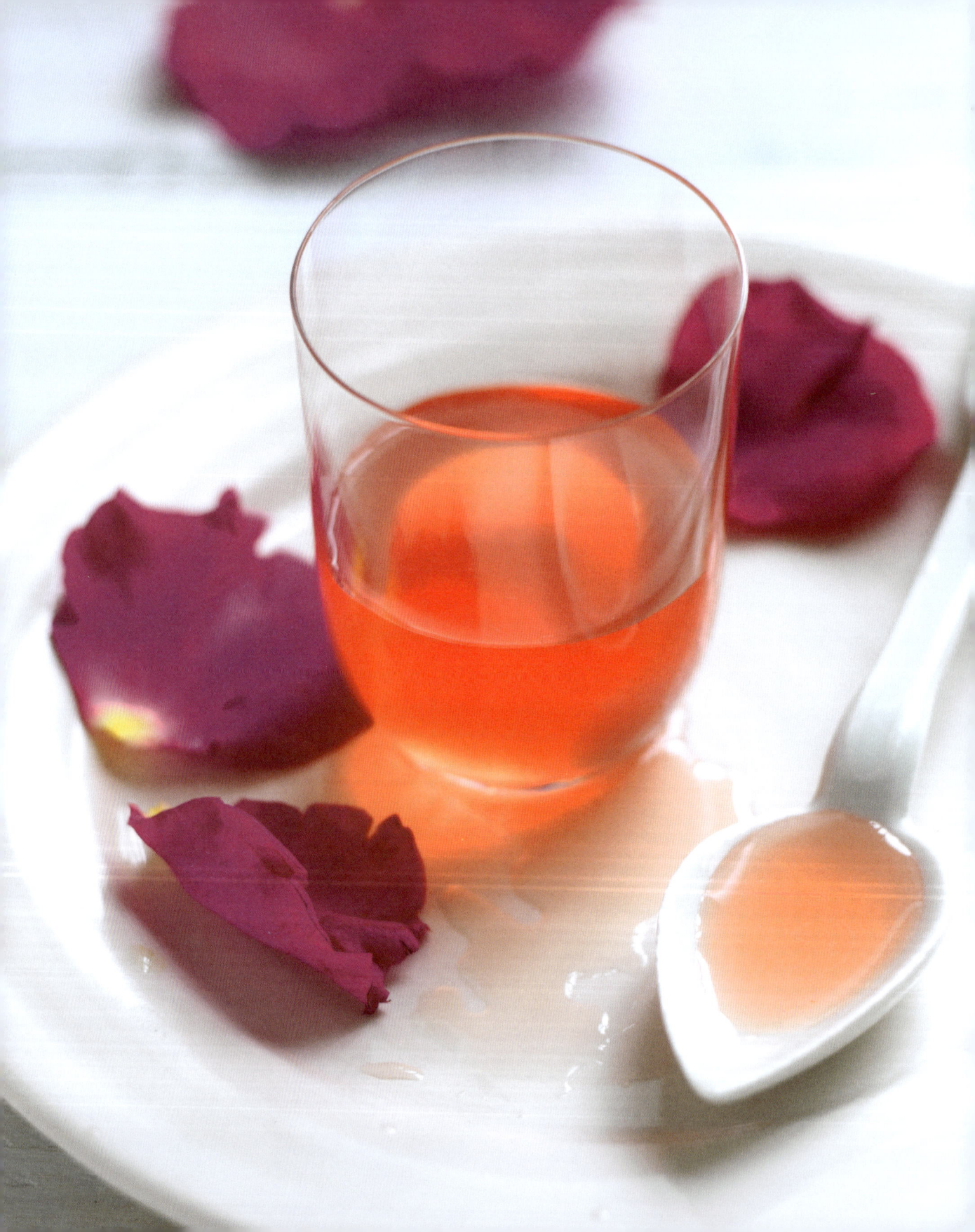

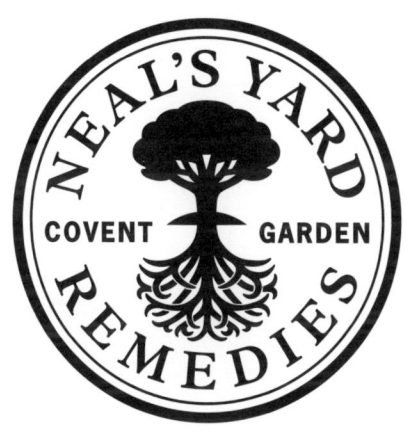

ESSENTIAL
HERBS

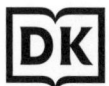

CONTENTS

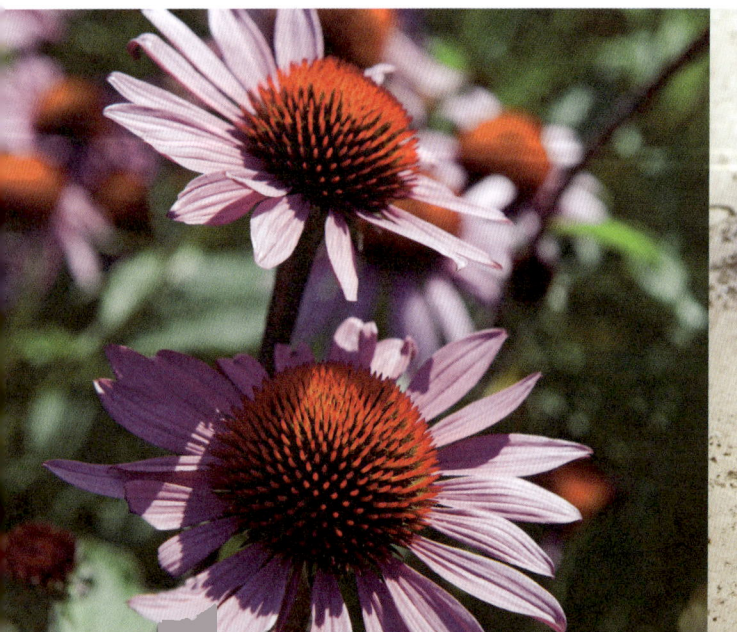

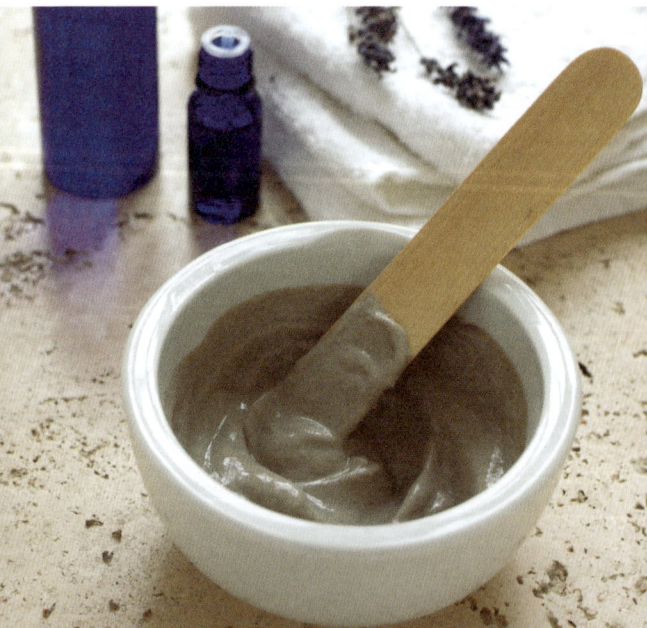

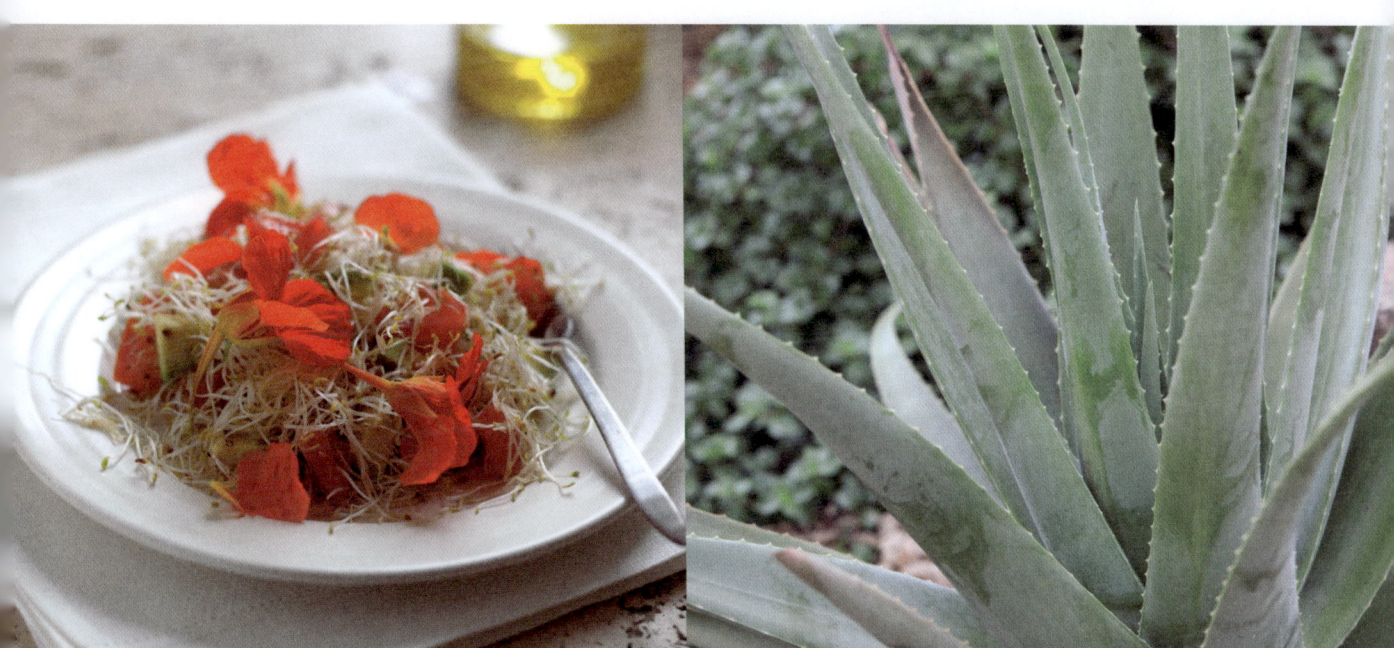

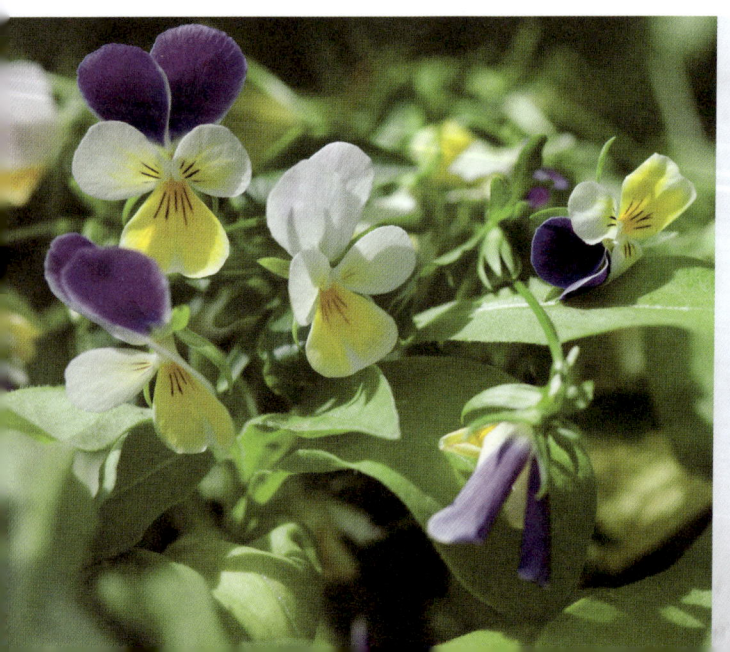
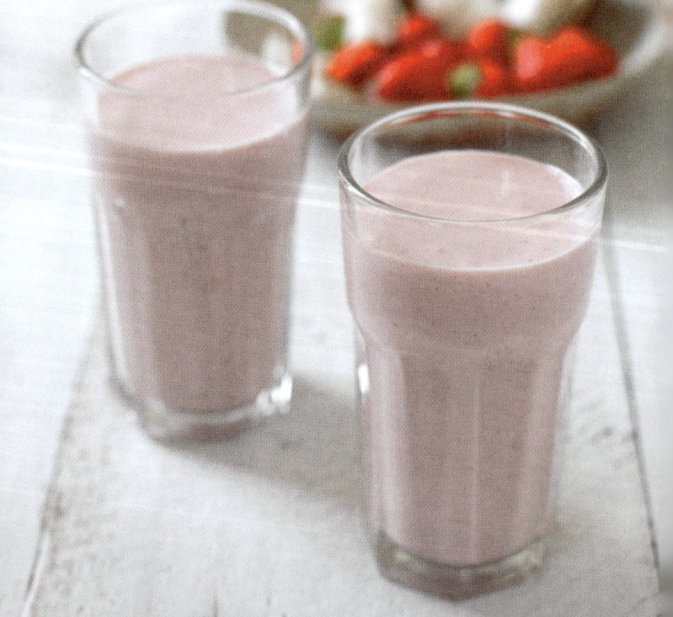

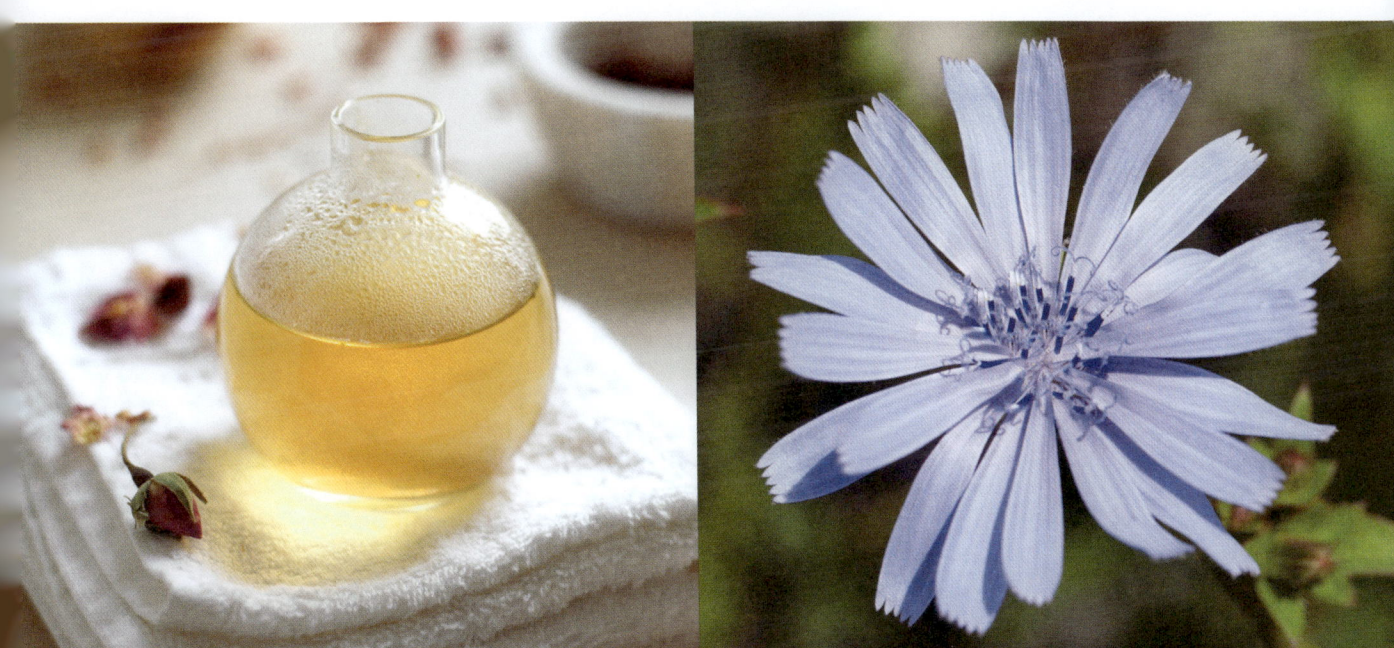

INTRODUCTION

According to the World Health Organization, herbal remedies are the most widespread system of medicine used in the world. In many developed countries that knowledge was almost lost, but the last couple of decades have seen a renewed interest in herbal remedies, and more and more people are recognizing the many benefits of using them to treat themselves and their family.

Used appropriately, herbs can be a satisfying part of a more holistic lifestyle, and many herbs are of course the starting point of much of the modern medicine used today. When used with common sense, herbal remedies are a safe and effective form of home help. If we can treat colds, flu, or minor injuries in the early stages we can often prevent the development of something more serious and avoid using conventional drugs with their risk of side-effects

Learning which herbs work for us enables us to learn more about the plants that surround us, as well as our own healing processes. However, some herbs are not suitable for everyone or at every stage of life (during pregnancy, for example); if in any doubt you should always consult a medical practitioner.

We have "tried and tested" all the recipes in this book, so we can promise they are delicious as well as being good for you. We are excited to have the opportunity to introduce you to some more unusual plants and flavors so you can be more adventurous while trusting that your health and well-being will benefit.

Neal's Yard Remedies has over thirty years of expertise and passion in creating wonderful, natural hair and skin care products and we are delighted to share some of our favorite ways of using herbs to heal and nurture your skin. Enjoy creating and using your own herbal remedies!

Susan Curtis, Natural Health Director,
Neal's Yard Remedies

CONSULTANT'S NOTE

Hippocrates, the father of medicine, wrote: "Let food be thy medicine, and medicine be thy food." Many herbs described in this book are used both as tasty foods and as medicines, and the delicious recipes provide new ideas for combining healthy ingredients. Although the herbal medicines have not yet all been researched by modern science, most have stood the test of time. You should always see your doctor for serious health problems, but I hope this book will help readers treat and prevent minor illnesses, and understand treatments prescribed by their herbalist.

Dr. Merlin Willcox MRCGP MCPP

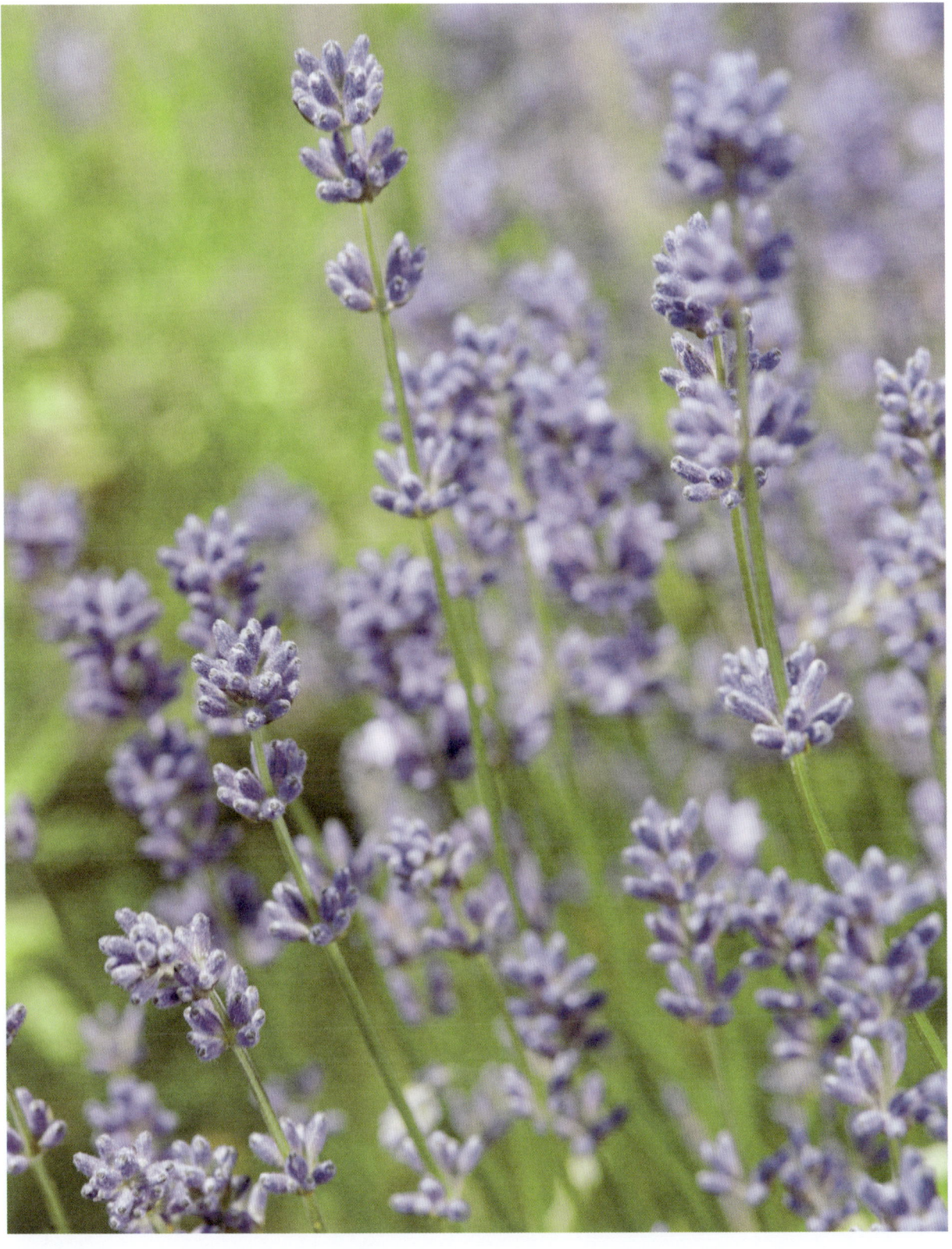

REMEDY CHOOSERS

This chapter is designed to help you find a selection
of herbs to treat a range of ailments quickly and easily.
Use the charts in conjunction with the A–Z (pp.34–171)
to choose the best remedies for your needs.

SKIN, HAIR & NAILS

Our skin acts as a physical barrier between our bodies and the world around us. The herbs shown in this chart all help alleviate skin-related ailments, along with those more closely associated with hair and nails. For long-term skin, hair, and nail health, maintain a healthy diet and manage possible underlying factors (see opposite).

Common name	BURDOCK	OATS	CALENDULA	GOTU KOLA	HORSETAIL	ST. JOHN'S WORT	LAVENDER
Scientific name	*Arctium lappa*	*Avena sativa*	*Calendula officinalis*	*Centella asiatica*	*Equisetum arvense*	*Hypericum perforatum*	*Lavandula angustifolia*
How to use	Take as a decoction of the root or as a powder.	Take as an infusion, apply to skin as a scrub or tincture, or use as a decoction in the bath.	Take as an infusion, or apply to skin as a powder, lotion, ointment, or tincture.	Take as an infusion, or apply to skin as a powder, lotion, ointment, or tincture.	Take as a decoction or apply to skin as a paste.	Take as an infusion or tincture, or apply to skin as a macerated oil.	Take as an infusion, dilute essential oil, or apply to skin as a lotion or in an ointment.
SKIN — ACNE	✓	✓	✓	✓			✓
ATHLETE'S FOOT	✓					✓	
ECZEMA	✓	✓	✓	✓	✓	✓	✓
HIVES							
INSECT BITES							✓
PSORIASIS	✓	✓	✓			✓	
ROSACEA			✓	✓			
HAIR & NAILS — BRITTLE NAILS				✓	✓		
DAMAGED HAIR					✓		✓
DANDRUFF			✓				
FUNGAL NAIL INFECTION			✓				
Caution		Use gluten-free oats if gluten intolerant (see p.59 for full guidance).	Avoid internal use during pregnancy.	Do not take for more than 6 weeks without a break. Can cause sensitivity to light.	Avoid if taking diuretics or lithium. Do not use for more than 4 weeks continuously without medical guidance (see p.76 for further advice).	Avoid during pregnancy. May interact with prescription medication; seek professional guidance before using (see p.92 for full guidance).	

NOTES

• Identifying possible underlying causes of skin, hair, and nail ailments is key to managing symptoms. Make sure your diet includes plenty of vitamins and minerals, reduce sugar intake, and drink plenty of water. Other factors, such as emotions, sleep, hormones, genetic factors, and sun exposure, may also play a part.

• For severe or long-lasting symptoms, seek medical advice.

• Unless otherwise stated, all tinctures and essential oils are diluted as advised in the herb's A–Z entry. For further guidance, see pp.176–177.

• If you are or may be pregnant, check herbs in the A–Z (pp.34–171) to ensure that they are safe for use.

• Test any external treatments on a small patch of skin before using to check for any possible adverse reaction.

CHAMOMILE	ROSEMARY	CHICKWEED	THYME	RED CLOVER	NETTLE	SUPPORTING ADVICE
Matricaria recutita	*Rosmarinus officinalis*	*Stellaria media*	*Thymus vulgaris*	*Trifolium pratense*	*Urtica dioica*	
Take as an infusion, or apply to skin as a tincture.	Take as an infusion or tincture, dilute essential oil, or add to lotion or ointment.	Take as an infusion, apply maceration to skin, or add to a cream or ointment.	Take as an infusion, dilute essential oil and apply to skin in a lotion.	Take as an infusion, or apply to skin as a lotion or in an ointment.	Take leaf as an infusion.	
✓				✓	✓	Take equal parts burdock root, red clover, gotu kola, and echinacea as a tea or tincture. Exfoliate twice weekly, cleanse with witch hazel, and moisturize.
✓			✓		✓	Calendula can be taken both internally (as a tincture or tea) or externally (p.300). Neem soap (p.301) and foot balm (p.321) can also provide relief.
✓		✓		✓	✓	Combine lavender and chamomile essential oils (p.177) to treat inflamed skin. Use chickweed to relieve itching. Avoid potential stressors.
✓					✓	Chamomile and nettle act as antihistamines. Take either herb as a tea or tincture, or apply externally.
			✓	✓	✓	Apply lavender oil undiluted onto the bite to reduce itching.
✓		✓		✓		Psoriasis can be exacerbated by stress (pp.30–31).
✓	✓		✓	✓		Apply clay masks, such as witch hazel and lavender (p.313) or rose (p.316), to cleanse and tighten pores, followed by a toner (pp.309–310) to regulate sebum. Rosacea can be exacerbated by stress (pp.30–31).
	✓					Soak horsetail leaves in apple cider vinegar for 2–3 weeks, then strain and use as a nail soak twice a week.
	✓			✓		Use lavender and rosemary conditioner (pp.340–341).
	✓		✓		✓	Use a thyme and cider rinse (p.338).
			✓			Combine calendula with pau d'arco as a tea or tincture. Internal treatments for athlete's foot (see above) may also help.
Avoid if allergic to the Compositae (daisy) family.	Avoid taking therapeutic doses during pregnancy.	May cause nausea and vomiting if taken in large amounts.	Avoid taking therapeutic doses during pregnancy (a small amount in food is fine; see p.148 for full guidance).	Avoid during pregnancy. May interact with blood-thinning medication; seek professional guidance before using.		

DIGESTION & GUT HEALTH

Gut health is closely linked to our overall well-being, so it is important to keep the digestive system in good working order. This chart includes herbs that can stimulate or calm digestion, along with those that support healthy gut bacteria. These herbs may be taken together or individually to treat mild ailments and discomfort as and when required.

Common name	MARSH-MALLOW	CHICORY	GLOBE ARTICHOKE	MEADOW-SWEET	FENNEL	LICORICE	CHAMOMILE
Scientific name	*Althaea officinalis*	*Cichorium intybus*	*Cynara cardunculus*	*Filipendula ulmaria*	*Foeniculum vulgare*	*Glycyrrhiza glabra*	*Matricaria recutita*
How to use	Add to food or take as capsules, infusion, or tincture.	Add to food or take as an infusion or tincture.	Add to food or take as capsules or infusion.	Take as an infusion or fluid extract.	Add to food or take as an infusion, tincture or decoction.	Add to food or take as capsules, infusion, or tincture.	Take as an infusion or tincture.
AILMENTS							
BAD BREATH	✓	✓	✓		✓		
BLOATING	✓	✓	✓		✓		✓
CONSTIPATION		✓	✓		✓	✓	
CRAMPING				✓	✓		✓
DIARRHEA				✓			
GASTRITIS	✓			✓		✓	✓
IBS	✓	✓	✓	✓			✓
INDIGESTION	✓		✓	✓	✓	✓	✓
LIVER DISORDERS		✓	✓				
NAUSEA		✓	✓	✓			
PREBIOTICS	✓	✓	✓				
STOMACH ACHE							✓
STOMACH ULCERS	✓			✓		✓	✓
TRAPPED GAS				✓	✓		
Caution				Avoid during pregnancy, if taking blood thinners, or if sensitive to aspirin.	Essential oil should not be taken internally except under professional advice.	Avoid if taking blood pressure medication. Avoid during pregnancy (see p.86 for full guidance).	Avoid if allergic to the Compositae (daisy) family.

NOTES

• If symptoms do not clear up in a couple of days, or if you experience any severe symptoms, such as difficulty swallowing, bleeding, persistent change in bowel function, or sudden weight loss, seek medical advice immediately.

• Unless otherwise stated, all tinctures and essential oils are diluted as advised in the herb's A–Z entry. For further guidance, see pp.176–177.

• If you are or may be pregnant, check herbs in the A–Z (pp.34–171) to ensure that they are safe for use.

LEMON BALM	PEPPERMINT	SENNA	DANDELION	SLIPPERY ELM	GINGER	SUPPORTING ADVICE
Melissa officinalis	*Mentha x piperita*	*Senna alexandrina*	*Taraxacum officinale*	*Ulmus rubra*	*Zingiber officinale*	
Take as an infusion.	Take as an infusion or as a tea.	Take as an infusion, tincture, powder, or capsules.	Take root as a decoction or tincture.	Take as a powder, as capsules or lozenges, or mixed into a paste.	Add to food, or take as a decoction or tincture.	
	✓					Gargle peppermint or ginger tea to treat any possible infection. Other herbs shown here all help support the health of the mouth's microbiome, reducing the likelihood of bad breath in future.
	✓				✓	Drink fennel and peppermint tea 2-3 times a day and eat fermented foods (p.250) to support healthy gut bacteria, which can help reduce bloating.
		✓	✓			Eat high-fiber foods and drink plenty of fluids, including relaxing chamomile tea.
✓	✓				✓	Use a hot water bottle. Drink chamomile, fennel, and meadowsweet tea to help reduce symptoms.
				✓		Drink plenty of fluids to ensure electrolyte balance.
✓	✓			✓	✓	Avoid medications like aspirin as they can irritate the gut lining and make symptoms worse.
	✓	✓	✓	✓		See above for remedies for IBS-related bloating and cramping.
✓	✓			✓	✓	Avoid tea, coffee, alcohol, spicy foods, and eating late at night. Smoking and stress (pp.30–31) can also exacerbate symptoms.
			✓			Combine dandelion root with milk thistle as a tincture or capsules; together, these act as a liver tonic, stimulating bile flow and offering a mild laxative effect.
✓	✓		✓		✓	Drink an infusion of lemon and ginger in hot water in the morning to reduce nausea and support digestion.
						The roots of these herbs all have a prebiotic effect, supporting a healthy gut and immune system which, in turn, encourages brain health.
	✓					Combine chamomile and fennel as a tea or tincture.
						Smoking, alcohol, stress (pp.30–31), and a poor diet can all exacerbate symptoms.
	✓					
	Do not use essential oil for children under five.	See p.137 for full safety guidance.	Use under medical supervision if suffering from gallstones.		Avoid if taking blood-thinning medication (see p.170 for full guidance).	

CIRCULATION

Herbal remedies can be used alongside a heart-healthy diet and plenty of exercise to support and strengthen the cardiovascular system. These remedies are intended to help prevent illness and treat mild symptoms; for sudden cardiac issues or if symptoms are severe, seek medical advice immediately.

	YARROW	GARLIC	CAYENNE OR CHILE PEPPER	HAWTHORN	GINKGO	WITCH HAZEL	OLIVE
Common name							
Scientific name	Achillea millefolium	Allium sativum	Capsicum annuum	Crataegus laevigata	Ginkgo biloba	Hamamelis virginiana	Olea europaea
How to use	Take as an infusion or tincture.	Add to food, or take as powder or capsules.	Add to food, or add drops of tincture to an ointment and apply externally.	Take as an infusion or tincture.	Take as an infusion, capsules, or tincture.	Take as an infusion or apply distillate, ointment, or cream.	Take leaf as an infusion, tincture, or as capsules.
ANEMIA				✓			
CHILBLAINS			✓		✓		
COLD EXTREMITIES			✓		✓		
FLUID RETENTION							
HIGH BLOOD PRESSURE	✓	✓		✓			✓
HIGH CHOLESTEROL		✓					✓
LOW BLOOD PRESSURE			✓				
PILES	✓					✓	
PALPITATIONS				✓			
VARICOSE VEINS					✓	✓	
Caution	Avoid during pregnancy. Can lower blood pressure (see p.36 for full guidance).	Do not use if taking blood-thinning medication (see p.43 for full guidance).	Avoid touching the eyes or any cuts after handling. Wash hands thoroughly after use.	Seek professional advice before use (see p.68 for full guidance).	Seek professional advice if taking blood pressure medication or any other prescribed medication.		High doses of olive oil (1–4 tbsp) can have a laxative effect.

AILMENTS (row-group label)

NOTES

• Family history, smoking, obesity, alcohol consumption, and physical inactivity can all increase the risk of cardiovascular issues. Minimize the risks by maintaining a healthy diet and a doctor-recommended exercise program.

• If you experience symptoms of angina, or if symptoms are otherwise severe, seek medical advice immediately.

• Unless otherwise stated, all tinctures and essential oils are diluted as advised in the herb's A–Z entry. For further guidance, see pp.176–177.

• If you are or may be pregnant, check herbs in the A–Z (pp.34–171) to ensure that they are safe for use.

	ROSEMARY	DANDELION	LINDEN	NETTLE	CRAMP BARK	GINGER	SUPPORTING ADVICE
	Rosmarinus officinalis	*Taraxacum officinale*	*Tilia cordata*	*Urtica dioica*	*Viburnum opulus*	*Zingiber officinalis*	
	Take as an infusion or use as essential oil.	Take leaf as an infusion or tincture.	Take as an infusion or tincture.	Take as an infusion or tincture.	Take as a tincture.	Add to food or take as capsules.	
				✓			Increase the amount of vitamin C in your diet (p.180, p.208); this will boost the body's ability to absorb iron.
						✓	Drink ginkgo and ginger together as a warming tea, or add a few drops of chile tincture and ginger essential oil to an ointment or rub.
						✓	Drink ginkgo and ginger together as a warming tea. Wear gloves and socks. Apply heat pads.
		✓		✓			Drink dandelion leaf tea; dandelion is high in potassium and acts as a diuretic, helping to lower high blood pressure (exacerbated by fluid retention) and reduce swelling around the ankles.
	✓	✓	✓	✓	✓		Combine yarrow, hawthorn, and linden as a tea. Identify possible causes, such as diet (high in fat and salt) and stress (pp.108–109). Seek professional advice before taking herbal remedies for high blood pressure.
						✓	Eat a Mediterranean diet, including foods like globe artichokes, along with anti-inflammatory foods such as ginger and oats.
							Chile (added to food or taken as a tincture) and licorice (taken as a tea) both act as stimulants, helping raise blood pressure.
					✓		Combining dandelion root with milk thistle as a tea or tincture can help keep bowels soft. Alternatively, eat 1 tbsp flaxseeds (soaked overnight) each morning for a similar result.
			✓				Hawthorn and linden can both help strengthen the heart; combine with motherwort and lemon balm if the palpitations are caused by anxiety (pp.30–31) or an overactive thyroid.
	✓						
	Avoid taking therapeutic doses during pregnancy.	Use under medical supervision if suffering from gallstones.	Avoid during pregnancy. Seek professional guidance before taking for high blood pressure.		Avoid during pregnancy or while breastfeeding except under professional supervision.	Avoid if taking blood-thinning medication, or if suffering from peptic ulcers or gallstones.	

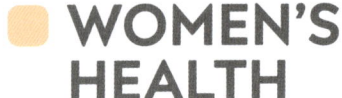

WOMEN'S HEALTH

The ever-changing bodily rhythms of puberty, fertility, and menopause can bring with them a wide range of needs and challenges. This chart includes a selection of key herbs that can help you cope with these different issues using natural remedies.

	Common name	BLACK COHOSH	LADY'S MANTLE	DANG GUI	BEARBERRY	WILD YAM	ST. JOHN'S WORT	LEMON BALM
	Scientific name	*Actaea racemosa*	*Alchemilla xanthochlora*	*Angelica sinensis*	*Arctostaphylos uva-ursi*	*Dioscorea villosa*	*Hypericum perforatum*	*Melissa officinalis*
	How to use	Take as an infusion, decoction, or capsules.	Take as an infusion or tincture.	Take as an infusion, tincture, or capsules.	Take as an infusion or tincture.	Take as an infusion, tincture, or capsules.	Take as an infusion, tincture, or capsules.	Take as an infusion, tincture, or capsules.
AILMENTS	BLADDER PROBLEMS				✓	✓		
	HEAVY PERIOD		✓					
	HOT FLASHES	✓		✓		✓		
	INFERTILITY			✓				
	MENOPAUSAL SYMPTOMS	✓		✓		✓		✓
	PMS		✓	✓			✓	✓
	PERIOD PAIN	✓		✓		✓		✓
	Caution	Avoid during pregnancy. See p.38 for full guidance.		Avoid taking during heavy periods as the herb can enhance blood flow.	Avoid during pregnancy, while breastfeeding, or if suffering from kidney disease. See p.56 for full guidance.	Saponin (a chemical compound found in wild yam) may cause nausea in sensitive individuals.	Avoid during pregnancy. May interact with prescription medication (including the contraceptive pill). See p.92 for full guidance.	

NOTES

• Family history, environmental factors, sugar consumption, thyroid health, and stress levels all play a role in fluctuating hormones and symptoms.

• The herbs in this chart can be taken as and when needed, or regularly to improve the overall condition. For persistent problems, consult an experienced herbalist. If symptoms worsen, seek medical advice.

• Unless otherwise stated, all tinctures and essential oils are diluted as advised in the herb's A–Z entry. For further guidance, see pp.176–177.

• If you are or may be pregnant, check herbs in the A–Z (pp.34–171) to ensure that they are safe for use.

RASPBERRY LEAF	SAGE	SCHISANDRA	RED CLOVER	CRAMP BARK	AGNUS CASTUS	SUPPORTING ADVICE
Rubus idaeus	*Salvia officinalis*	*Schisandra chinensis*	*Trifolium pratense*	*Viburnum opulus*	*Vitex agnus-castus*	
Take as an infusion or tincture.	Take as an infusion, tincture, or capsules.	Take as an infusion or tincture.	Take as an infusion, tincture, or capsules.	Take as an infusion or tincture.	Take as a tincture or decoction.	
		✓		✓		See p.180, p.201, and p.227 for recipes that support the urinary system.
✓		✓		✓	✓	Take either lady's mantle or raspberry leaf in the first instance to help reduce bleeding, as both herbs have astringent properties. Blood loss may result in a lack of energy; increase iron intake (through diet, herbs, or supplements) if that is the case.
	✓	✓	✓			All the herbs listed contain plant-based estrogens, which help reduce menopausal sweating; sage may be the best option given its wide availability.
✓					✓	Avoid caffeine. Use stress-reducing remedies (pp.30–31). A good diet, including plenty of vitamins B6 and E, fatty acids, and zinc, can help. Difficulty with conception can be due to a number of factors; consult your medical provider for advice and support.
	✓	✓			✓	Combine black cohosh, dang gui, schisandra, sage, and angus castus as a tea or tincture to help ease menopausal symptoms and strengthen the nervous system. See above for advice relating to hot flashes.
		✓	✓		✓	Combine anxiety-reducing herbs (pp.30–31) with dang gui and angus castus as a tincture to help reduce PMS-related symptoms. Evening primrose and multivitamins containing vitamins B6 and C, zinc, chromium, and calcium can also be helpful. For acne, see pp.12–13. For fluid retention, see pp.16–17.
✓		✓	✓	✓		Prepare a massage oil using one of the herbs shown and massage abdomen. A cramp bark tincture, taken 3–4 times daily, can help relieve discomfort from menstrual cramps. Evening primrose can also provide relief. Increase intake of vitamin B6.
Avoid during early stages of pregnancy; use only in third trimester.	Avoid taking therapeutic doses during pregnancy or if epileptic.	Avoid during pregnancy, or if suffering from feverish chills or conditions involving heat. Large doses may cause heartburn.	Avoid during pregnancy, or while suffering feverish chills or conditions involving heat. Large doses may cause heartburn.	Avoid during pregnancy or while breastfeeding except under professional supervision.	Avoid if taking progesterone drugs and during pregnancy except under professional supervision. See p.166 for full guidance.	

MEN'S HEALTH

With evidence suggesting that men are more reluctant than women to visit their doctor when they have a health issue, the herbs shown here can offer an alternative form of treatment for a range of male-specific ailments. For severe or long-lasting issues, however, it is always advisable to speak to a medical professional.

Common name	GOTU KOLA	GINKGO	ST. JOHN'S WORT	GOJI	JAPANESE GINSENG	SCHISANDRA
Scientific name	*Centella asiatica*	*Ginkgo biloba*	*Hypericum perforatum*	*Lycium barbarum*	*Panax japonicus*	*Schisandra chinensis*
How to use	Take as an infusion, or apply to skin as a maceration.	Take as an infusion, tincture, or capsules.	Take as an infusion, tincture, or capsules.	Add to food, or take as a tincture or capsules.	Take as a decoction, tincture, or capsules.	Take as an infusion, tincture, or capsules.
AILMENTS — BLADDER URGENCY			✓			
ERECTILE DYSFUNCTION	✓	✓		✓	✓	
INFERTILITY						
LOW LIBIDO	✓			✓	✓	✓
MALE PATTERN BALDNESS	✓					
PROSTATE ENLARGEMENT						
Caution	Do not take for more than 6 weeks without a break. Can cause sensitivity to light.	Seek professional advice if taking blood pressure medication or any other prescribed medication.	Avoid during pregnancy. May interact with prescription medication. See p.92 for full guidance.	Avoid during colds or flu, if suffering from diarrhea, or if digestion is poor.	Do not take with drinks containing caffeine.	Avoid if suffering from feverish chills or conditions involving heat. Large doses may cause heartburn.

NOTES

Family history, environmental factors, sugar consumption, thyroid health, and stress levels all play a role in fluctuating hormones and symptoms.

• The herbs in this chart can be taken as and when needed, or regularly to improve the overall condition.

• For persistent problems, consult an experienced herbalist. If symptoms worsen, seek medical advice.

• Unless otherwise stated, all tinctures and essential oils are diluted as advised in the herb's A–Z entry. For further guidance, see pp.176–177.

SAW PALMETTO	PAU D'ARCO	DAMIANA	NETTLE	ASHWAGANDHA	SUPPORTING ADVICE
Serenoa repens	*Tabebuia impetiginosa*	*Turnera diffusa*	*Urtica dioica*	*Withania somnifera*	
Take as a tincture or capsules.	Take as a decoction, tincture, or capsules.	Take as an infusion or tincture.	Take root as a decoction.	Take as an infusion, tincture, or capsules.	
✓					Combine saw palmetto with bearberry and echinacea in a tincture to help treat bladder infections. This remedy can be used with treatments for prostate enlargement (see below), which can also be a cause of bladder urgency.
				✓	Gotu kola, ginkgo, goji, and Japanese ginseng all act as stimulants, and can be taken either as a tea or tincture. Relaxants like ashwagandha or valerian can also help counter psychological or physical causes of erectile dysfunction, depending on the individual.
✓		✓			These herbs help to both stimulate the male reproductive system and restore the nerves, reducing anxiety. A good diet, including plenty of vitamins B6 and E, fatty acids, and zinc, plays an important role in sperm formation.
✓		✓		✓	Combine saw palmetto and ashwagandha as a tincture to enhance sexual stamina. Maca can also invigorate the body (p.182).
✓			✓		In addition to the herbs listed, rosemary-based conditioners and oils (p.340, p.342) can enhance hair growth. Zinc (found in pumpkin seeds) can also help.
✓	✓		✓		Combine saw palmetto and nettle root as a tincture or as capsules in the first instance. Zinc can also help treat prostate enlargement.
May interfere with blood-thinning medication; seek professional guidance before using.	Large doses may cause nausea or gastrointestinal upset.	May reduce iron absorption.			

COUGHS & COLDS

Early treatment is the key to preventing coughs, colds, and flu from becoming too serious or developing complications. This chart is not comprehensive, but it does contain key herbs that boost the immune system, including garlic and echinacea, along with those that can help combat a fever and reduce catarrh.

Common name	YARROW	GARLIC	MARSH-MALLOW	ECHINACEA	EUCALYPTUS	LICORICE	HYSSOP
Scientific name	*Achillea millefolium*	*Allium sativum*	*Althaea officinalis*	*Echinacea purpurea*	*Eucalyptus globulus*	*Glycyrrhiza glabra*	*Hyssopus officinalis*
How to use	Take as an infusion or tincture.	Add to food, or take as a tincture or capsules.	Take leaf as an infusion or root as a maceration.	Take as an infusion, decoction, or tincture.	Take as an inhalation in steam, or rub salve on chest.	Take as a decoction, syrup, or tincture, or drink diluted in a tincture.	Take as an infusion, tincture, syrup, or macerated oil as a chest rub.
BRONCHITIS		✓	✓		✓	✓	✓
CATARRH		✓	✓	✓	✓		✓
CHEST INFECTION		✓		✓	✓	✓	
COLDS	✓	✓		✓	✓		
COUGH: CHESTY		✓		✓	✓	✓	✓
COUGH: DRY		✓	✓			✓	
FEVER	✓			✓			✓
FLU	✓	✓		✓	✓	✓	✓
WHOOPING COUGH		✓	✓	✓	✓	✓	✓
Caution	Avoid during pregnancy. Can lower blood pressure (see p.36 for full guidance).	Can cause gastric irritation in some people (see p.43 for full guidance).		High doses can occasionally cause nausea and dizziness.	Do not use oil on babies or very young children. Avoid taking the essential oil internally (see p.77 for full guidance).	Avoid if taking blood pressure medication. Avoid during pregnancy (see p.86 for full guidance).	Avoid during pregnancy. In high doses the essential oil can trigger epileptic seizures; speak to a medical professional before using.

AILMENTS

NOTES

• The herbs shown in this chart all work best if you take the opportunity to rest and reduce excess stress in your life while you recover.

• If symptoms become serious or do not clear up in a couple of days, seek medical advice.

• Unless otherwise stated, all tinctures and essential oils are diluted as advised in the herb's A–Z entry. For further guidance, see pp.176–177.

• If you are or may be pregnant, check herbs in the A–Z (pp.34–171) to ensure that they are safe for use.

ELECAMPANE	RIBWORT PLANTAIN	ELDERBERRY	ELDERFLOWER	THYME	MULLEIN	SUPPORTING ADVICE
Inula helenium	*Plantago lanceolata*	*Sambucus nigra*	*Sambucus nigra*	*Thymus vulgaris*	*Verbascum thapsus*	
Take as a decoction, tincture, or syrup.	Take as an infusion and a juice, or use diluted in a tincture or syrup.	Take as a decoction, syrup, or tincture.	Take as an infusion or gargle.	Take as an infusion or syrup, gargle, or use the essential oil in a chest rub.	Take as an infusion or tincture.	
✓	✓			✓	✓	Combine hyssop macerated oil with eucalyptus and thyme essential oils to use as a chest rub (see p.94).
✓	✓			✓	✓	Combine equal parts hyssop, thyme, and mullein with honey to make a syrup. This can help soothe lungs, loosen phlegm, and clear mucus.
		✓		✓		Try echinacea-based recipes (see p.213 and pp.222–223); the antibacterial herbs used in these recipes (which also include elder and thyme) help support the immune system and expel phlegm from the lungs.
		✓	✓	✓		Combine equal parts of yarrow, elderflower, and peppermint in an infusion with honey for relief from cold symptoms.
✓	✓	✓	✓	✓		Use single herbs separately, or blend equal parts thyme and elecampane in a tincture to help clear infection. Ribwort plantain helps dry mucous membranes, while licorice can be used to soothe and expel phlegm.
		✓	✓	✓	✓	Licorice and elder-based cordials and syrups (see p.204) can soothe and provide relief from a dry cough.
			✓			Combine equal parts yarrow, linden, and elderflower in a tea.
		✓	✓			Combine equal parts yarrow, elderflower, and peppermint in a tea to help bring down temperature and relieve flu symptoms.
	✓	✓		✓		Combine licorice and elderberry as a syrup to soothe the sore throat associated with whooping cough. If the cough is severe, or if you suspect a child may be suffering from whooping cough, seek medical advice immediately.
Avoid during pregnancy and while breastfeeding.		Excessive consumption of fresh berries can have a laxative effect.		Avoid taking therapeutic doses during pregnancy (a small amount in food is fine; see p.148 for full guidance).		

EAR, NOSE & THROAT

It's never pleasant to have to deal with a blocked nose, sore throat, or earache, but the right remedy can go a long way to easing the discomfort and getting you on the road to recovery. Pair these herbs with the treatments shown on pp.22–23 to help alleviate the wider symptoms of colds and flu.

	Common name	GARLIC	MARSHMALLOW	ECHINACEA	EUCALYPTUS	LICORICE	HYSSOP
	Scientific name	*Allium sativum*	*Althaea officinalis*	*Echinacea purpurea*	*Eucalyptus globulus*	*Glycyrrhiza glabra*	*Hyssopus officinalis*
	How to use	Add to food or take as capsules.	Take as an infusion or maceration.	Take as a decoction or tincture at first sign of symptoms.	Take as a decoction, use as an inhalation or essential oil in steam, or rub salve on chest.	Take as a decoction, syrup, or tincture, or use diluted to drink.	Take as an infusion, tincture, syrup, or use macerated oil as a chest rub.
NOSE	BLOCKED NOSE	✓		✓	✓		
	RUNNY NOSE			✓			
	SINUSITIS	✓			✓		✓
EAR	EARACHE	✓					
	EAR INFECTION	✓		✓			
	TINNITUS	✓					
THROAT	LARYNGITIS		✓				
	SORE THROAT		✓	✓		✓	
	TONSILLITIS		✓	✓			
	Caution	Can cause gastric irritation in some people (see p.43 for full guidance).		High doses can occasionally cause nausea and dizziness. Seek professional advice before using if taking immunosuppressant medication.	Do not use oil on babies or very young children. Avoid taking the essential oil internally (see p.77 for full guidance).	Avoid during pregnancy or if you have high blood pressure. Do not take for prolonged periods except under professional advice.	Avoid if taking blood pressure medication. Avoid during pregnancy (see p.94 for full guidance).

NOTES
- The herbs shown in this chart all work best if you take the opportunity to rest and reduce excess stress in your life while you recover.

- If symptoms become serious or do not clear up in a few days, seek medical advice.

- Unless otherwise stated, all tinctures and essential oils are diluted as advised in the herb's A–Z entry. For further guidance, see pp.176–177.

- If you are or may be pregnant, check herbs in the A–Z (pp.34–171) to ensure that they are safe for use.

RIBWORT PLANTAIN	SAGE	ELDER	THYME	MULLEIN	SUPPORTING ADVICE
Plantago lanceolata	*Salvia officinalis*	*Sambucus nigra*	*Thymus vulgaris*	*Verbascum thapsus*	
Take as an infusion, or use diluted in a tincture to drink.	Take as an infusion, or use diluted in a tincture to drink or gargle.	Take berries as a decoction, syrup, or tincture and flowers as an infusion, syrup, or tincture.	Take as an infusion or tincture, or inhale leaves or essential oil in steam.	Take as an infusion, or apply warm infused oil to outer ear.	
✓		✓		✓	Use echinacea and elderberry winter guard recipe (p.222) or inhale eucalyptus and thyme essential oils in steam. Ribwort plantain (taken as a tea or tincture) can help dry mucous membranes.
✓	✓		✓	✓	Take ribwort plantain as a tea or tincture to help dry mucous membranes, along with an echinacea and thyme tincture or elderberry syrup to help clear infection.
✓		✓			Address contributing factors, such as a tooth infection or allergens (dust mites, for instance), and avoid mucous-forming foods, such as dairy. If sinusitis is not due to these factors, use a eucalyptus oil nasal spray or inhale the oil in steam to clear the sinuses.
			✓	✓	Warm a bottle of mullein oil by placing it in a bowl of hot water, then add a few drops of the warmed oil to a cotton ball and apply to the outer ear.
		✓	✓	✓	Place a hot water bottle on the affected ear to provide comfort while waiting for herbs to work.
		✓			Traditionally, ginkgo has been used to increase blood circulation to the ear and reduce symptoms of tinnitus.
	✓		✓		Gargle with either green- or purple-leaved sage tea to help relive symptoms and soothe the voice.
	✓	✓	✓		Take either thyme and licorice or elderberry syrup to soothe the throat. Propolis pastilles may also help.
✓		✓	✓		Dilute rose hip syrup and freeze it into ice pops to soothe the throat.
	Avoid taking therapeutic doses during pregnancy or if epileptic.	Excessive consumption of fresh berries can have a laxative effect.	Avoid taking therapeutic doses during pregnancy (a small amount in food is fine; see p.148 for full guidance).		

FIRST AID

A number of herbs have the ability to help prevent infection, heal wounds, soothe insect bites, and stop bleeding. They can provide fast and effective relief for minor first aid conditions that can be dealt with at home. However, they should not be used as a substitute for professional first aid care when needed.

	Common name	GARLIC	ALOE VERA	CALENDULA	ECHINACEA	WITCH HAZEL	ST. JOHN'S WORT	LAVENDER
	Scientific name	*Allium sativum*	*Aloe vera*	*Calendula officinalis*	*Echinacea purpurea*	*Hamamelis virginiana*	*Hypericum officinalis*	*Lavandula angustifolia*
	How to use	Take fresh cloves as food.	Use fresh gel from the plant.	Take as an infusion or tincture, use as a wash, or add to a cream.	Take as an infusion or tincture, use as a wash, or add to a cream.	Take as an infusion or apply to cloth and use as a cold compress.	Take as an infusion or tincture, or apply undiluted as a macerated oil.	Use essential oil externally.
AILMENTS	BOILS	✓		✓	✓	✓		✓
	BRUISES					✓		
	BURNS		✓	✓			✓	✓
	COLD SORES						✓	✓
	CUTS			✓	✓	✓		
	HAY FEVER				✓			
	HEADACHES							✓
	INSECT BITES		✓		✓			✓
	MILD PAIN				✓			✓
	NOSEBLEEDS					✓		
	SCRATCHES			✓	✓	✓		✓
	SPLINTERS					✓		
	SPRAINS					✓		
	SUNBURN		✓				✓	✓
	Caution		Avoid internal use during pregnancy.	Avoid internal use during pregnancy.	Avoid if taking immuno-suppressant medication. High doses can occasionally cause nausea and dizziness.		Avoid during pregnancy. May interact with prescription medication. Can cause light sensitivity (see p.92 for full guidance).	

NOTES

- The treatments shown in this chart are intended for minor injuries. If you are in any doubt about the severity of the injury or the treatment required, seek urgent medical advice.

- Unless otherwise stated, all tinctures and essential oils are diluted as advised in the herb's A–Z entry. For further guidance, see pp.176–177.

- If you are or may be pregnant, check herbs in the A–Z (pp.34–171) to ensure that they are safe for use.

- Test any external treatments on a small patch of skin before using to check for any possible adverse reaction.

CHAMOMILE	RIBWORT PLANTAIN	COMFREY	SLIPPERY ELM	CRAMP BARK	SUPPORTING ADVICE
Matricaria recutita	*Plantago lanceolata*	*Symphytum officinale*	*Ulmus rubra*	*Viburnum opulus*	
Take as an infusion or tincture, or use essential oil.	Use fresh juice from the leaves or take as an infusion.	Apply a decoction to skin or use ointment.	Mix with water into a paste to make a poultice.	Use as a tincture or decoction.	
✓			✓		Apply a warm slippery elm poultice to draw the boil to the surface in the first instance.
		✓			Apply a cold compress of witch hazel and comfrey.
✓					Cool with running water. Add 5 drops each St. John's wort and calendula tinctures to cold water and pour over.
					Add either lavender and melissa essential oils or St. John's wort macerated oil to a cream and apply to the skin. Alternatively, drink lemon balm–infused tea.
✓	✓				Add 5 drops each echinacea and calendula tinctures to cold water and pour over to reduce risk of infection.
✓					Combine nettle and chamomile as an infusion or tincture.
✓				✓	Combine cramp bark with feverfew as a tincture or tea and drink regularly throughout the day.
✓	✓		✓		Remove any insect sting from the skin and clean thoroughly. If a bull's-eye rash or flu-like symptoms appear, seek medical advice.
✓				✓	The herbs shown are used to fight infection and reduce inflammation, thus helping reduce pain.
					Pinch nose above nostrils and tilt head forward. Apply a witch hazel and yarrow compress.
✓	✓				Keep wound clean.
			✓		Apply slippery elm as a poultice to draw splinter out of the skin. Clean wound with witch hazel.
		✓			Apply a witch hazel and comfrey compress.
✓					Combine St. John's wort macerated oil with a few drops lavender essential oil and apply externally.
Avoid if allergic to the Compositae (daisy) family.		For external use only. Avoid during pregnancy (see p.141 for full guidance).		Avoid during pregnancy or while breastfeeding except under professional supervision.	

MUSCLES & JOINTS

Most problems associated with muscles and joints develop over the course of several years, and can be the result of many factors, including poor posture and dietary, environmental, and emotional stressors. Healing can take time, but the right combination of herbal medicines can help ease the pain and aid recovery.

	Common name	BLACK COHOSH	WILD CELERY	CAYENNE OR CHILE PEPPER	TURMERIC	MEADOWSWEET	ST. JOHN'S WORT
	Scientific name	*Actaea racemosa*	*Apium graveolens*	*Capsicum annuum*	*Curcuma longa*	*Filipendula ulmaria*	*Hypericum perforatum*
	How to use	Take as an infusion, tincture, or capsules.	Use as a decoction, massage afflicted areas with essential oils, juice stems, or add to food.	Add drops of tincture to an ointment or massage oil.	Use as a decoction, tincture, powder, or capsules.	Take as a fluid extract or dilute tincture to use with a compress.	Take as an infusion, tincture, capsules, or infused oil.
AILMENTS	ARTHRITIS	✓	✓	✓	✓	✓	
	BACK ACHE	✓			✓		✓
	BROKEN BONE						
	INFLAMMATION	✓	✓		✓	✓	✓
	MUSCULAR ACHES	✓		✓			
	NEURALGIA	✓		✓		✓	✓
	OSTEOARTHRITIS				✓		
	PAIN RELIEF	✓		✓		✓	✓
	RESTLESS LEG	✓					
	SCIATICA	✓	✓				✓
	SPRAIN			✓			✓
	SWELLING		✓				
	Caution	Avoid during pregnancy (see p.38 for full guidance).	Avoid using seeds if pregnant. Do not take essential oil internally unless under professional supervision.	Avoid touching the eyes or any cuts after handling. Wash hands thoroughly after use.	Avoid therapeutic doses during pregnancy (a small amount in food is fine; see p.69 for full guidance).	Avoid during pregnancy, if taking blood thinners, or if sensitive to aspirin.	Avoid during pregnancy. May interact with prescription medication (see p.92 for full guidance).

NOTES

• Where possible and appropriate, gentle manipulation and exercise can alleviate symptoms and aid recovery. Simple dietary changes (avoiding refined sugars, eating organic and whole grain foods, and increasing your intake of omega 3 and essential fatty acids) can also help.

• For severe or long-lasting symptoms, seek medical advice.

• Unless otherwise stated, all tinctures and essential oils are diluted as advised in the herb's A–Z entry. For further guidance, see pp.176–177.

• If you are or may be pregnant, check herbs in the A–Z (pp.34–171) to ensure that they are safe for use.

	JUNIPER	DOG ROSE	ROSEMARY	WHITE WILLOW BARK	COMFREY	CRAMP BARK	SUPPORTING ADVICE
	Juniperus communis	*Rosa canina*	*Rosmarinus officinalis*	*Salix alba*	*Symphytum officinale*	*Viburnum opulus*	
	Add essential oil to ointment.	Take rose hips as an infusion or syrup.	Take as an infusion, tincture, or use the infused oil.	Take as an infusion, decoction, tincture, or capsules.	Apply externally as an infused oil, ointment, or compress.	Take as an infusion, tincture, capsules, or use as a cream or ointment.	
	✓		✓	✓	✓		Add turmeric and black pepper to food to increase intake of plant-based nutrients. Juniper essential oil (along with cypress, black pepper, and ginger essential oils) can be used as massage oil.
			✓			✓	Massage with St. John's wort cream, drops of chile tincture, or rosemary essential oil. Apply heat pads. Try back- and core-strengthening exercises.
					✓		Eat mineral-rich plants like oats and kelp. Drink nettle and horsetail tea to encourage healing.
		✓	✓	✓			Add turmeric to food, as this has an anti-inflammatory effect, and avoid inflammatory foods such as red meat. Combine dog rose and meadowsweet as a tea, or white willow bark and devil's claw as a decoction. Use juniper and rosemary essential oils as massage oil 2–3 times daily.
	✓	✓	✓			✓	Combine juniper, rosemary, and ginger essential oils as a massage oil and massage into affected area.
				✓		✓	Drink chamomile tea and take a combined willow and valerian tincture. If the cause is viral, take St. John's wort and lemon balm as a tea or tincture.
	✓	✓	✓		✓		Drink rose hip, ginger, and turmeric tea 2–3 times daily. Combine St. John's wort and arnica macerated oil with a few drops of juniper and rosemary essential oils and massage into the affected area.
	✓			✓			Muscle and joint pain can be caused by inflammation; see above for suitable herbal remedies.
						✓	Can be due to a magnesium or iron deficiency; take a supplement if necessary. Take an infusion or tincture of lemon balm, skullcap, and linden half an hour before bed.
						✓	Take cramp bark decoction or tincture 3-4 times daily to relax the muscles around the affected nerve. Add 2 drops rosemary essential oil to 1 fl oz (30 ml) St. John's wort macerated oil and massage into the sciatic area.
				✓	✓		Elevate the injury. Apply ice and a comfrey compress.
				✓	✓		Elevate the injury. Apply a cold compress made with an infusion of comfrey and willow bark.
	Avoid during pregnancy (see p.97 for full guidance).		Avoid taking therapeutic doses during pregnancy.	Avoid during pregnancy or if allergic to aspirin.	For external use only. Avoid during pregnancy (see p.141 for full guidance).	Avoid during pregnancy or while breastfeeding except under professional supervision.	

MEMORY, MIND & EMOTIONS

Provided that any underlying causes are properly understood and addressed, herbal remedies can provide short-term solutions for a range of emotional and mental challenges. When combined with other treatments, including talking therapies, breath work, and gentle exercises, herbs may help improve your mental state over the longer term.

Common name	OATS	ST. JOHN'S WORT	LAVENDER	MOTHER-WORT	CHAMOMILE	LEMON BALM	PASSION-FLOWER
Scientific name	*Avena sativa*	*Hypericum perforatum*	*Lavandula angustifolia*	*Leonurus cardiaca*	*Matricaria recutita*	*Melissa officinalis*	*Passiflora incarnata*
How to use	Take as an infusion, tincture, or as food.	Take as an infusion, tincture, or as food.	Take as an infusion or tincture, or use as a massage oil.	Take as an infusion, tincture, or capsules.	Take as an infusion or tincture, or use as a diluted essential oil.	Take as an infusion or tincture, or use as a diluted essential oil.	Take as an infusion, tincture, or capsules.

AILMENTS

Ailment	OATS	ST. JOHN'S WORT	LAVENDER	MOTHER-WORT	CHAMOMILE	LEMON BALM	PASSION-FLOWER
ANXIETY	✓	✓	✓	✓	✓	✓	✓
BRAIN FOG						✓	
DEPRESSION	✓	✓	✓			✓	
EMOTIONAL SHOCK	✓		✓	✓	✓	✓	
EXHAUSTION		✓				✓	
HEADACHES			✓		✓	✓	✓
MIGRAINES						✓	✓
NERVOUS TENSIONS	✓	✓	✓		✓	✓	✓
RESTLESSNESS	✓					✓	
SLEEPLESSNESS			✓		✓	✓	✓
STRESS	✓	✓	✓	✓	✓	✓	
Caution	Use gluten-free oats if gluten intolerant (see p.59 for full guidance).	Avoid during pregnancy. May interact with prescription medication (see p.92 for full guidance).		Avoid during pregnancy and heavy periods. Seek professional advice before using with a heart condition.	Avoid if allergic to the Compositae (daisy) family.		May cause drowsiness.

NOTES

• Mental health is complex, and can be influenced by a range of contributing factors including family history, diet and lifestyle choices, social considerations, and stress levels. If symptoms are severe or long-lasting, seek medical advice and professional support.

• Unless otherwise stated, all tinctures and essential oils are diluted as advised in the herb's A–Z entry. For further guidance, see pp.176–177.

• If you are or may be pregnant, check herbs in the A–Z (pp.34–171) to ensure that they are safe for use.

ROSEMARY	SKULLCAP	LINDEN	VALERIAN	VERVAIN	ASHWAG-ANDHA	SUPPORTING ADVICE
Rosmarinus officinalis	*Scutellaria lateriflora*	*Tilia cordata*	*Valeriana officinalis*	*Verbena officinalis*	*Withania somnifera*	
Take as an infusion, tincture, or use as a diluted essential oil.	Take as an infusion, tincture, tea, or capsules.	Take as an infusion or tincture.	Take as an infusion, tincture, or capsules.	Take as an infusion or tincture.	Take as a decoction, fluid extract, powder, or capsules.	
	✓	✓	✓	✓	✓	Reduce caffeine intake; substitute with chamomile or lemon balm tea.
✓						Ginkgo and gotu kola can also be used to alleviate symptoms. Plant-based estrogens can also help if the brain fog is a result of low estrogen levels.
✓	✓		✓	✓		A combination of St. John's wort and vervain as a tea or tincture may help alleviate symptoms of mild depression. Oats have traditionally been served at breakfast to improve stamina and boost spirits.
	✓		✓			Valerian tincture can particularly help calm the nerves. Flower remedies (such as Neal's Yard Remedies Five Flower Remedy) can also be used for shock.
					✓	Address any vitamin deficiency and rest as needed. Ashwagandha can provide adrenal support, take time out to fully rest and recover.
✓	✓	✓		✓		A passionflower, lavender, or lemon balm tincture is recommended in the first instance.
✓	✓		✓			Combine passionflower and skullcap with feverfew as an infusion and take 3 times daily. Identify and avoid potential triggers, such as allergens.
✓	✓	✓	✓	✓	✓	Oats, vervain, and alfalfa can help reduce tension and increase the body's intake of B-vitamins.
	✓		✓			Drink lemon balm and skullcap tea during the day.
	✓		✓		✓	Before bed, drink passionflower and chamomile tincture (p.218) or try a lavender and aloe vera bath (p.328). Take a valerian tincture at night if you are still unable to sleep.
	✓	✓	✓	✓		Drink lemon balm and skullcap tea during the day to aid relaxation. Take ashwagandha capsules at night to support the adrenal glands (reducing the release of stress hormones).
Avoid taking therapeutic doses during pregnancy.		Avoid during pregnancy. Seek professional advice before taking for high blood pressure.	May enhance effects of sleep-inducing drugs.	Avoid during pregnancy. Excess use may cause vomiting.	Avoid during pregnancy.	

PREGNANCY & CHILDBIRTH

Herbal remedies have been used for centuries to aid with pregnancy and childbirth. While care should be taken to check that herbs are safe for use during pregnancy or breastfeeding (see note, opposite), they can provide a natural solution for a range of pre- and postpartum ailments and challenges.

		CALENDULA	WITCH HAZEL	ST. JOHN'S WORT	JASMINE	LAVENDER	CHAMOMILE	ALFALFA
	Common name							
	Scientific name	*Calendula officinalis*	*Hamamelis virginiana*	*Hypericum perforatum*	*Jasminum officinale*	*Lavandula angustifolia*	*Matricaria recutita*	*Medicago sativa*
	How to use	Use as a bath infusion, ointment, or cream.	Apply as a cream or cold compress, or take as an infusion.	Take as an infusion or tincture, or use a macerated oil externally.	Use as a massage oil.	Use as a massage oil.	Take as an infusion or tincture, or use as massage oil.	Take as food, infusion, or tincture.
AILMENTS	AID BREASTFEEDING							✓
	AID LABOR				✓		✓	
	ANEMIA							
	CRACKED NIPPLES	✓		✓				
	CRAMPS					✓	✓	
	HEMORRHOIDS	✓	✓				✓	
	HEARTBURN					✓	✓	
	NAUSEA					✓	✓	
	POSTPARTUM PAIN RELIEF	✓	✓	✓		✓	✓	✓
	STRETCH MARKS			✓		✓		
	SWOLLEN ANKLES							✓
	THRUSH	✓				✓	✓	
	URINARY INFECTIONS	✓						
	VARICOSE VEINS		✓					
	Caution	Avoid internal use during pregnancy.		Avoid during pregnancy. May cause sensitivity to light and interact with prescription drugs.	Avoid during breastfeeding or pregnancy as it can stimulate contractions.		Avoid if allergic to the Compositae (daisy) family.	Avoid during early stages of pregnancy; use only in third trimester.

NOTES

• The herbs listed in this chart are generally fit for use during pregnancy and/or breastfeeding, but do consult an experienced herbalist if unsure. Many herbs listed elsewhere in this book should be avoided during pregnancy; always check the advice given in the A–Z (pp.34–171) before use.

• For persistent problems, consult a midwife or OB/GYN. If symptoms worsen, seek medical advice.

• Unless otherwise stated, all tinctures and essential oils are diluted as advised in the herb's A–Z entry. For further guidance, see pp.176–177.

RASPBERRY LEAF	DANDELION	NETTLE	CRAMP BARK	GINGER	SUPPORTING ADVICE
Rubus idaeus	*Taraxacum officinale*	*Urtica dioica*	*Viburnum opulus*	*Zingiber officinalis*	
Take as an infusion or tincture.	Take as an infusion or tincture.	Take as an infusion or tincture.	Take as a decoction or tincture.	Take as food, infusion, or tincture.	
✓		✓			In addition to these herbs, fennel seed can help increase milk supply and reduce colic in babies.
✓			✓		Take raspberry leaf daily three months prior to birth. Combine jasmine and clary sage essential oils as massage oil to relieve back ache during labor. Combine chamomile and rose essential oils as aromatherapy to relieve anxiety and pain.
	✓	✓		✓	Increase iron intake by eating leafy vegetables, including nettles (p.234); nettle and rose hip tea can be drunk daily throughout pregnancy to boost iron levels. Dandelion root has also been shown to contain iron.
					Apply calendula as an ointment to the affected area.
			✓		Increase calcium intake.
				✓	Drink slippery elm, chamomile, and lavender as a tea.
✓				✓	Inhaling aromatic, citrus-smelling herbs, such as lemon balm, on a tissue may relieve symptoms, while chamomile can help aid digestion.
					Combine ¾oz (20 g) each oats, calendula, St. John's wort, and shepherd's purse to a muslin bag and add to a bath to infuse. This soothing blend can aid the healing of the perineum or a C-section wound.
					Add a few drops of lavender essential oil to either coconut oil, vitamin E cream, or wheat germ oil and massage into the affected area.
	✓	✓			Speak to a midwife. Avoid standing for long periods and rest with feet elevated. Drink dandelion-leaf tea to help lower blood pressure. Support stockings may help.
					Apply live yogurt or a calendula and lavender rinse to the affected area. Avoid tight or nylon underwear. Eat garlic to encourage growth of healthy bacteria.
	✓	✓			Drink cranberry juice, or a tea made with equal parts dandelion leaf, nettle, and corn silk. Prebiotic foods and herbs (pp.14–15) can also help.
✓					Eat foods high in vitamins C and E and zinc to strengthen the blood vessels. Massage olive oil infused with horse chestnut (p.114) into the affected area.
Avoid during early stages of pregnancy; use only in third trimester.	Seek medical advice before use if suffering from gallstones.		Seek professional guidance before use during pregnancy.	Avoid if taking blood-thinning medication, or if suffering from peptic ulcers or gallstones.	

A–Z OF HERBS

Discover more than 100 of the most useful medicinal herbs for natural health and well-being. Find out what each herb can be used for, how to use them to cure common ailments at home, and how to grow, forage, and harvest them for yourself.

Achillea millefolium
YARROW

Native to Europe and western Asia, yarrow was traditionally used to treat wounds, although it was also once used in Germany and the Nordic countries as an alternative to hops in beer-making. Today it is valued for its astringent and anticatarrhal properties, and is used in remedies for colds and urinary disorders. It is widely naturalized in North America, New Zealand, and Australia.

PARTS USED Leaves, flowers, essential oil
MAIN CONSTITUENTS Volatile oil, isovalerianic acid, asparagine, salicylic acid, sterols, flavonoids
ACTIONS Astringent, diaphoretic, diuretic, peripheral vasodilator, digestive stimulant, restorative for menstrual system, febrifuge
ESSENTIAL OIL anti-inflammatory, anti-allergenic

HOW TO USE
INFUSION Drink 1 cup (1–2 tsp herb per cup of boiling water) 3 times a day to encourage sweating and reduce fevers; combines well with peppermint for common colds. One cup stimulates the appetite.
TINCTURE Take 20–40 drops (1–2 ml) 3 times daily, usually with herbs such as couch grass or buchu, for urinary disorders.
FRESH LEAVES A single leaf inserted in the nostril will rapidly stop a nosebleed.
OINTMENT Apply to minor cuts and grazes.
MASSAGE OIL Add 10 drops of yarrow oil to 5 tsp (25 ml) of infused St. John's wort oil to make a rub for hot, inflamed joints.
STEAM INHALATION Use 1 tbsp fresh flowers in boiling water to ease hay fever symptoms. Inhale the steam for at least 2–3 minutes.

HOW TO SOURCE
GROW Prefers a well-drained position in full sun, but is tolerant of a wide range of conditions. Sow seeds in spring. Propagation by root division is best in spring or fall. It can easily become invasive.
FORAGE Generally found in pasture, hedges, or among grass in meadows throughout Europe.
HARVEST Gather leaves and aerial parts in summer, and flowers when they appear.

CAUTION Avoid during pregnancy. Can lower blood pressure. Essential oils should not be taken internally without professional advice. In rare cases can cause skin rashes, and prolonged use can increase skin photosensitivity.

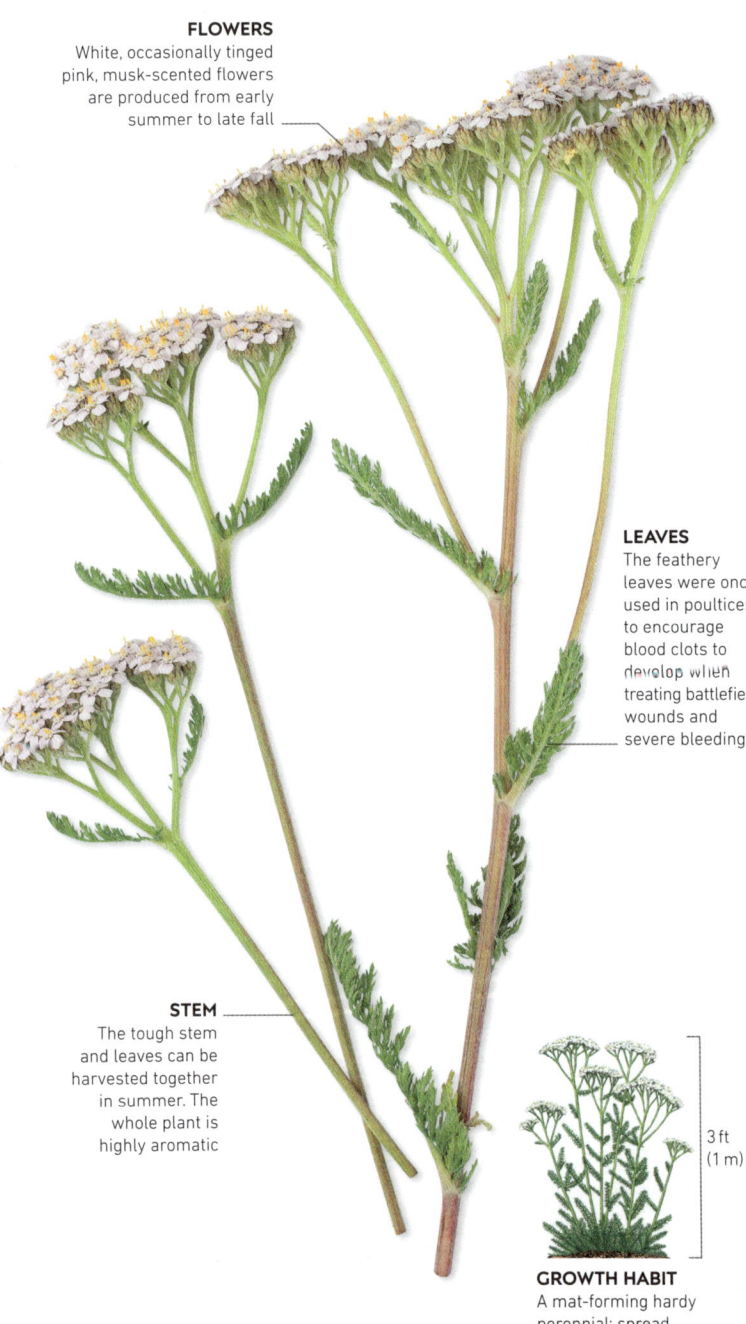

FLOWERS
White, occasionally tinged pink, musk-scented flowers are produced from early summer to late fall

LEAVES
The feathery leaves were once used in poultices to encourage blood clots to develop when treating battlefield wounds and severe bleeding

STEM
The tough stem and leaves can be harvested together in summer. The whole plant is highly aromatic

3 ft (1 m)

GROWTH HABIT
A mat-forming hardy perennial; spread 2–8 in (5–20 cm).

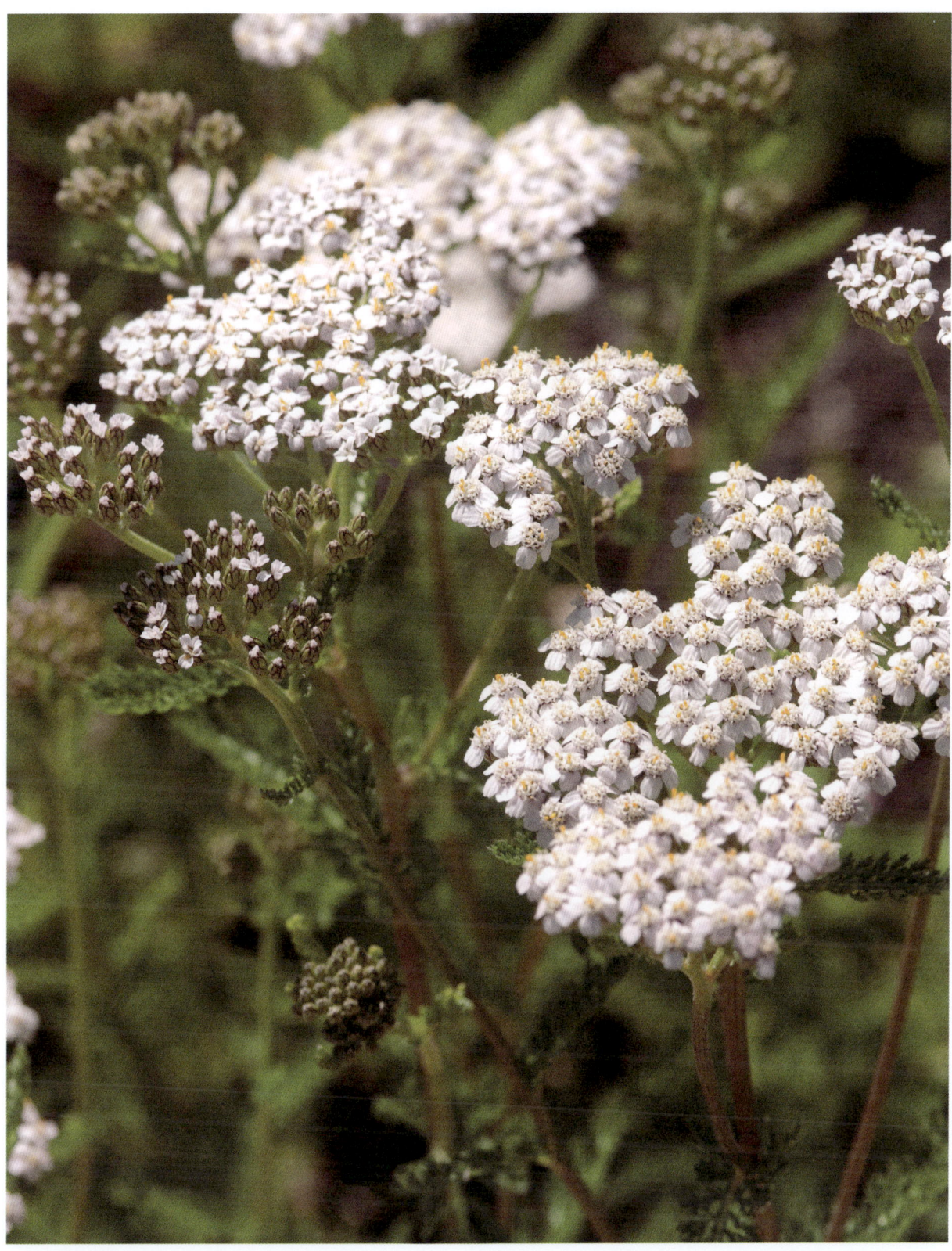

Actaea racemosa
BLACK COHOSH

FLOWER BUD
When in bloom in late summer, the fragrant flowers are fluffy and white, and sometimes described as being like a bottle brush

LEAVES
When fully unfurled, the elegant, divided basal leaves are as much as 36 in (90 cm) in length, making this plant a distinctive addition to a woodland garden

6 ft
(2 m)

GROWTH HABIT
Erect, clump-forming woodland perennial with a spread of 24 in (60 cm).

Originally found in Canada and the eastern parts of the US, black cohosh was a favorite remedy with Native Americans. It was used for a range of gynecological disorders, snakebites, fevers, and rheumatism. It has been used in Europe since the 19th century, and is also known as *Cimicifuga racemosa*. Some cases of liver damage have been reported, and it is restricted in some countries.

PARTS USED Root and rhizome
MAIN CONSTITUENTS Cinnamic acid derivatives, chromone, isoflavones, tannins, triterpene glycosides, salicylic acid
ACTIONS Antispasmodic, anti-arthritic, anti-inflammatory, antirheumatic, mild analgesic, relaxing nervine, relaxes blood vessels, emmenagogue, diuretic, sedative, antitussive, hypotensive, hypoglycemic

HOW TO USE

TINCTURE Take 20–40 drops in a little water 3 times daily for period pain; combine with an equal amount of motherwort tincture and take 3 times daily for hot flashes, night sweats, and emotional upsets associated with menopause. Take 20 drops 3 times daily with an equal amount of valerian to support treatments for high blood pressure.
DECOCTION Use ½ oz (15 g) of the root in 1½ pints (900 ml) of water simmered for 15 minutes—twice daily for rheumatic pains, lumbago, facial neuralgia, sciatica, or tendonitis.
TABLETS/CAPSULES Use for menopausal problems or rheumatic disorders; follow dosage directions on the pack. It is best not to take more than 40–80 mg daily.
SYRUP Combine 1 cup of a decoction (made as above) with 1 cup of sugar or ¾ cup honey, bring to a boil, and simmer gently for 5–10 minutes to make a syrup. Take in 1 tsp (5 ml) doses every 2–3 hours for whooping cough and bronchitis.

HOW TO SOURCE

GROW Prefers moist, fertile soil in dappled or partial shade. Sow ripe seeds in a cold frame and transplant to 3½ in (7 cm) pots; plant in final positions in late spring.
FORAGE Found in woodland areas in North America and some parts of Europe.
HARVEST Dig mature roots in fall.

CAUTION Do not exceed recommended dosage. May rarely cause liver problems. Do not use if you have a history of liver disease; if in doubt, consult your doctor. Avoid during pregnancy.

Agastache rugosa
PURPLE GIANT HYSSOP

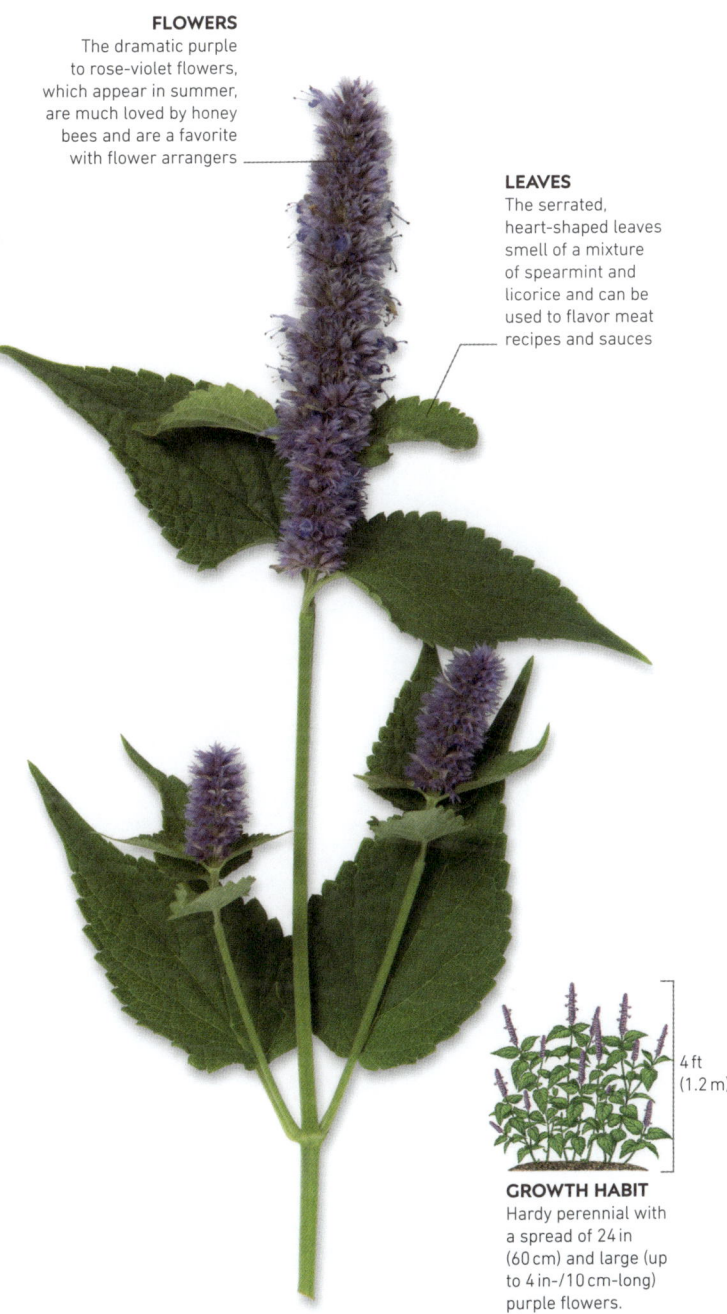

FLOWERS
The dramatic purple to rose-violet flowers, which appear in summer, are much loved by honey bees and are a favorite with flower arrangers

LEAVES
The serrated, heart-shaped leaves smell of a mixture of spearmint and licorice and can be used to flavor meat recipes and sauces

GROWTH HABIT
Hardy perennial with a spread of 24 in (60 cm) and large (up to 4 in-/10 cm-long) purple flowers.

4 ft (1.2 m)

Native to eastern Asia, including parts of India, China, and Japan, purple giant hyssop is also known as Korean mint. It is one of two species that are known as *huo xiang* in Chinese medicine, and which have been used for at least 1,500 years. *Huo xiang* is largely taken for digestive problems associated with nausea, vomiting, and poor appetite.

PARTS USED Aerial parts, essential oil
MAIN CONSTITUENTS Volatile oil (incl. methyl chavicol, anethole, anisaldehyde, limonene, pinene, linalool)
ACTIONS Antibacterial, antifungal, febrifuge, carminative, diaphoretic

HOW TO USE

INFUSION Drink 1 cup (1–2 tsp aerial parts per cup of boiling water) 1–2 times a day for abdominal bloating and indigestion.
LOTION/OINTMENT Use 1 cup of infusion to bathe ringworm patches, or make into an ointment and apply 2–3 times daily. Alternatively, add 10 drops of the essential oil to 1 tbsp (15 ml) of almond oil.
TINCTURE Take 10–40 drops in a little water to relieve nausea.
DECOCTION In traditional Chinese medicine it is combined in decoctions with such herbs as *huang qin* (baikal skullcap, *Scutellaria baicalensis*) and *lian qiao* (forsythia fruits, *Forsythia suspensa*) for acute diarrhea.
PATENT REMEDIES Included in various Chinese patent formulae, such as *huo xiang zheng qi san* (powder for dispelling turbidity with giant hyssop) which is used to clear "dampness." Follow the dosage directions on the package.

HOW TO SOURCE

GROW Prefers well-drained, fertile soil with well-rotted organic matter in full sun. Can be grown from seeds planted in 3 in (7 cm) pots and transplanted to their final growing position when large enough to handle.
FORAGE Unlikely to be found growing wild beyond its native habitat, although cultivated plants that then self-seed are possible. Collect leaves throughout the growing season and use in any recipe that requires mint. They can also be infused to make a refreshing tea.
HARVEST The aerial parts are gathered in summer before flowering.

CAUTION In Chinese medicine it should be avoided in cases of fever. Avoid therapeutic doses in pregnancy.

Agrimonia eupatoria
AGRIMONY

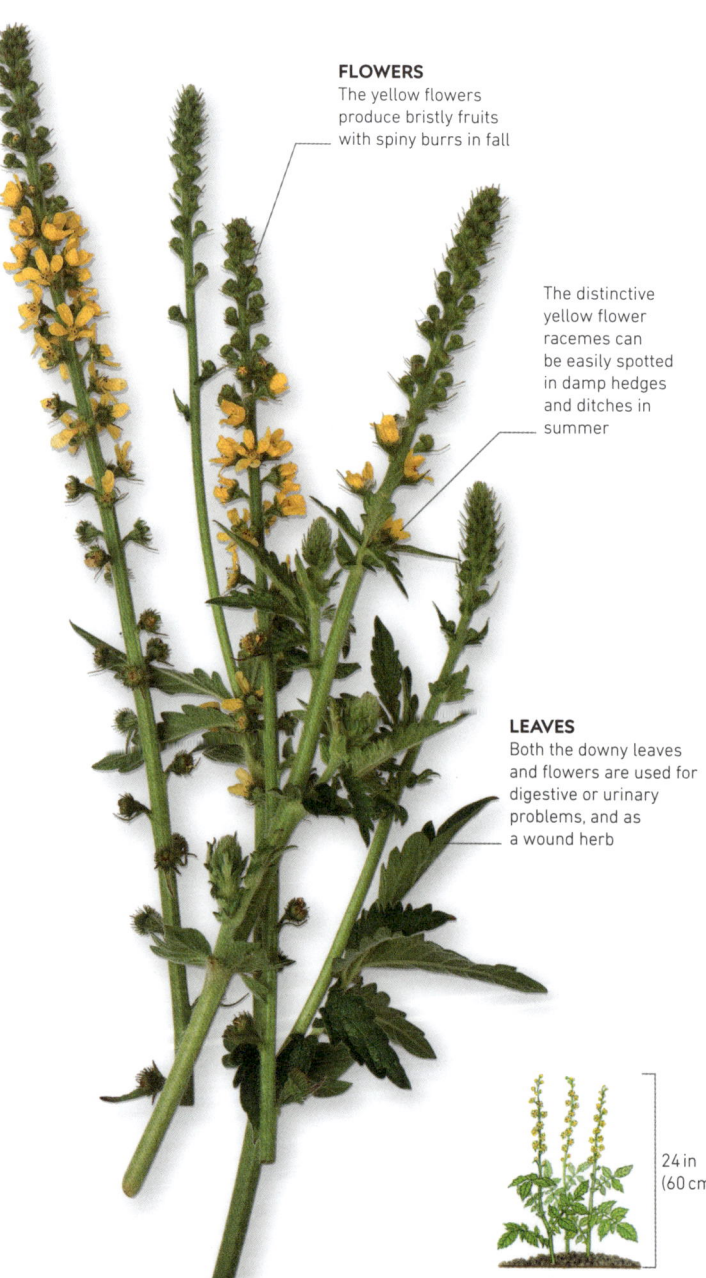

FLOWERS
The yellow flowers produce bristly fruits with spiny burrs in fall

The distinctive yellow flower racemes can be easily spotted in damp hedges and ditches in summer

LEAVES
Both the downy leaves and flowers are used for digestive or urinary problems, and as a wound herb

24 in (60 cm)

GROWTH HABIT
Perennial with hairy upright stems; spread 8–12 in (20–30 cm).

Widely found in Europe, western Asia, and northern Africa, agrimony has been used as a medicinal herb since ancient times. Originally used for eye problems and diarrhea or dysentery, it later became a favorite wound herb on the battlefield, and is used today for urinary disorders and poor digestion. A related Chinese variety, *Agrimonia pilosa*, is used in similar ways in East Asia.

PARTS USED Aerial parts
MAIN CONSTITUENTS Tannins, coumarins, volatile oil, flavonoids, minerals (incl. silica), vitamins B and K
ACTIONS Astringent, diuretic, tissue healer, hemostatic, cholagogue, tonic, vulnerary, some antiviral activity reported

HOW TO USE

INFUSION Drink 1 cup (1–2 tsp herb per cup of boiling water) 3 times daily to improve sluggish digestion or to help strengthen the digestive system in cases of food intolerance. Agrimony is an ideal herb for children with diarrhea (consult an herbalist for children's dosage), and can also be taken by nursing mothers to dose babies.
LOTION Use a standard infusion to bathe cuts, scrapes, skin sores, weeping eczema, and varicose ulcers. It can be applied several times daily.
GARGLE Use 1 cup of above infusion as a gargle for hoarseness, sore throats, and laryngitis.
TINCTURE Take 20–80 drops (1–4 ml) 3 times daily for cystitis, urinary infections, or incontinence. For severe or persistent urinary symptoms, seek urgent medical advice to avoid potential kidney damage.

HOW TO SOURCE

GROW Prefers damp, fertile soil, and will tolerate partial shade or full sun. Sow the seeds in a cold frame in fall or spring and transplant them when they are large enough to handle.
FORAGE Commonly found on wasteland or in damp hedges. It is easily noticeable because of its tall bright yellow flower spikes. Gather the whole aerial parts in summer.
HARVEST Gather in summer while in flower.

CAUTION This astringent herb is best avoided if constipated.

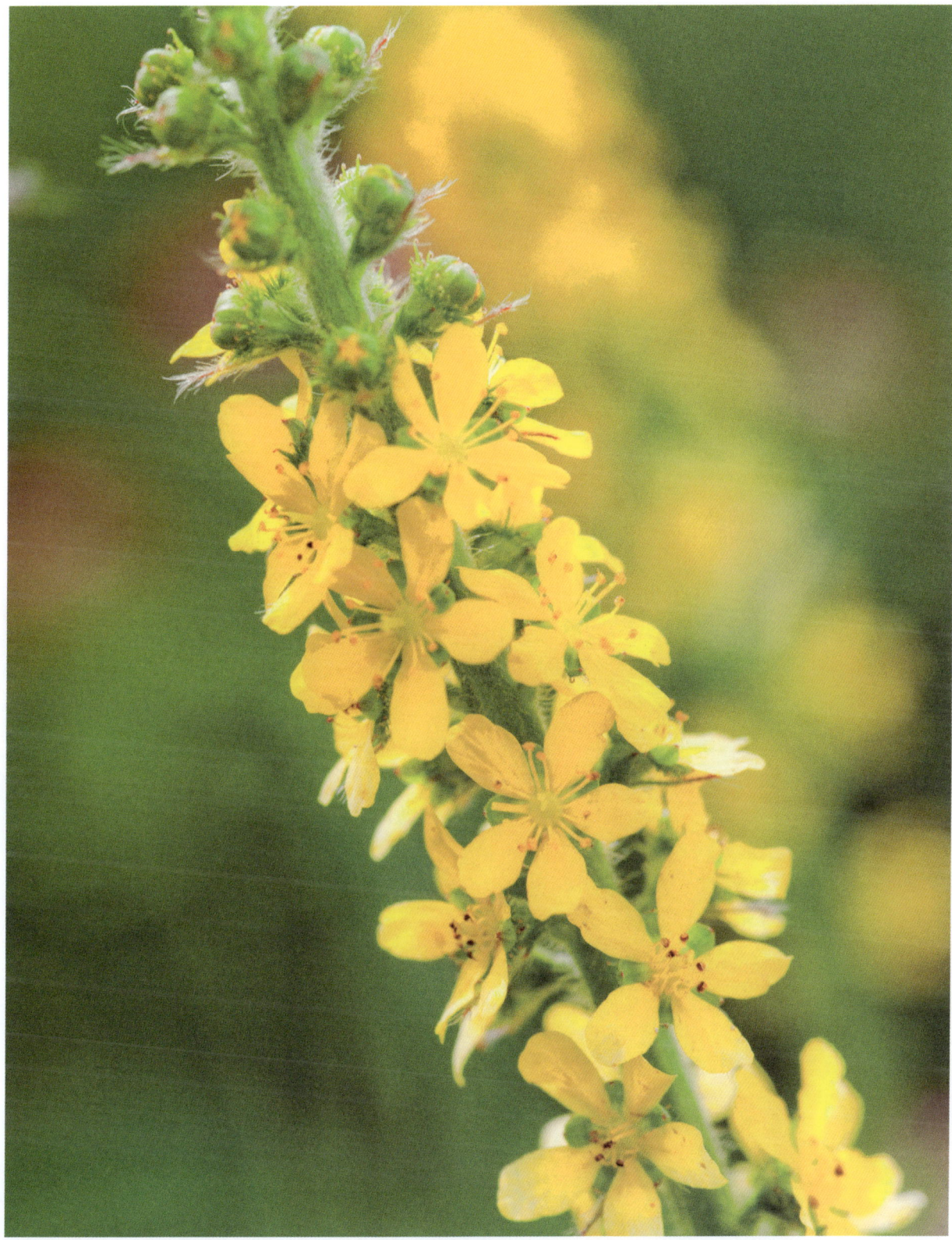

Alchemilla xanthochlora
LADY'S MANTLE

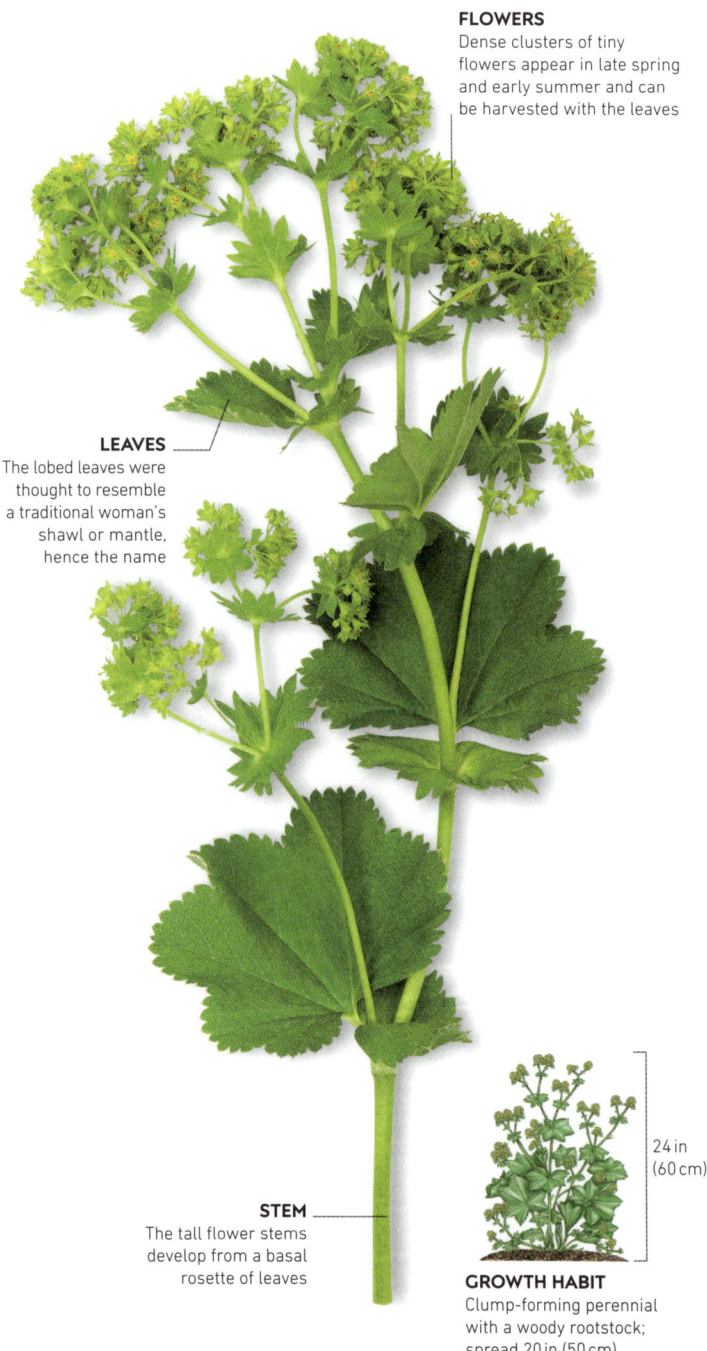

FLOWERS
Dense clusters of tiny flowers appear in late spring and early summer and can be harvested with the leaves

LEAVES
The lobed leaves were thought to resemble a traditional woman's shawl or mantle, hence the name

STEM
The tall flower stems develop from a basal rosette of leaves

24 in
(60 cm)

GROWTH HABIT
Clump-forming perennial with a woody rootstock; spread 20 in (50 cm).

As its name suggests, lady's mantle has a long tradition of gynecological uses and has been a remedy for menstrual irregularities, heavy menstrual bleeding, and to ease childbirth. The plant originated in northern Europe and mountainous regions further south. In recent years, it has become a popular garden plant highly valued by flower arrangers for its flower stems.

PARTS USED Aerial parts
MAIN CONSTITUENTS Tannins, salicylic acid, saponins, phytosterols, volatile oil, bitter principle
ACTIONS Astringent, menstrual regulator, digestive tonic, anti-inflammatory, wound herb

HOW TO USE

INFUSION Drink 1 cup (2 tsp herb per cup of boiling water) up to 5 times a day for acute diarrhea or gastroenteritis, or to ease heavy menstrual bleeding or period pain.
TINCTURE Take 20–40 drops (1–2 ml) 3 times daily to help regulate the menstrual cycle or, if combined with the same quantity of St. John's wort, to ease period pains.
LOTION/DOUCHE Use the infusion above externally as a wash to bathe weeping eczema or skin sores.
GARGLE 1 cup of above infusion can be used as a gargle for sore throats, laryngitis, or as a mouthwash for mouth ulcers.
CREAM/OINTMENT/PESSARIES Apply night and morning for vaginal discharges or itching. Insert 1 pessary at night. If symptoms do not improve in 2–3 days, seek medical advice.

HOW TO SOURCE

GROW A hardy, clump-forming perennial, lady's mantle prefers moist, well-drained soil in full sun or dappled shade. The round, finely toothed leaves can have up to 11 distinct lobes. It can be grown from seed sown directly in spring or by division in spring or summer. Lady's mantle will self-seed enthusiastically.
FORAGE Found throughout northern Europe and the mountainous regions of central and southern Europe. It can also be found self-seeding outside gardens in other areas throughout the summer.
HARVEST Gather the whole aerial parts throughout the summer.

Allium sativum
GARLIC

Garlic is believed to have originated in southwest Siberia, but spread to much of Europe and Asia in ancient times. It has been used as a medicinal herb for at least 5,000 years, and is now known to reduce the risk of further heart attacks, as well as lower blood cholesterol levels. Also a strong antibiotic, garlic is used to treat colds, catarrh, and respiratory infections.

PARTS USED Bulb
MAIN CONSTITUENTS Volatile oil (incl. allicin, alliin, and ajoene); enzymes; vitamins A, B, C, and E; minerals (incl. selenium and germanium); flavonoids
ACTIONS Antibiotic, expectorant, diaphoretic, hypotensive, antithrombotic, hypolipidemic, hypoglycemic, antihistaminic, anthelmintic

HOW TO USE

JUICE Take up to 1 tsp (5 ml) of juice in honey or water twice a day to combat infections, arteriosclerosis, or to reduce the risk of thrombosis.
FRESH CLOVES Rub the cut side of a fresh clove on acne pustules at night. Eat 2–3 cloves in cooked food each day to improve the cardiovascular system, lower cholesterol, or help prevent colds and flu.
CAPSULES Take 1 capsule before meals (check dosage on the package) to help prevent seasonal infections.
TINCTURE Take 40–80 drops (2–4 ml) in water 3 times daily for cardiovascular problems, respiratory disorders, or fungal infections.
POWDER For anyone who has suffered a heart attack, take up to 1 level teaspoon each day stirred into water or fruit juice to help prevent further attacks.

HOW TO SOURCE

GROW Prefers a warm site in deep, fertile, well-drained soil in full sun. Plant bulbs or individual cloves 2–4 in (5–10 cm) deep in the soil in fall or winter.
FORAGE May be found growing wild in warm areas, but generally only likely to occur in cultivation.
HARVEST Gather the bulbs in late summer and early fall and air-dry before storing in frost-free conditions.

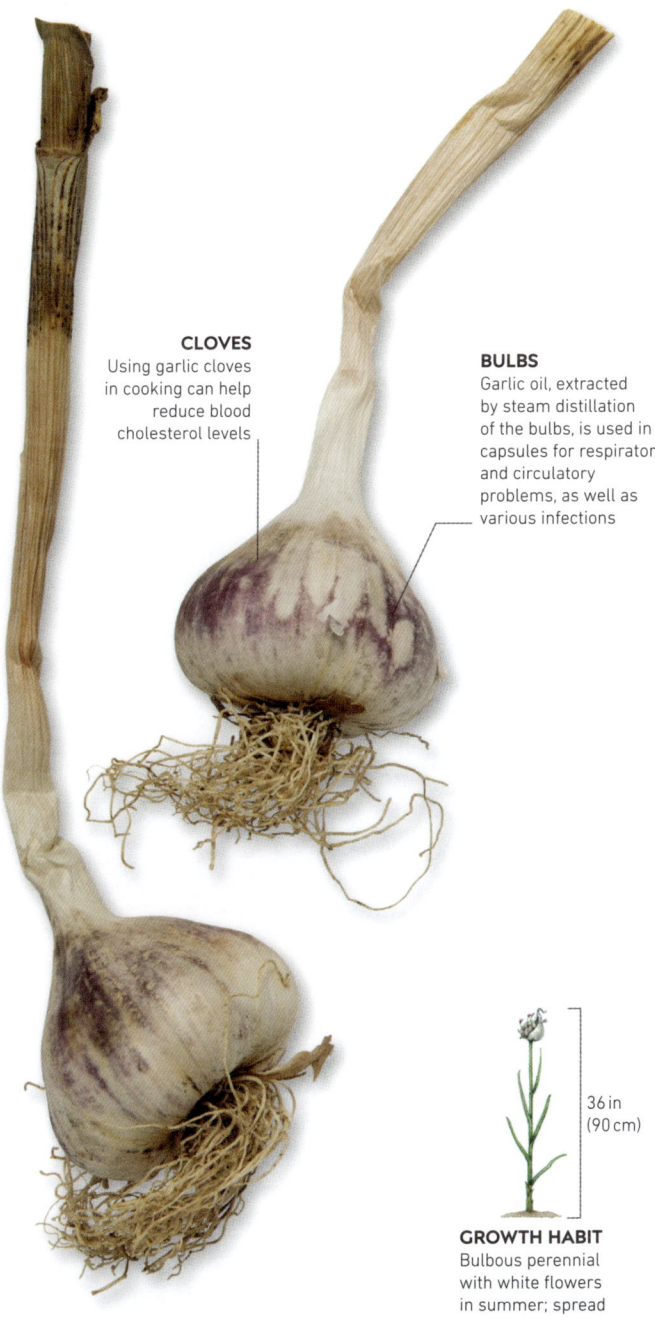

CLOVES
Using garlic cloves in cooking can help reduce blood cholesterol levels

BULBS
Garlic oil, extracted by steam distillation of the bulbs, is used in capsules for respiratory and circulatory problems, as well as various infections

36 in (90 cm)

GROWTH HABIT
Bulbous perennial with white flowers in summer; spread 9–12 in (23–30 cm).

CAUTION Garlic oil is a skin irritant and should only be taken in capsules. Garlic can cause gastric irritation in some people. Avoid consuming large quantities if taking blood-thinning medication.

Aloe vera
ALOE VERA

Native to tropical Africa, where it has been used as an antidote to poison arrow wounds, aloe vera reached Europe in ancient times and was well known to the Greeks and Romans as a wound herb. The sap is cooling and healing and for centuries has been used to treat burns, inflammation, and skin ulcers, while the whole leaf is purgative. Internal use is restricted in some countries.

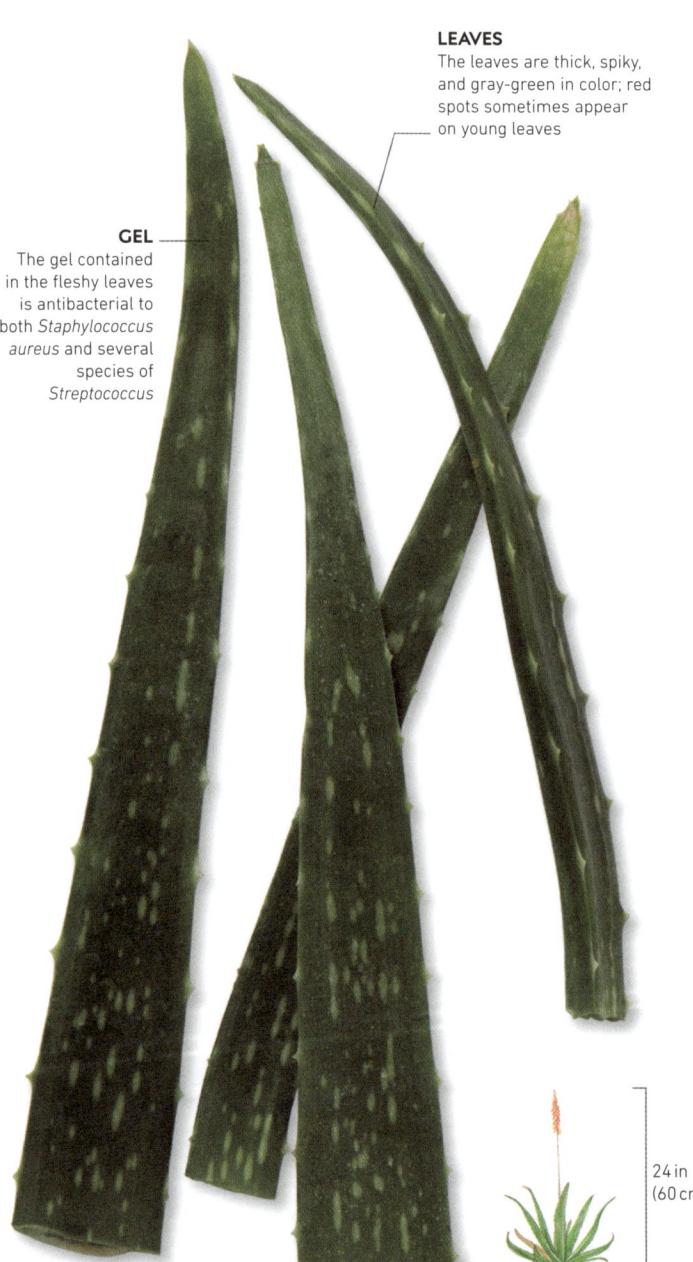

LEAVES
The leaves are thick, spiky, and gray-green in color; red spots sometimes appear on young leaves

GEL
The gel contained in the fleshy leaves is antibacterial to both *Staphylococcus aureus* and several species of *Streptococcus*

24 in
(60 cm)

GROWTH HABIT
Frost-tender, evergreen perennial with an indefinite spread.

PARTS USED Leaves, gel
MAIN CONSTITUENTS Anthraquinone glycosides (incl. aloin and aloe-emodin), resins, polysaccharides, sterols, saponins, chromones
ACTIONS Purgative, cholagogue, wound healer, tonic, demulcent, antibacterial, antifungal, styptic, sedative, anthelmintic

HOW TO USE

FRESH GEL Split open a leaf and use the gel directly, or scrape it out with a blunt knife. Apply directly to burns, sunburn, dry skin, wounds, fungal infections, diaper rash, shingles, ringworm, insect bites, allergic rashes, eczema, or any itchy skin condition.
TINCTURE Made from the whole pulped leaf. Take 1 tsp (5 ml) 3 times daily for constipation or take 10–60 drops (0.5–3 ml) 3 times daily for poor appetite or to stimulate bile flow in sluggish digestion.
CAPSULES Commercially made from powdered leaf. Use in 100–500 mg doses for constipation.
HAIR RINSE Combine 2 tsp (10 ml) of gel with ½ cup of standard chamomile infusion (p.176) and use as a conditioner.

HOW TO SOURCE

GROW Prefers well-drained sandy soil in full sun with a moderate summer water supply and dry winters. Usually propagated by breaking off and replanting the small offsets that appear on mature plants, but can be grown from seeds sown in spring or early summer at 70°F (21°C). Grown as a houseplant in temperate areas; benefits from being kept outside in warm summers.
FORAGE Likely to be found growing wild in tropical regions only. Easily confused with many related, generally larger, species that grow outside in warmer regions.
HARVEST Collect the gel and leaves from plants as required throughout the year.

CAUTION Do not take aloe vera internally during pregnancy.

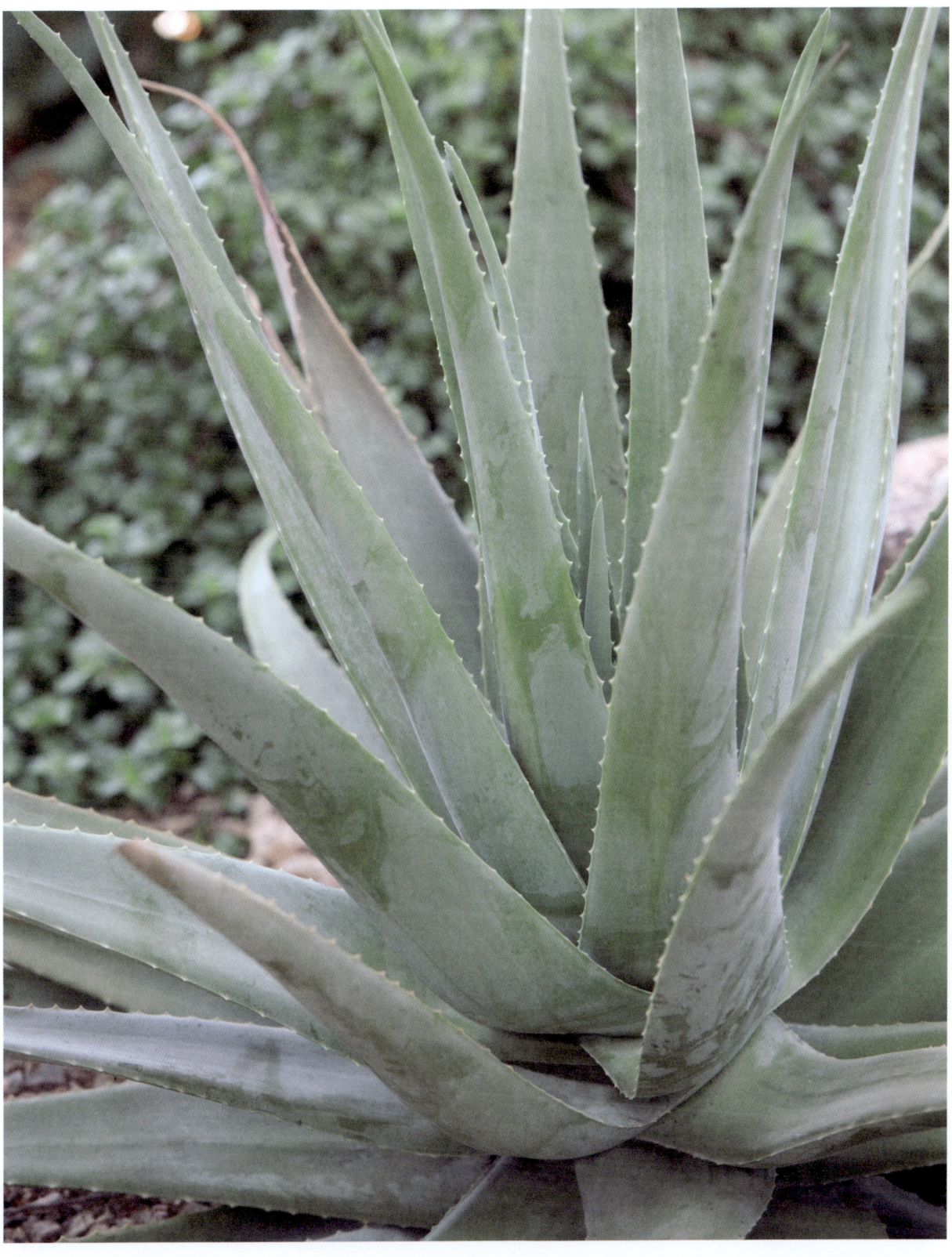

Aloysia triphylla
LEMON VERBENA

FLOWERS
Tiny white or pale lilac
flowers appear in summer,
which is generally when
the leaves are harvested

LEAVES
The leaves are
steam-distilled to
make an essential
oil, which is used
in aromatherapy
for digestive and
nervous problems

STEM
The woody parts of the
plant need protection in
winter if grown outside
in cold areas

GROWTH HABIT
Half-hardy deciduous
shrub with a spread
of 10 ft (3 m).

10 ft
(3 m)

Originally found growing in rocky areas
of Chile and Argentina, lemon verbena
is now cultivated worldwide both as a
highly aromatic garden ornamental and
for use in perfumery. It is also used in
cooking to give a strong lemony taste to
desserts, marinades, and fruit drinks. It
is traditionally regarded as both soothing
and uplifting, so is used in restorative teas.

PARTS USED Leaves, essential oil
MAIN CONSTITUENTS Volatile oil (incl. citral, nerol,
and geraniol)
ACTIONS Sedative, carminative, antispasmodic,
febrifuge, stimulates liver and gall bladder function,
some antifungal activity (to *Candida albicans*) reported

HOW TO USE

INFUSION Use ½ tsp dried leaves per cup (p.176)
after meals for flatulence or at night for insomnia.
Combine with dandelion leaves and drink 3 times
daily to improve liver function. Can be used to ease
feverish conditions in children; consult an herbalist
for advice on dosage.
BATHS Add 1 cup of above infusion to bath water
to ease stress and tension.
MASSAGE OIL True lemon verbena oil is difficult
to obtain, as it is often adulterated with other
lemon-scented oils. Use 5 drops in 1 tbsp (15 ml)
of almond oil as a massage for cramps, indigestion
anxiety, insomnia, or other stress-related conditions.

HOW TO SOURCE

GROW Prefers full sun and moist but well-drained
soil. Usually propagated by heeled softwood cuttings
in summer; it also self-seeds if it sets fruit after a hot
summer. It is not frost-hardy, so in colder areas is best
grown in containers and over-wintered under glass.
Alternatively, cut back to the wood, keep dry, and
protect with fleece or straw lagging in winter (it
should survive temperatures as low as 5°F/-15°C).
FORAGE Unlikely to be found growing wild outside
South America, although self-seeding in warmer
areas is possible.
HARVEST Collect the leaves in summer.

CAUTION Prolonged use or large internal doses can
cause gastric irritation. The oil can irritate sensitive
skin and is photosensitizing, so avoid bright sunlight
if using it externally.

Althaea officinalis
MARSHMALLOW

Originally found in coastal areas of Europe, marshmallow is now widely naturalized. The plant's botanical name comes from the Greek verb, *altho* (to heal), and it has been valued for its soothing and healing action, both internally and externally, for at least 3,500 years. As well as being used medicinally, both the root and leaves can be eaten as vegetables.

PARTS USED Root, leaves, flowers
MAIN CONSTITUENTS Root: asparagine, mucilage, polysaccharides, pectin, tannins
Leaves: mucilage, flavonoids, coumarin, salicylic, and other phenolic acids
ACTIONS Root: demulcent, expectorant, diuretic, wound herb
Leaves: expectorant, diuretic, demulcent
Flowers: expectorant

HOW TO USE

MACERATION Soak 1 oz (30 g) of root in 1 pint (600 ml) of cold water overnight and strain: the result can often be very thick and mucilaginous and may need further dilution. Take ½–1 cup 3 times daily for acid reflux, gastric ulceration, cystitis, and dry coughs.
POULTICE Make a paste from 1 tsp of powdered root mixed with a little water and use on boils, abscesses, ulcers, or poorly healing infected wounds.
OINTMENT Use to draw pus, splinters, or thorns.
INFUSION Drink 1 cup (1–2 tsp dried leaves per cup of boiling water) 3 times daily for bronchitis, bronchial asthma, or pleurisy.
SYRUP Make a syrup by combining 1 pint (600 ml) of a standard infusion of fresh flowers with 1 lb (450 g) of honey or syrup; bring to a boil and simmer gently for 10–15 minutes. Take 1 tsp (5 ml) doses as required.

HOW TO SOURCE

GROW Prefers fertile, moist, well-drained soil in full sun; tolerates other conditions. Sow seed in trays of compost in midsummer and transplant to 3 in (7.5 cm) pots when large enough to handle. Plant the following spring. Alternatively, divide plants in fall. Can self-seed enthusiastically in ideal conditions.
FORAGE Likely to be found in ditches, riversides, tidal zones, and pond margins, especially in coastal areas. Gather the flowers in summer to make a cough syrup, or the leaves during the growing period. The root can be boiled as a vegetable.
HARVEST Dig the root in fall. Cut the aerial parts as the plant starts to flower.

FLOWERS
The pale pink flowers bloom in summer: a traditional French recipe combines them with the flowers of corn poppy (*Papaver rhoeas*), sweet violet (*Viola odorata*), and mullein in a tisane des quatre fleurs

LEAVES
The leaves can be cooked and eaten like cabbage, or the leaf tips eaten in salads

6 ft
(1.8 m)

GROWTH HABIT
Upright perennial with a spread of 24–36 in (60–90 cm).

Angelica archangelica
ANGELICA

Native to northern Europe, angelica is a statuesque plant with striking flower heads in summer. It reputedly takes its medieval Latin name (*herba angelica*) from a belief that it protects against evil spirits, and has been used for a wide range of ailments for centuries. The stems are also used in cooking, and the essential oil is used as a food flavoring.

SEEDS
The essential oil, extracted from the seeds or root, is widely used as a food flavoring and in many aperitifs and liqueurs

PARTS USED Leaves, root, essential oil
MAIN CONSTITUENTS Volatile oil (incl. phellandrene, pinene, borneol, linalool, and limonene), iridoids, resin, coumarins (incl. bergapten and angelicin), valeric acid, tannins
ACTIONS Antispasmodic, diaphoretic, anti-inflammatory, expectorant, carminative, diuretic, antibacterial, digestive stimulant, pectoral, tonic

HOW TO USE

INFUSION Drink 1 cup (1 tsp herb per cup boiling water) of leaves for indigestion.
DECOCTION Take ½–1 cup of a root decoction, made by simmering ½oz (15 g) of root in 1 pint (600 ml) of water for 5 minutes, for any cold condition where increased body heat is required, including arthritic and rheumatic problems in the elderly, poor circulation, or weak digestion.
TINCTURE Take 60 drops (3 ml) 3 times daily of the leaf tincture for bronchitis or flatulent digestion. Take 20–40 drops (1–2 ml) of the root tincture 3 times daily for bronchial catarrh, chesty coughs, digestive disorders including chronic indigestion and loss of appetite, or as a liver stimulant.
MASSAGE OIL Use 5 drops in 1 tbsp (15 ml) of almond oil as a chest rub for bronchitis and coughs or to massage arthritic joints.

HOW TO SOURCE

GROW Prefers deep, fertile, moist soil in sun or partial shade. Surface-sow seeds when ripe or in spring. Thin out seedlings as required when they are large enough to handle. Self-seeds in the right conditions.
FORAGE Found in damp, grassy places in northern and eastern Europe and into Asia.
HARVEST Gather leaves and stems in early summer, year-old roots in fall, and seeds as they ripen.

STEM
The stems can be candied and used in cake decorations and cooking

8 ft
(2.5 m)

GROWTH HABIT
Robust biennial or short-lived perennial; spread 4 ft (1.2 m).

CAUTION Avoid during pregnancy. Do not take therapeutic doses in pregnancy, or if diabetic, unless under professional guidance. Avoid exposure to sun if using externally (phototoxic).

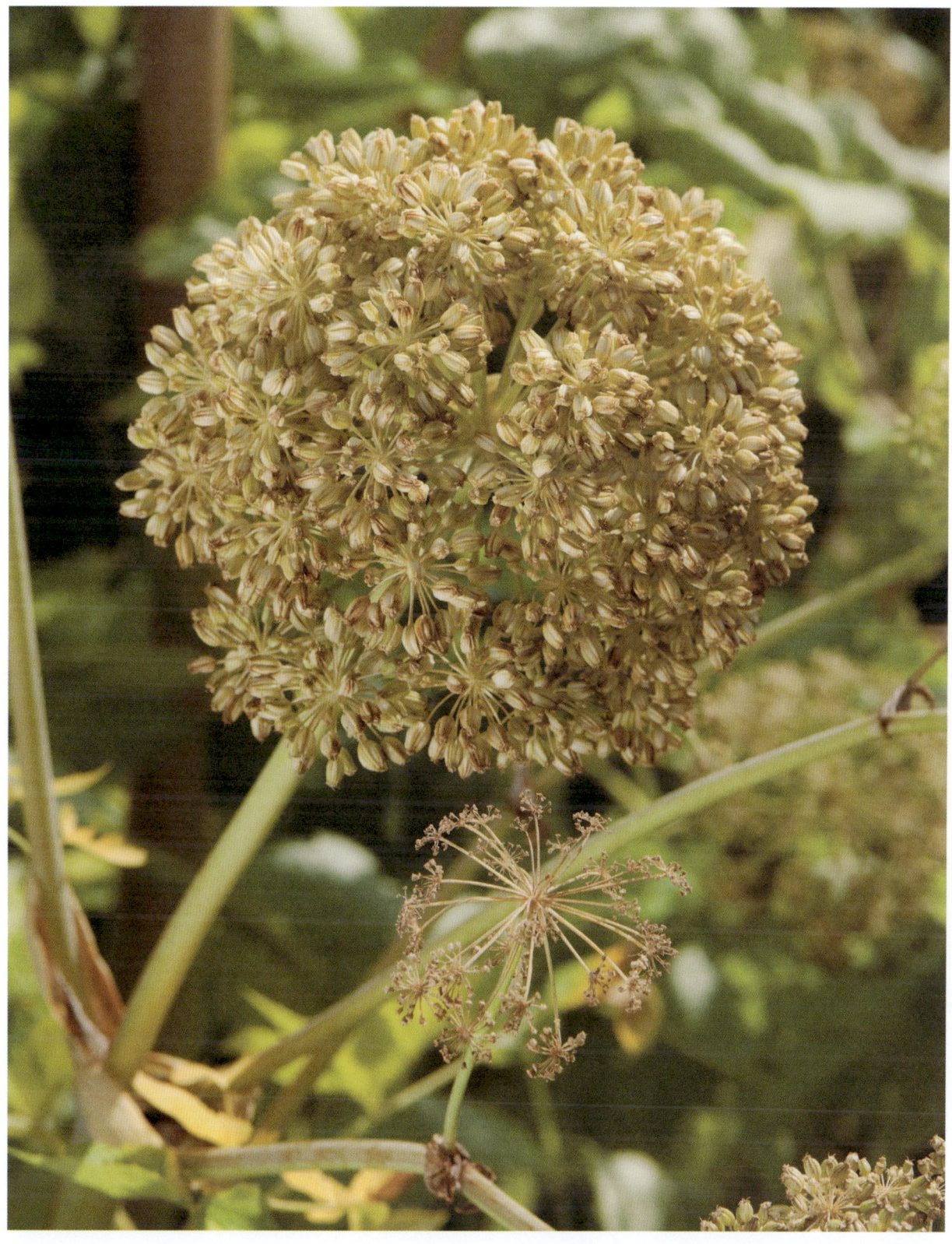

Angelica sinensis
DANG GUI

Native to China and Japan, dang gui has been used for thousands of years as a Chinese remedy for women's health and cardiac conditions. These days it is often used as a heart and liver tonic, and can help improve menstrual function, increase blood circulation to the pelvis, relieve arthritic pain, and speed up the metabolism.

PARTS USED Root
MAIN CONSTITUENTS Phytosterols, ferulic acid, fixed oils, coumarins (angelol and angelicone)
ACTIONS Anti-inflammatory, antiarrhythmic, antifungal, antibacterial, antiviral, regulates uterine function, mild laxative

HOW TO USE

DECOCTION Make a decoction (p.176) by heating 1–2 tsp (4–12 g) of dried root in 1 pint (600 ml) of water for 15 minutes. Take ½–1 cup 3 times daily as a urinary antiseptic and gentle laxative.
TINCTURE To treat period pain, take 20–60 drops (1–3 ml) of tinctured root in a little hot water 3 times daily from 5 days before the period is due to start until it has finished. Dang gui can also be combined with other herbs in tincture form to treat mild palpitations and liver disorders.

HOW TO SOURCE

GROW Prefers deep, moist, well-drained fertile soil, ideally at a high altitude. The plant grows best in cold temperatures no lower than 23°F (–5°C). Seedlings can be planted straight into the ground in a shady spot during spring or fall. The plant flowers from August to September.
FORAGE Found in semi-shady woodlands and high altitudes in damp areas of Korea, Japan, and China.
HARVEST Gather the roots in late fall.

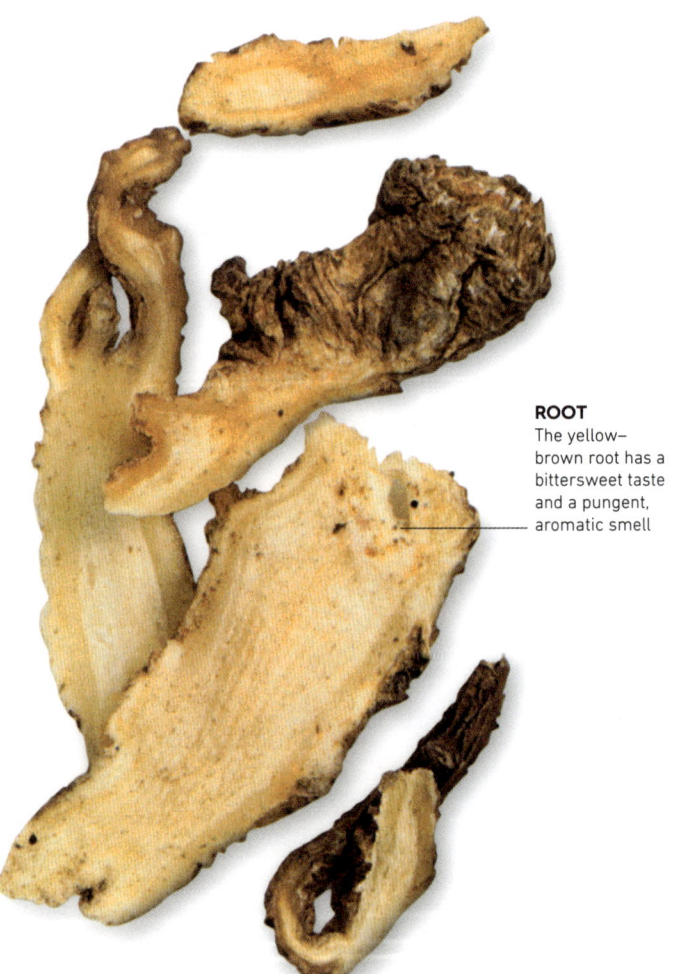

ROOT
The yellow–brown root has a bittersweet taste and a pungent, aromatic smell

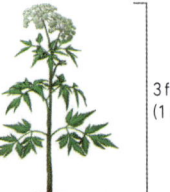

GROWTH HABIT
Herbaceous perennial; spread 28 in (70 cm).

3 ft (1 m)

CAUTION Avoid if you have a bleeding disorder, heavy periods, diarrhea, or abdominal swelling.

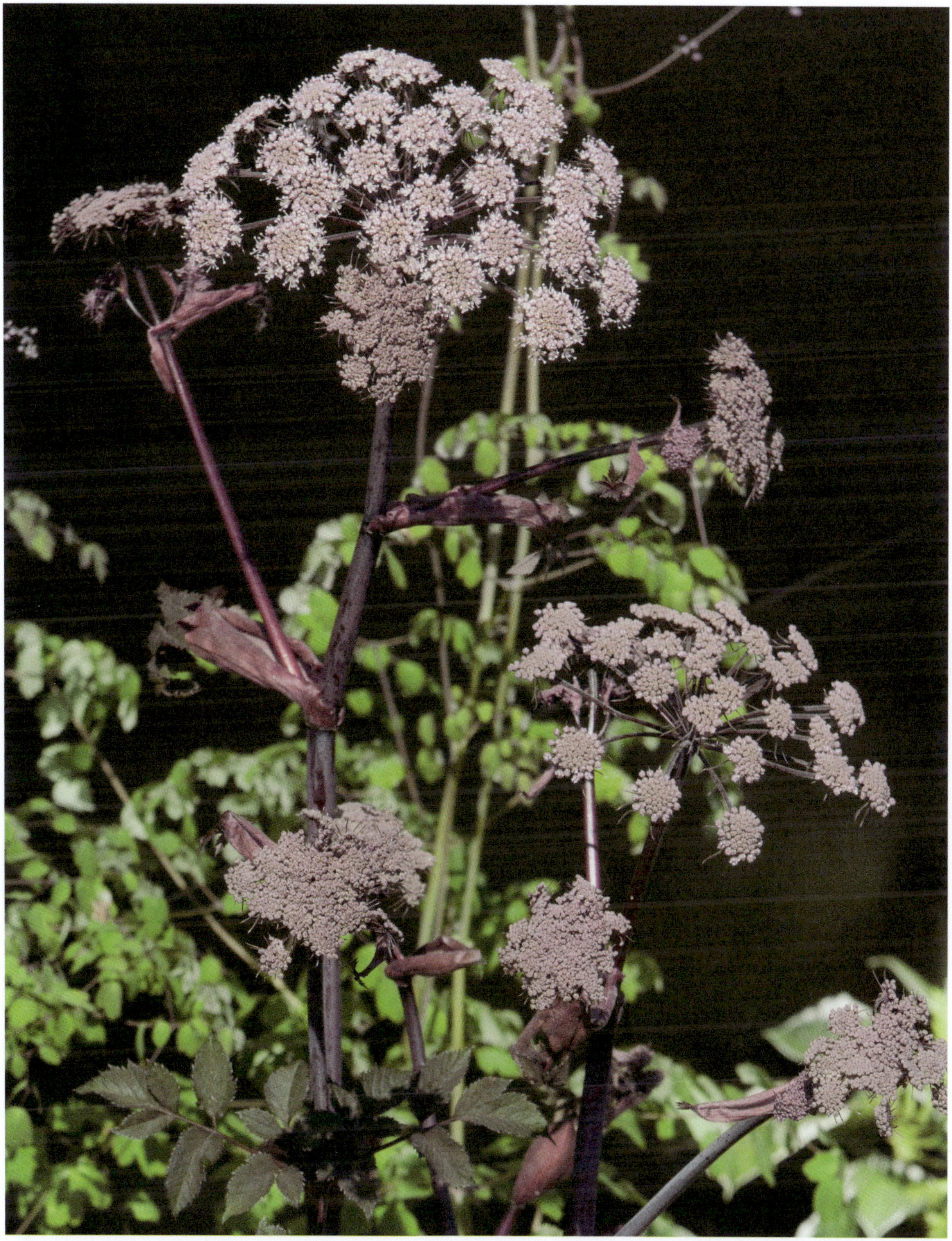

Apium graveolens
WILD CELERY

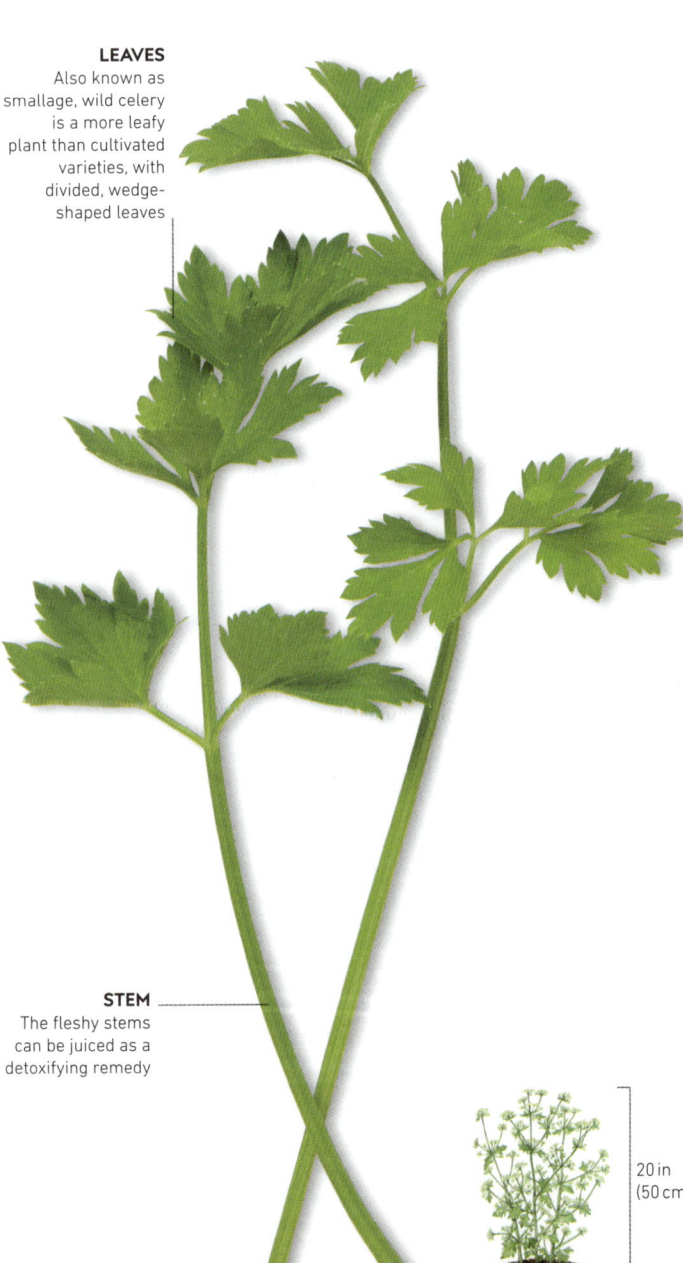

LEAVES
Also known as smallage, wild celery is a more leafy plant than cultivated varieties, with divided, wedge-shaped leaves

STEM
The fleshy stems can be juiced as a detoxifying remedy

20 in (50 cm)

GROWTH HABIT
Biennial with a bulbous root; spread 6–12 in (15–30 cm).

Native to Europe, the Mediterranean region, and western Asia, celery has long been cultivated as a vegetable and cooked or used raw in dishes such as Waldorf salad (celery, walnuts, and apple). Medicinally, the seeds and essential oil of celery are used mainly for urinary and arthritic disorders, and also to help clear uric acid from joints affected by gout.

PARTS USED Seeds, stalks, essential oil
MAIN CONSTITUENTS Volatile oil (incl. limonene, apiole, selinene, and phthalides), coumarins, furanocoumarins, flavonoids, minerals (incl. iron, phosphorus, and potassium)
ACTIONS Antirheumatic, sedative, urinary antiseptic, diuretic, carminative, hypotensive, antispasmodic, galactagogue, anti-inflammatory, encourages elimination of uric acid, antifungal activity reported

HOW TO USE

DECOCTION Use ½oz (15 g) of seeds to 1 pint (600 ml) of water, simmer for 10 minutes and take in ½–1 cup doses 3 times daily for rheumatic disorders, gout, rheumatoid arthritis, and urinary tract inflammations.
MASSAGE OIL Use 20 drops (1 ml) oil in 4 fl oz (120 ml) of almond oil and massage into the abdomen for indigestion, flatulence, and liver congestion. Use also for sciatica, rheumatism, and arthritis.
FOOTBATH Add 20 drops (1 ml) oil to a bowl of warm water to soak feet or toe joints with very painful gout.
JUICE Liquidize the stalks (ribs) and leaves and drink in 1 cup doses as a remedy for debility and nervous exhaustion.

HOW TO SOURCE

GROW Prefers moist, well-drained soil in full sun. Plant the seeds in seed trays in spring, cover with a thin layer of topsoil, and place in a heated propagator or on a warm window sill. Transfer to 3 in (7.5 cm) pots, and when 4 in (10 cm) tall, plant in final growing positions 12 in (30 cm) apart.
FORAGE It is recommended to grow your own. Grows wild in coastal areas. In the wild, the leaves can be confused with deadly hemlock or water dropwort, the latter having an unpleasant smell when crushed.
HARVEST Pick the cultivated variety as a vegetable in the first year; collect the seeds when ripe in the second summer.

CAUTION Do not use seeds if pregnant. Do not use cultivated seeds medicinally, as they are often treated with fungicides. Do not take the essential oil internally unless under professional supervision.

Aralia racemosa
AMERICAN SPIKENARD

Traditionally used for a range of ailments including rheumatism, coughs, indigestion, asthma, and blood poisoning, American spikenard is found in many parts of the United States, from the Midwest to the eastern seaboard. The herb is known to encourage sweating and is detoxifying, but has otherwise been poorly researched.

PARTS USED Root
MAIN CONSTITUENTS Volatile oil, tannins, glycosides, diterpenes
ACTIONS Expectorant, diaphoretic, warming stimulant, detoxifying

HOW TO USE

DECOCTION Take ½ cup of a decoction made from ½oz (15 g) dried root in 1 pint (600 ml) of water 3 times daily for rheumatic disorders.
SYRUP Combine 1 cup of strained decoction with 1 cup of sugar or honey, bring to a boil, and simmer gently for 5–10 minutes to make a syrup. Take in 1 tsp (5 ml) doses every 2–3 hours for coughs including bronchitis and whooping coughs.
LIQUID EXTRACT Take 30–60 drops (1.5–3 ml) 3 times daily in a little water for rheumatic disorders, lumbago, and similar aches and pains.
POULTICE Mix ½oz (15 g) of powdered root into a paste with a little water, spread on gauze, and use as a poultice for skin conditions including eczema.

HOW TO SOURCE

GROW Prefers partial shade, but tolerates sun. Sow the seeds where you want to grow them in fall or in winter in a cold frame or unheated greenhouse; transplant into final positions the following spring.
FORAGE Largely found in woodland areas in the Midwest and eastern US and southern Canada; unlikely to occur growing wild in other areas. As well as their medicinal applications, the roots can be used in teas or to flavor beer.
HARVEST Dig up the roots in summer or fall.

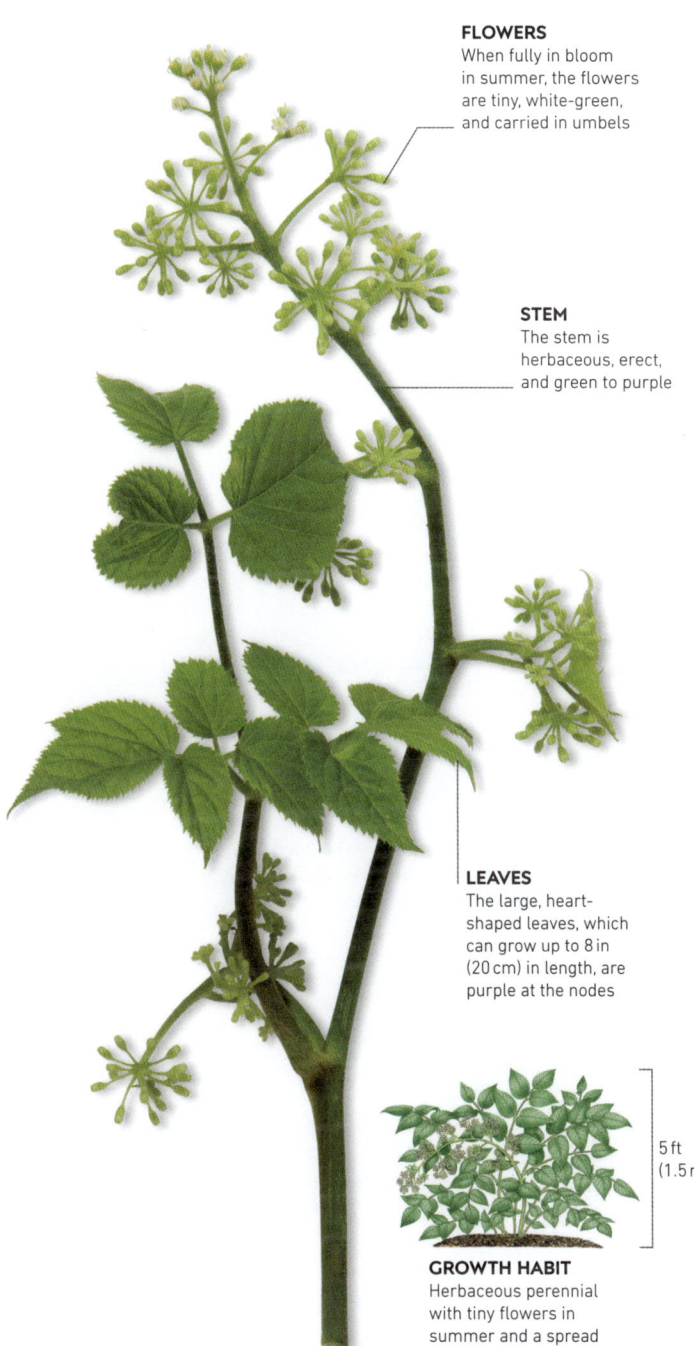

FLOWERS
When fully in bloom in summer, the flowers are tiny, white-green, and carried in umbels

STEM
The stem is herbaceous, erect, and green to purple

LEAVES
The large, heart-shaped leaves, which can grow up to 8 in (20 cm) in length, are purple at the nodes

5 ft
(1.5 m)

GROWTH HABIT
Herbaceous perennial with tiny flowers in summer and a spread of 2–6 ft (60 cm–2 m).

CAUTION Avoid during pregnancy.

Arctium lappa
BURDOCK

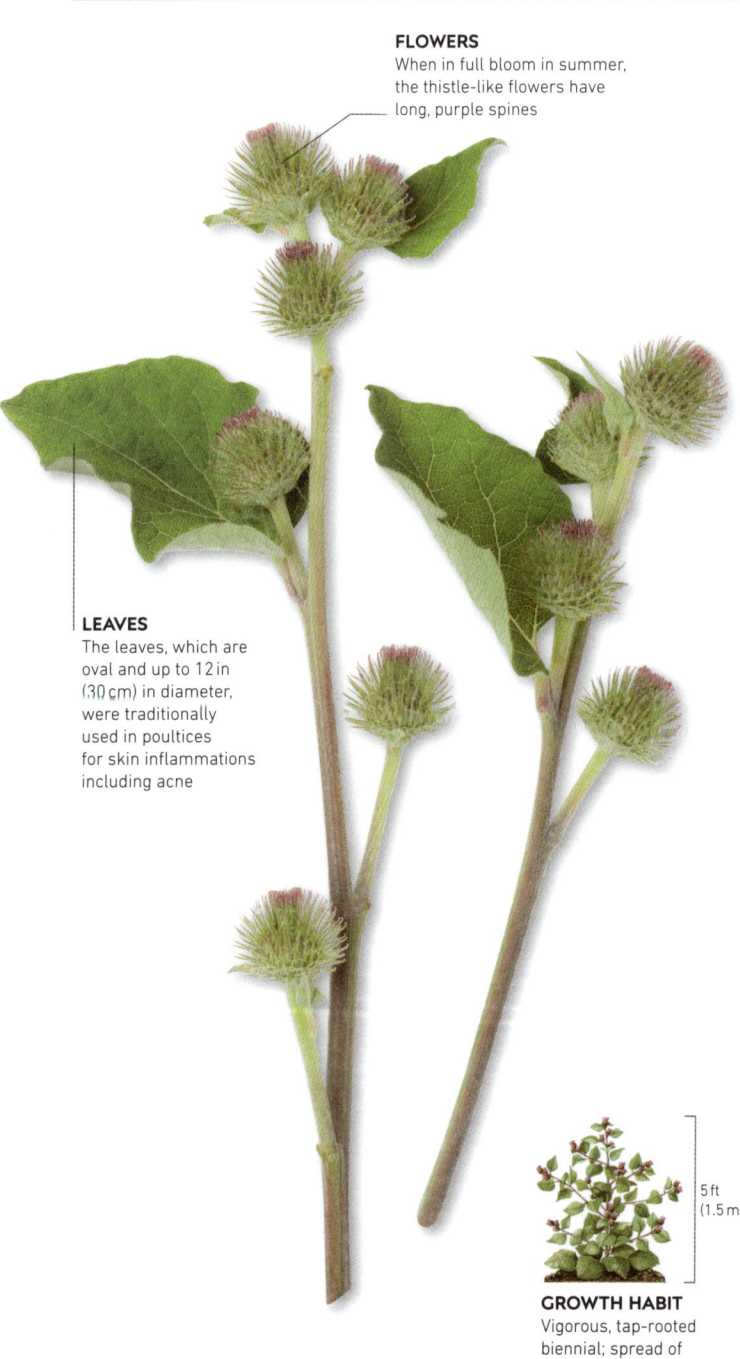

FLOWERS
When in full bloom in summer, the thistle-like flowers have long, purple spines

LEAVES
The leaves, which are oval and up to 12 in (30 cm) in diameter, were traditionally used in poultices for skin inflammations including acne

GROWTH HABIT
Vigorous, tap-rooted biennial; spread of up to 3 ft (1 m).

5 ft (1.5 m)

Native to Europe and Asia, burdock is largely regarded as a cleansing remedy that helps rid the body of toxins, including heavy metals, and is generally used for skin problems, arthritic conditions, and infections. The root and leaves are traditionally used in Europe, while the seeds are preferred in Chinese medicine and are often included in remedies for common colds.

PARTS USED Root, leaves, seeds
MAIN CONSTITUENTS Leaf/root: bitter glycosides (incl. arctiopictrin), flavonoids (incl. arctin), tannins, volatile oil, antibiotic polyacetylenes, resin, mucilage, inulin, alkaloids, sesquiterpenes
Seeds: essential fatty acids, vitamins A, B2
ACTIONS Root: cleansing, mild laxative, diuretic, diaphoretic, antirheumatic, antiseptic, antibiotic
Leaves: mild laxative, diuretic Seeds: febrifuge, anti-inflammatory, antibacterial, hypoglycemic

HOW TO USE

ROOT DECOCTION Make an infusion (p.176) of 1 tsp root per cup boiling water. Drink ½–1 cup 3 times daily for skin disorders, including persistent boils, sores, psoriasis, and dry eczema. Use a cup of the mix as a wash for acne and fungal skin infections including athlete's foot or ringworm.
INFUSION Take 1 wineglass of a standard leaf infusion (p.176) before meals as a mild digestive stimulant to combat indigestion.
SEED DECOCTION Take 1 standard decoction of the seeds up to 3 times daily for feverish colds and infections with sore throat and cough; it is often combined with honeysuckle flowers or forsythia berries.
TINCTURE Take 1–2 tsp (5–10 ml) root tincture 3 times daily to detoxify the system in arthritic conditions, for urinary stones and gravel, or to stimulate digestion. Usually used in combination with other herbs.
POULTICE Use a root poultice for skin sores and leg ulcers.

HOW TO SOURCE

GROW Prefers moist, neutral to alkaline soil in full sun to partial shade. Sow the seeds where you want to grow them in spring. Self-seeds prolifically and can be invasive. Harvest the plant before the fruits are ripe to reduce the spread.
FORAGE Easily spotted in hedges and waste areas in Europe and western Asia.
HARVEST The root is generally collected in late summer and the leaves when the plant is just starting to flower; the seeds should be gathered when ripe in fall.

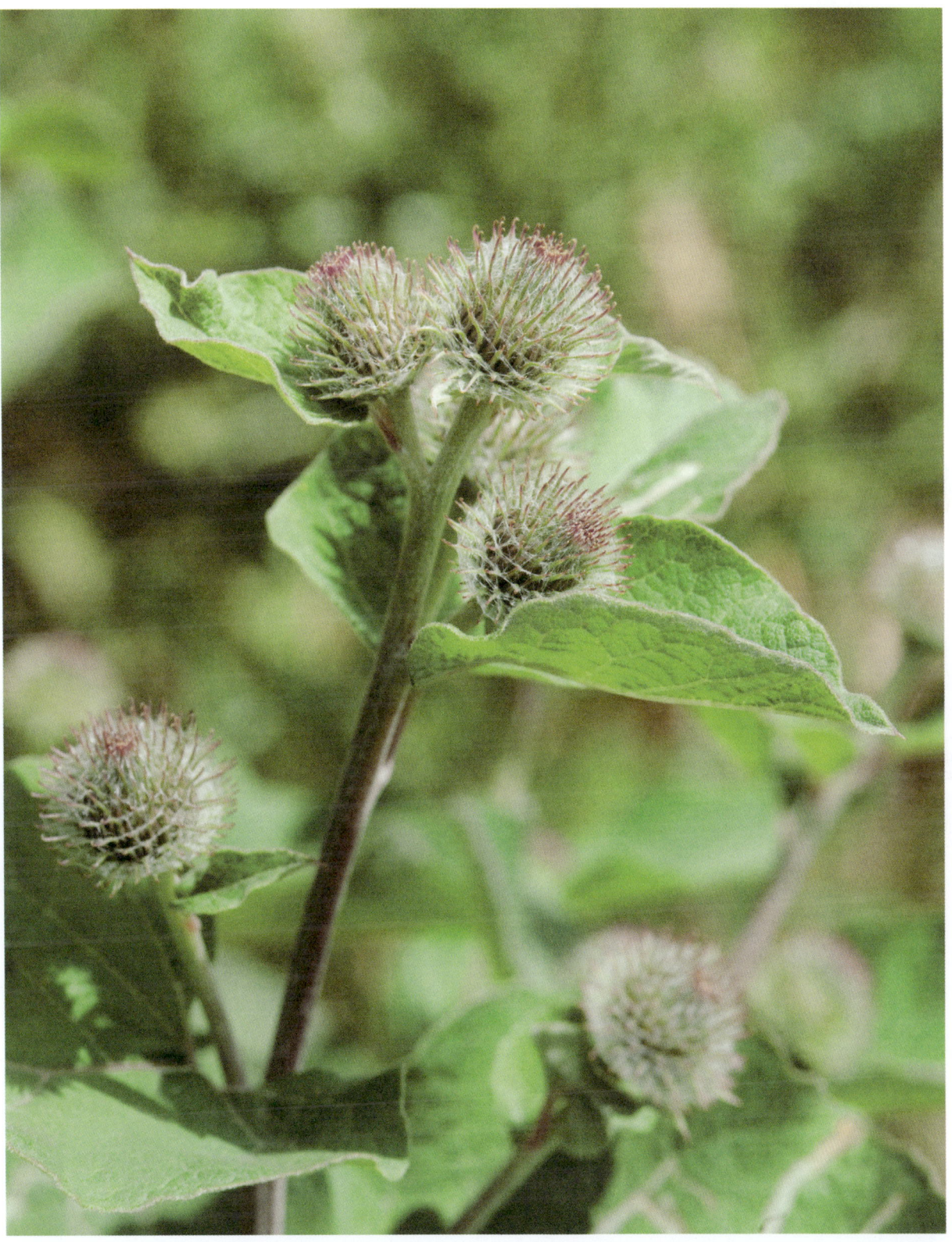

Arctostaphylos uva-ursi
BEARBERRY

Native to moorland in Europe, Asia, and North America, this plant's fruits are a favorite food for bears—hence its common name, bearberry or uva-ursi (in Latin, literally "grape-bear"). It is highly regarded by herbalists as a urinary antiseptic largely due to the presence of chemicals called hydroquinones, which help disinfect the urinary tract.

PARTS USED Leaves, berries
MAIN CONSTITUENTS Hydroquinones (incl. arbutin), ursolic acid, tannic acid, gallic acid, phenolic glycosides, flavonoids, volatile oil, resin, tannins
ACTIONS Astringent, antibacterial, demulcent, urinary antiseptic, possibly diuretic, hemostatic, oxytocic, tonic

HOW TO USE

INFUSION Drink 1 cup (1–2 tsp herb per cup of boiling water) of leaves 3 times daily for cystitis, urethritis, or burning pain when urinating. It is often combined with couch grass or cleavers. For any severe or persistent urinary symptoms, you should seek urgent medical advice to avoid any potential damage to the kidneys.
TINCTURE Take 40–80 drops (2–4 ml) 3 times daily for urinary problems or leucorrhea (a white or yellow vaginal discharge).
TABLETS Available commercially, often in combination with dandelion, as a remedy for fluid retention. Follow the directions on the package.

HOW TO SOURCE

GROW A moorland plant, it prefers moist, fertile, acidic soil in partial or dappled shade, and makes good ground cover in the right conditions. Requires lime-free (ericaceous) soil. Sow seeds in a cold frame in fall and pot as soon as the seedlings are large enough to handle.
FORAGE Found in moorland areas. The leaves can be harvested in summer. The berries are edible and can be gathered in fall and made into jellies and jams.
HARVEST The leaves are mainly collected in spring or summer, and the berries are collected in fall.

LEAVES
The small leaves need to be gathered and dried individually for use in remedies for cystitis and other urinary problems

FLOWERS
The bell-shaped flowers have 5 white or pink petals that curl in around the narrow center of the flower. They appear in late spring/early summer

6 in (15 cm)

GROWTH HABIT
Creeping, mat-forming, evergreen shrub with bell-shaped flowers; spread 36 in (90 cm) or more.

CAUTION Do not take during pregnancy, while breastfeeding, or if suffering from kidney disease. It should not be taken for more than 10 consecutive days without professional advice. Large doses may cause nausea and vomiting.

Artemisia absinthium
WORMWOOD

An extremely bitter herb, wormwood is largely used today as a digestive stimulant. Native to Europe, it was once a popular remedy for treating parasitic worms, as its name implies, and is still occasionally used in this way today. Its botanical name highlights a link to the French drink, absinthe, a favorite with the 19th-century avant garde that was highly addictive.

PARTS USED Leaves, flowering tops
MAIN CONSTITUENTS Volatile oil (incl. sesquiterpene lactones, thujone, and azulenes), bitter principle, flavonoids, tannins, lignan, silica, antibiotic polyacetylenes, inulin, hydroxycoumarins
ACTIONS Bitter digestive tonic, anthelmintic, uterine stimulant, cholagogue, choleretic, carminative, anti-inflammatory, immune stimulant

HOW TO USE

NB: Use only under medical supervision
TINCTURE Take 1 drop on the tongue to stimulate the digestion and combat any late-afternoon chocolate cravings.
MACERATION Add ½ level tsp of dried herb to 1 cup of cold water, steep overnight, strain, and drink in the morning for poor appetite, hepatitis, sluggish digestion, bloating, and stagnant liver syndromes.
COMPRESS Soak a cloth in a strained maceration and apply to bruises and insect bites.
WASH Use 1 cup of strained maceration as a wash for scabies or other parasitic skin infections.
FLUID EXTRACT Take 40 drops (2 ml) well diluted with water on an empty stomach for parasitic worms; repeat fortnightly.

HOW TO SOURCE

GROW Prefers well-drained, fertile soil in full sun, but tolerates poor, dry soil. Sow seeds in a cold frame in fall or spring and transplant to their final positions when large enough to handle. Alternatively, divide clumps in spring or take heeled semi-ripe cuttings in midsummer.
FORAGE Found in hedges and waste areas in Europe, central Asia, and parts of the US; gather the leaves in summer.
HARVEST Cut aerial parts while flowering.

CAUTION Avoid if pregnant or if blood pressure is high. Do not take for more than four to five weeks at a time. Take only under professional supervision and do not exceed stated dosages.

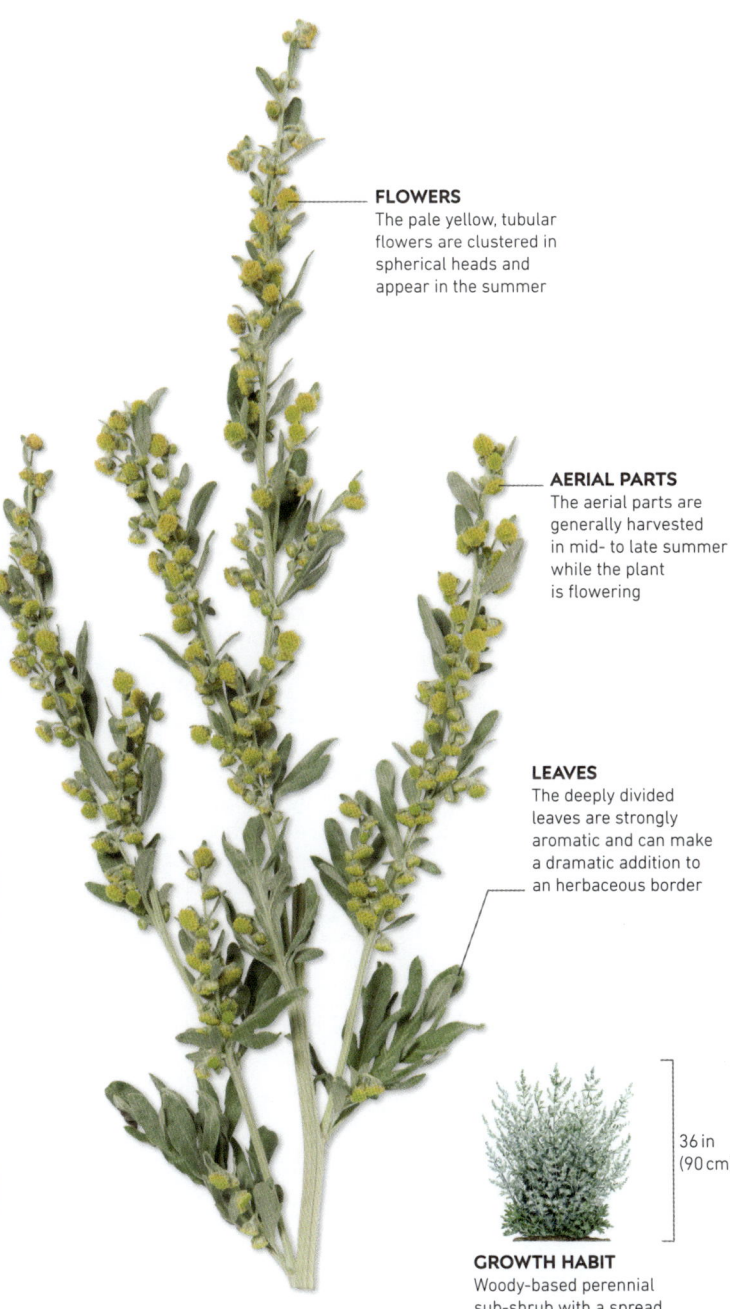

FLOWERS
The pale yellow, tubular flowers are clustered in spherical heads and appear in the summer

AERIAL PARTS
The aerial parts are generally harvested in mid- to late summer while the plant is flowering

LEAVES
The deeply divided leaves are strongly aromatic and can make a dramatic addition to an herbaceous border

36 in
(90 cm)

GROWTH HABIT
Woody-based perennial sub-shrub with a spread of 24–36 in (60–90 cm).

Astragalus membranaceus
ASTRAGALUS

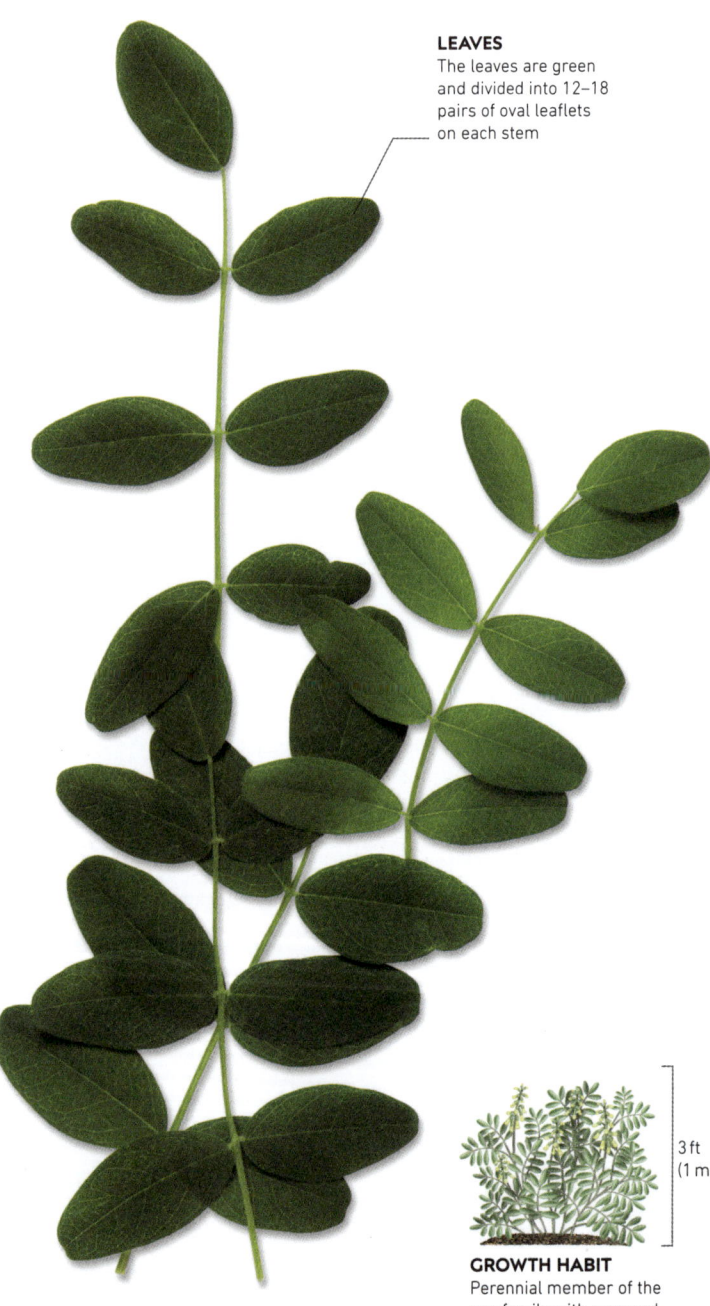

LEAVES
The leaves are green and divided into 12–18 pairs of oval leaflets on each stem

GROWTH HABIT
Perennial member of the pea family with a spread of 12–16 in (30–40 cm).

3 ft (1 m)

One of China's most important medicinal herbs, astragalus—the English term is milk vetch—is generally used as a tonic for younger people (whereas ginseng is the preferred stimulant for older people). It is particularly effective at strengthening the immune system and boosting energy levels, and is also used to clear abscesses and ulcers.

PARTS USED Root parts
MAIN CONSTITUENTS Flavonoids (mainly isoflavones), saponins (incl. astragalosides), polysaccharides (astragalans), asparagine, sterols
ACTIONS Antispasmodic, adaptogenic, diuretic, cholagogue, antibacterial, hypoglycemic, nervous stimulant, hypotensive, immune stimulant

HOW TO USE

DECOCTION Generally used in combination with other herbs rather than by itself: typically ⅓–½oz (9–15 g) is added to Chinese tang, a therapeutic decoction generally taken once or twice a day. It is used with ginseng (*Panax ginseng*) for general debility and fatigue, or with dang gui for low energy, blood loss, or some types of pain.
TINCTURE Take 40–80 drops (2–4 ml) up to 3 times daily as a general tonic, to boost the immune system if suffering from fatigue with recurrent infections, or for conditions involving excess sweating.
CAPSULES Widely available in commercial products that are generally marketed as energy tonics. Follow the dosage directions on the pack

HOW TO SOURCE

GROW Prefers full sun. Scarify seeds before planting ½in (1 cm) deep and about 4 in (10 cm) apart in late winter/early spring in a prepared seed bed that contains sharp sand and is alkaline (above pH 7). Thin to 12 in (30 cm) apart and only water when the soil dries out, as astragalus does not like wet ground.
FORAGE Only likely to be found growing wild in northwest China and Mongolia.
HARVEST Dig the roots of four-year-old plants in fall.

CAUTION Avoid in conditions involving excess heat and in acute stages of infections; may interfere with immune-suppressant or blood-thinning drugs.

Avena sativa
OATS

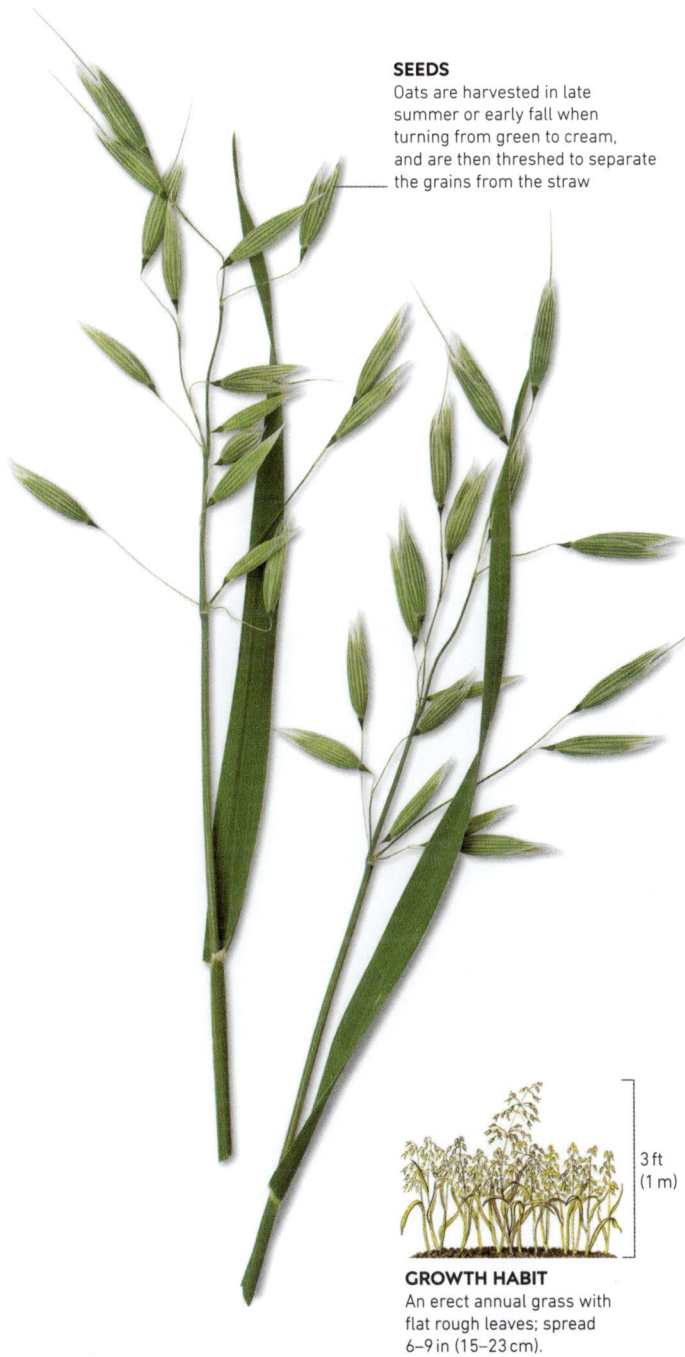

SEEDS
Oats are harvested in late summer or early fall when turning from green to cream, and are then threshed to separate the grains from the straw

GROWTH HABIT
An erect annual grass with flat rough leaves; spread 6–9 in (15–23 cm).

3 ft (1 m)

Native to northern Europe, oats are cultivated worldwide as a cereal crop. Both oatmeal and oat bran are readily available and used in savory dishes, oatmeal, or added to breakfast cereals. Oats, like the whole plant, are restorative for the nervous system, and can help reduce blood cholesterol levels. Traditionally the green, newly harvested whole plant was used medicinally.

PARTS USED Seeds, bran, oat straw (whole plant)
MAIN CONSTITUENTS Saponins, flavonoids, many minerals (incl. calcium), alkaloids, sterols, vitamins B1, B2, D, and E, carotene, silicic acid, protein (gluten), starch, fat
ACTIONS Antidepressant, restorative nerve tonic, diaphoretic, nutritive, reduces cholesterol levels, demulcent, vulnerary

HOW TO USE

TINCTURE This should ideally be made from the fresh green whole plant. Take 20 drops–1 tsp (1–5 ml) 3 times daily for nervous exhaustion, tension, anxiety, debility following illness, or depression. It combines well with vervain, wood betony, or valerian.
INFUSION Drink 1 cup (2 tsp herb per cup of boiling water) of oat straw as required as a restorative for the nervous system.
FACIAL SCRUB For dull, greasy skin or a tendency for acne, mix ½ cup of fine oatmeal with water to make a paste. Apply to the face and leave for 10 minutes before rinsing.
BATH Strain 1 pint (600 ml) of a standard decoction of the oat straw or whole grains into the bath to ease itching and eczema.

HOW TO SOURCE

GROW Prefers neutral or slightly acidic soil and cool, damp conditions, but will tolerate dry spells. Winter oats are sown in fall for a late summer harvest, or in spring as an early fall crop.
FORAGE Do not trespass in a farmer's crop, but self-seeding plants are often found in hedges or field margins. Forage for dried stems if they are not used for fodder. Wild oats are preferred by many herbalists as a more effective treatment.
HARVEST Harvest in late summer or early fall as the grains turn to pale cream.

CAUTION For those sensitive to gluten, decoctions or tinctures should be allowed to settle and then the clear liquid only decanted for use. Use gluten-free oats if gluten-intolerant.

Calendula officinalis
CALENDULA OR MARIGOLD

Traditionally said to lift the spirits and encourage cheerfulness, calendula (also known as marigold) is one of the most popular and versatile medicinal herbs in current use. It is widely available in commercial calendula ointments and creams, and is also used internally for digestive and gynecological problems or as a cleansing remedy for skin and rheumatic disorders.

PARTS USED Flower heads, essential oil
MAIN CONSTITUENTS Flavonoids, mucilage, triterpenes, volatile oil, bitter glycosides, resin, sterols, carotenes
ACTIONS Astringent, antibacterial, antifungal, anti-inflammatory, wound herb, mildly estrogenic, antispasmodic, menstrual regulator, tonic, cholagogue

HOW TO USE

Do not confuse with preparations made from French marigold (*Tagetes patula*).
INFUSION Drink 1 cup (1–2 tsp herb per cup boiling water) 3 times daily for inflammatory digestive disorders like gastritis, esophagitis, or colitis. Makes a suitable douche for vaginal thrush or as a mouthwash for gum disease.
CREAM/OINTMENT Use for minor cuts and scrapes, and any inflamed or dry skin: eczema, chapped hands, chilblains, sore nipples in breastfeeding, acne, minor burns and scalds, sunburn, etc. It is also helpful for fungal infections such as ringworm, thrush, and athlete's foot.
MACERATED OIL Use as an ointment on hemorrhoids or broken capillaries; add up to 20 percent lavender oil for sunburn.
TINCTURE Take 40 drops–1 tsp (2–5 ml) 3 times a day for menstrual problems, (irregular, heavy, or painful periods).

HOW TO SOURCE

GROW Prefers well-drained soil in a sunny site, but will tolerate partial shade. Sow seeds in fall or spring, and thin or transplant seedlings when large enough to handle. Can also be grown in containers. It flowers throughout the summer and self-seeds enthusiastically, so gather flowers regularly to avoid excessive seeding.
FORAGE Most likely to be found naturalized in Mediterranean areas in rocky places or cultivated sites and on wasteland; elsewhere, self-seeded plants outside gardens are possible, but less common.
HARVEST Collect flowers in summer.

CAUTION Avoid internal use of calendula during pregnancy.

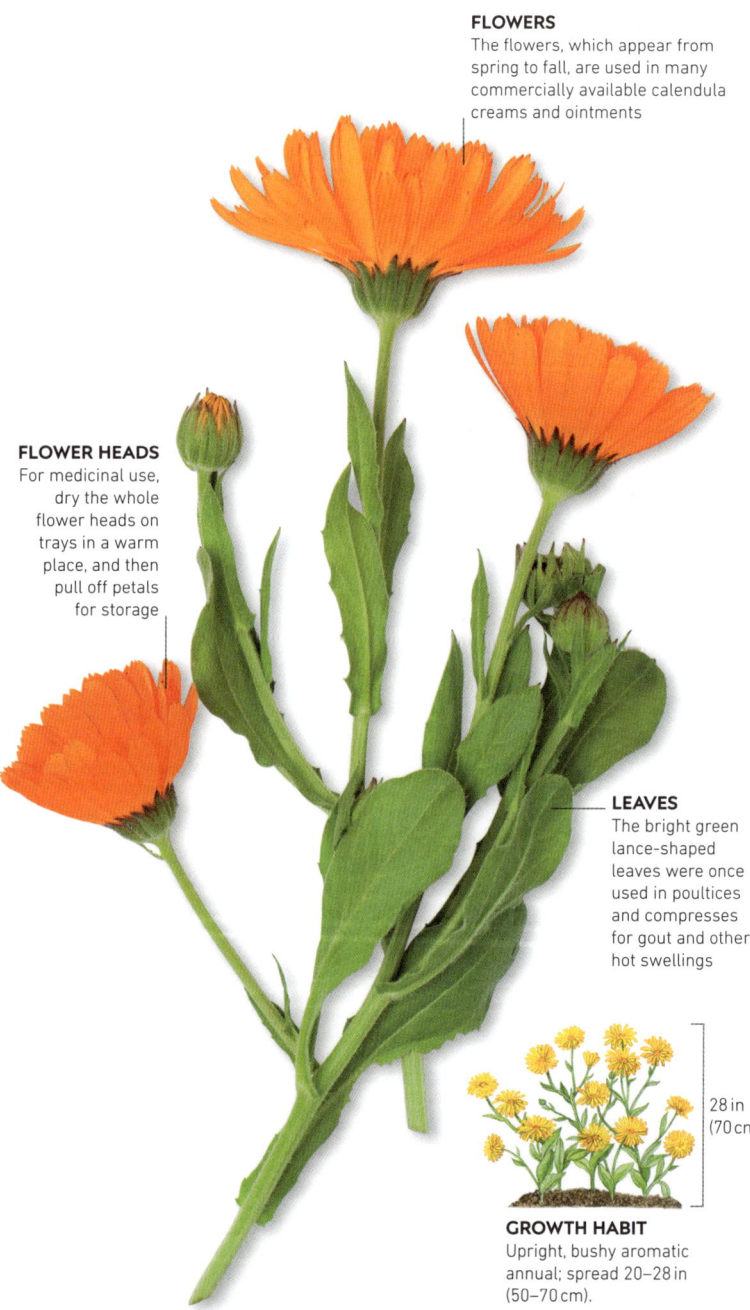

FLOWERS
The flowers, which appear from spring to fall, are used in many commercially available calendula creams and ointments

FLOWER HEADS
For medicinal use, dry the whole flower heads on trays in a warm place, and then pull off petals for storage

LEAVES
The bright green lance-shaped leaves were once used in poultices and compresses for gout and other hot swellings

28 in (70 cm)

GROWTH HABIT
Upright, bushy aromatic annual; spread 20–28 in (50–70 cm).

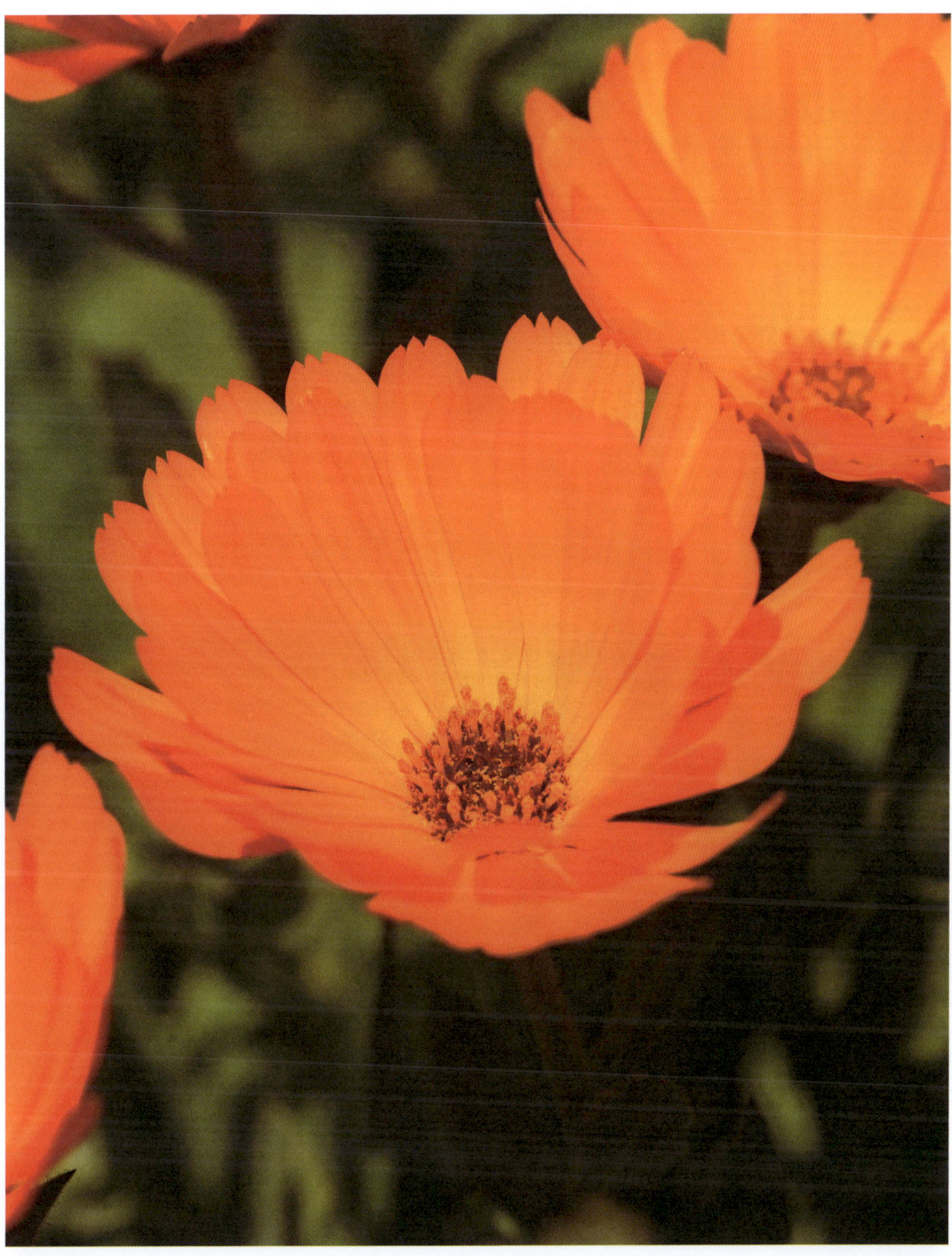

Capsicum annuum
CAYENNE OR CHILE PEPPER

Originally found in tropical regions of the Americas, cayenne was introduced into India and Africa by the Portuguese and reached Europe by the mid-16th century. It soon became an established culinary seasoning and medicinal herb. Today it is widely used as a warming remedy.

PARTS USED Fruit

MAIN CONSTITUENTS Capsaicin; carotenoids; fatty acids; flavonoids; vitamins A, B1, and C; volatile oil; sugars

ACTIONS Circulatory stimulant, diaphoretic, gastric stimulant, carminative, antiseptic, antibacterial Topically: counter-irritant, rubefacient

HOW TO USE

MACERATED OIL Heat 1 oz (30 g) of the powder, or 3–4 chopped fresh chiles, in 1 pint (600 ml) of sunflower oil in a bowl over a saucepan of simmering water (bain-marie) for 2 hours. Use as a massage oil for rheumatism, lumbago, arthritis, and so on, or to relieve pain from shingles.

TINCTURE Take 20 drops (1 ml) in a cup of warm water as a circulatory stimulant for cold hands and feet.

GARGLE Use 5–10 drops (¼–½ml) of tincture or a pinch (⅛ tsp) of cayenne powder to half a tumbler of warm water for sore throats or laryngitis.

DIET Add to food to treat low blood pressure.

HOW TO SOURCE

GROW Sow 2–3 seeds in each 3 in (7.5 cm) pot using good-quality compost. Plant when the soil temperature reaches 59°F (15°C) or, in temperate regions, pot into large containers and keep in a greenhouse.

FORAGE Grown in the tropics in America, Africa, and India, unlikely to be found growing wild outside these regions, but self-seeded plants that grow outside of gardens are possible.

HARVEST Gather the fruits when ripe in summer and dry immediately in the shade.

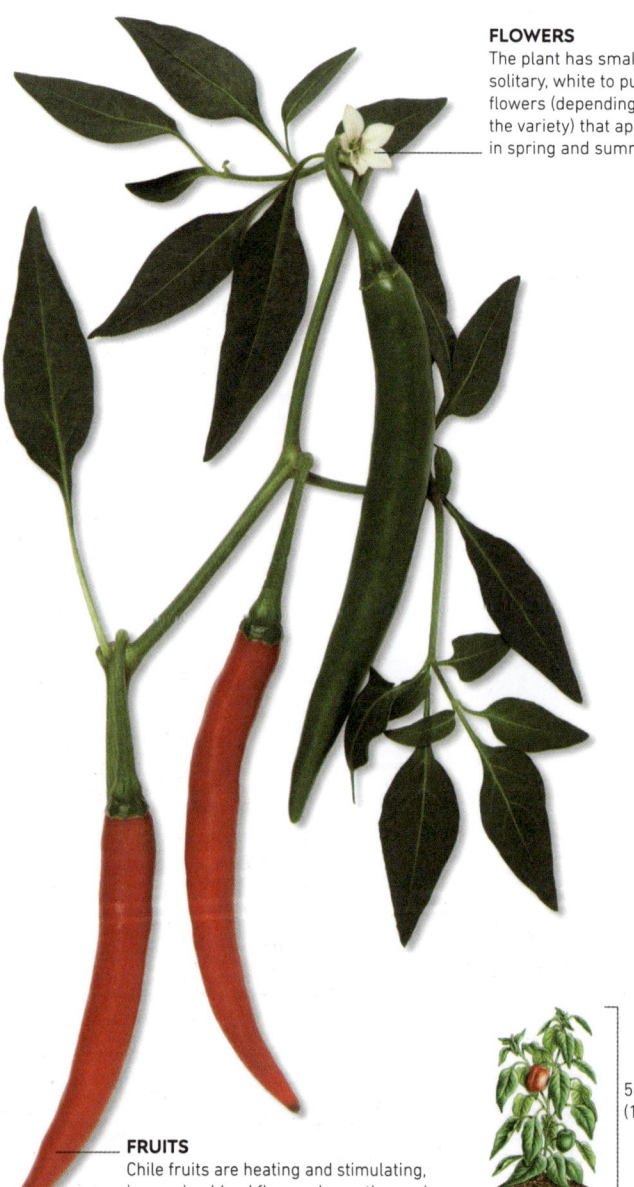

FLOWERS
The plant has small, solitary, white to purple flowers (depending on the variety) that appear in spring and summer

FRUITS
Chile fruits are heating and stimulating, increasing blood flow and sweating and stimulating digestion. Related varieties of Capsicum may be in different shapes

GROWTH HABIT
Bushy perennial shrub; spread 20 in–6 ft (50 cm–2 m).

5 ft (1.5 m)

CAUTION Do not exceed the stated dose: excess can lead to gastric irritation. Avoid touching the eyes or any cuts after handling cayenne, as it can sting. Compresses left on the skin for long periods can cause blistering.

Carum carvi
CARAWAY

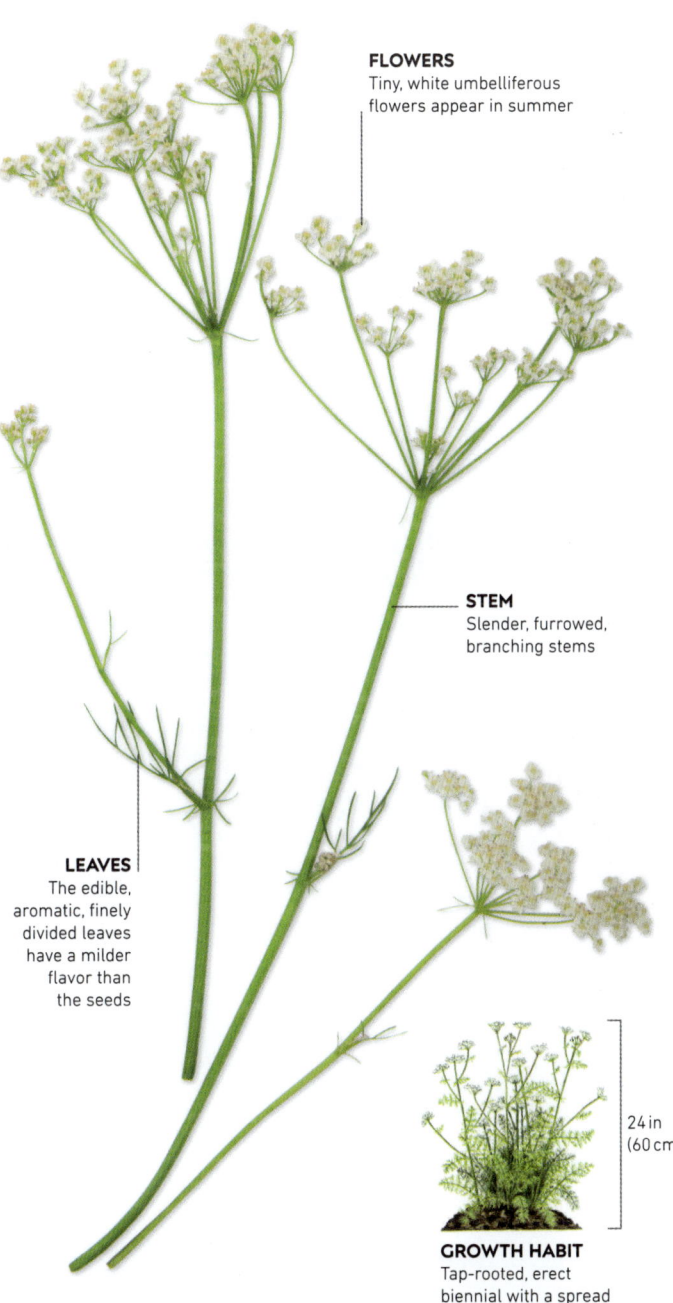

FLOWERS
Tiny, white umbelliferous flowers appear in summer

STEM
Slender, furrowed, branching stems

LEAVES
The edible, aromatic, finely divided leaves have a milder flavor than the seeds

24 in (60 cm)

GROWTH HABIT
Tap-rooted, erect biennial with a spread of 12 in (30 cm).

Native to Mediterranean regions, caraway is now naturalized in parts of Asia and North America. Cultivated commercially, the oil is used in pharmaceuticals and toiletries such as toothpastes and mouthwashes, and as a food flavoring. Like its relatives anise and fennel, caraway is used for digestive and respiratory disorders, and is popular for treating colic in infants.

PARTS USED Seeds, essential oil
MAIN CONSTITUENTS Volatile oil (mainly carvone and limonene), flavonoids, polysaccharides
ACTIONS Antispasmodic, carminative, antimicrobial, expectorant, galactogogue, emmenagogue, diuretic, tonic

HOW TO USE

INFUSION Pour 1 cup of boiling water over 1–2 tsp of crushed seeds. Drink 1 cup 3 times daily for menstrual cramps or colic in adults, or drink 1 cup a day to improve milk flow when breastfeeding. For children with gas or colic, reduce the dosage according to age. For children aged 1–2, use 2 tsp (10 ml) of a standard infusion diluted with 3½ fl oz (100 ml) of warm water per dose; for children aged 3–4, use 4 tsp (20 ml) of a standard infusion similarly diluted.
TINCTURE Take 60 drops–1 tsp (3–5 ml) of a tincture of the seeds 3 times daily for poor appetite or flatulence.
ESSENTIAL OIL Add 5 drops of essential oil to 1 tsp (5 ml) almond oil and use as a chest rub for bronchitis and productive coughs (a cough that produces phlegm, rather than a dry cough).

HOW TO SOURCE

GROW Prefers deep, fertile, well-drained soil and full sun. Sow seeds where you want them to grow in spring, and thin out seedlings to 3–4 in (7.5–10 cm) if required. The plant is biennial, flowering in its second year. Caraway requires a long, hot growing season to set seed, so it may not produce as many seeds in cooler areas.
FORAGE Found in grassy areas or wastelands. In warmer climates it will set seed in late summer; in cooler areas seeds are likely only if the summer has been hot.
HARVEST Collect ripe seeds in late summer.

CAUTION The essential oil can cause skin irritation.

Centella asiatica
GOTU KOLA

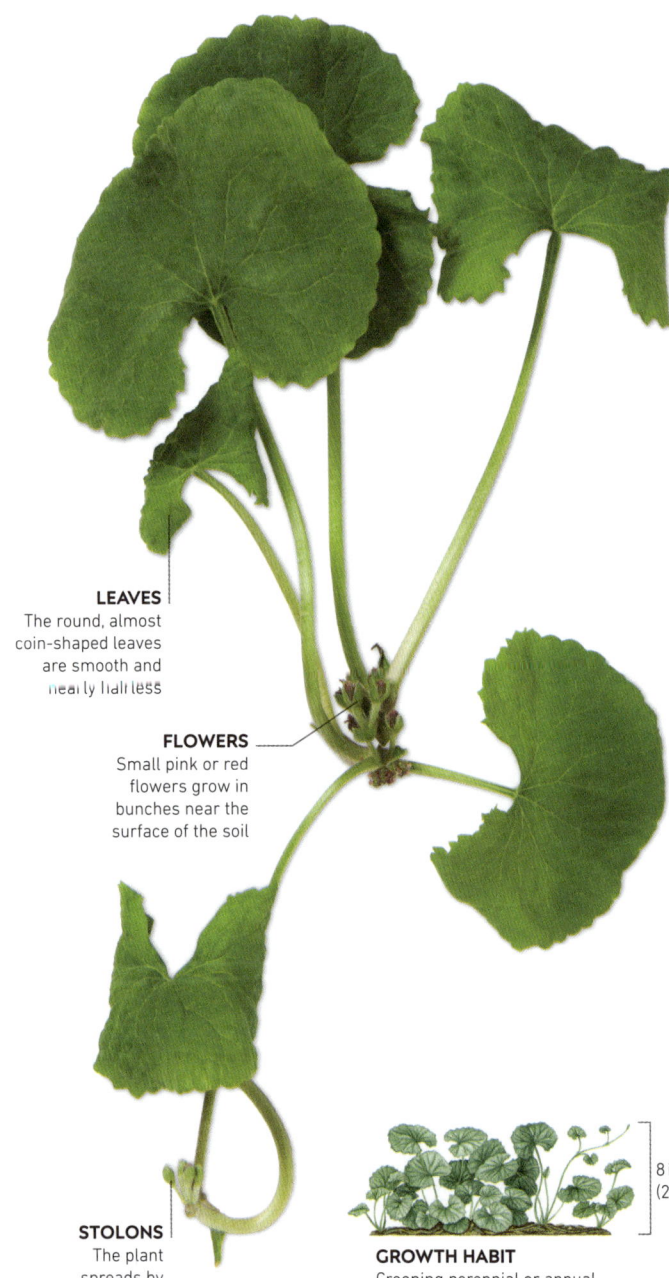

LEAVES
The round, almost coin-shaped leaves are smooth and nearly hairless

FLOWERS
Small pink or red flowers grow in bunches near the surface of the soil

STOLONS
The plant spreads by creeping stolons, or runners, that root at leaf nodes

GROWTH HABIT
Creeping perennial or annual rooting at nodes with clusters of kidney-shaped leaves; indefinite spread.

8 in
(20 cm)

Native to India, southeast Asia, and parts of northern Australia, gotu kola—a Sri Lankan name, which translates as "conical leaf"—is used as a fodder crop, as a vegetable or salad herb, and as a medicinal plant. In Ayurveda it is generally known as *brahmi* and used as a tonic remedy to improve longevity, memory, and intelligence. It is a restricted herb in some countries.

PARTS USED Whole plant
MAIN CONSTITUENTS Alkaloids (incl. hydrocotyline), terpenoid saponins, flavonoids, bitter principle, volatile oil
ACTIONS Tonic, antirheumatic, cleansing, adaptogen, relaxant, diuretic, laxative

HOW TO USE

INFUSION Use ½ tsp of the dried herb per cup of boiling water and take 1 cup daily for skin problems, rheumatism, or as a restorative for tiredness and depression.
TINCTURE Take 1 tsp (5 ml) in water daily for poor memory, inability to concentrate, or general exhaustion.
LOTION/OINTMENT Use on poorly healing wounds or skin ulcers.
FRESH LEAVES Traditionally given to Indian children to combat dysentery, or included in salads as a restorative tonic.
FLUID EXTRACT Take 20 drops in water up to 3 times daily for rheumatic disorders and poor venous circulation.
POWDER Used in Ayurvedic medicine to make a paste (mixed with a little water) and applied to eczema and skin sores.

HOW TO SOURCE

GROW Generally gathered in the wild, but can be grown in warmer areas from seeds sown directly in the spring. It prefers marshy ditches and riverbanks, so is best grown in partial shade in moist soil. It has an indefinite spread, so can make useful ground cover with the right growing conditions, but can become invasive.
FORAGE The whole plant can be gathered at any time where it is naturalized (parts of southern Africa, South America, the southern United States, and its native Asia).
HARVEST The whole plant matures in three months and is gathered—including the roots—throughout the year.

CAUTION Can occasionally cause photosensitivity. Do not take for more than six weeks without a break.

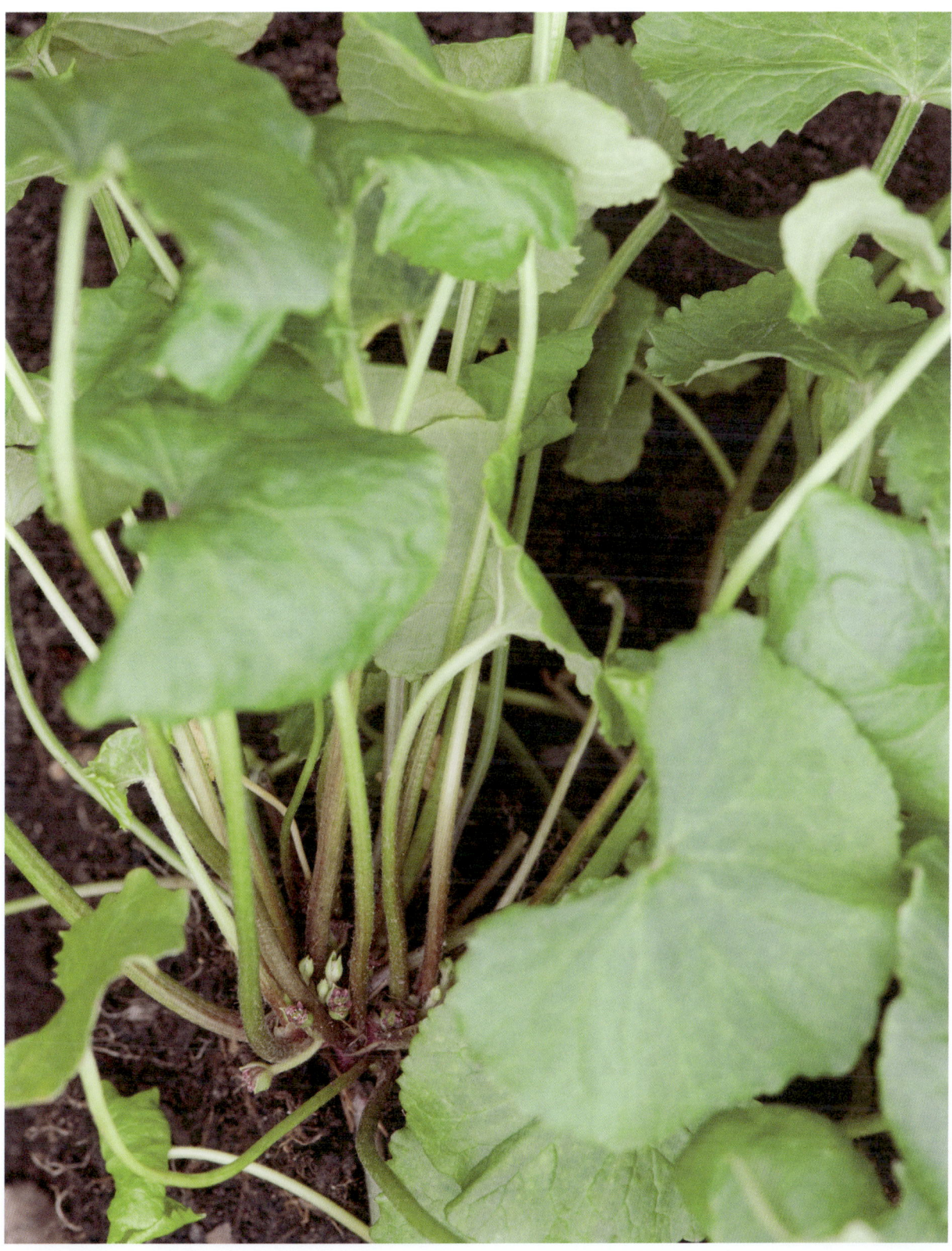

Cichorium intybus
CHICORY

Native to Mediterranean regions, chicory is now naturalized in many parts of Europe, North America, and Australia. It is cultivated as a vegetable—usually by producing chicons in complete darkness—and is also grown as a coffee substitute. The plant is extremely bitter, so it makes an excellent digestive stimulant and tonic, and is also a gentle laxative suitable for children.

PARTS USED Root, leaves, flowers
MAIN CONSTITUENTS Inulin (in the root), sesquiterpene lactones (lactucin and lactucopicrin), oligosaccharides, glycosides, vitamins, minerals
ACTIONS Laxative, diuretic, mild sedative, liver and digestive tonic

HOW TO USE

DECOCTION Drink ½–1 cup (2 tsp root per cup boiling water) 3 times daily as a stimulating tonic for the liver and digestive system. Use ½–1 cup of a quarter- to half-strength or less decoction 1–2 times a day for constipation. Chicory also contains oligosaccharides, which are probiotic and help maintain healthy gastrointestinal flora.
INFUSION Drink 1 cup (2 tsp leaves and flowers per cup of boiling water) 3 times daily to improve digestion.
TINCTURE Take 20–40 drops (1–2 ml) of the root tincture 3 times daily as an appetite stimulant.
FLUID EXTRACT Extracts have been successfully used for parasitic worm infections in sheep and cattle, although there is little research as to the effect on human parasites.

HOW TO SOURCE

GROW Prefers fertile, moist but well-drained, neutral to alkaline soil in full sun. Sow seeds in a cold frame in fall or spring and when the seedlings are established transplant them to final positions in rows at least 24 in (60 cm) apart. Dead-head the flowers regularly, as the plant can be a prolific self-seeder.
FORAGE Sometimes found in hedges and field borders, especially in southern Europe. The leaves can be collected during summer. They have a bitter taste and can be boiled to improve their flavor.
HARVEST Lift the roots in early spring in the second year.

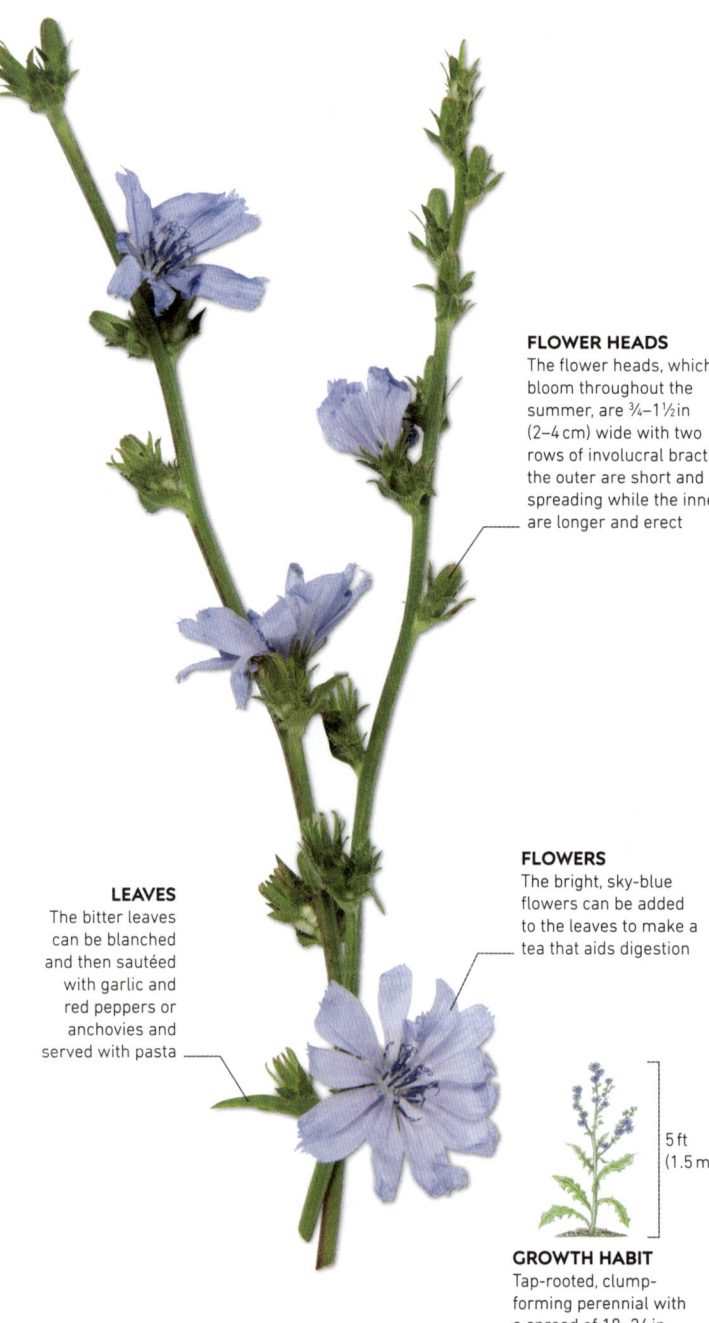

FLOWER HEADS
The flower heads, which bloom throughout the summer, are ¾–1½ in (2–4 cm) wide with two rows of involucral bracts: the outer are short and spreading while the inner are longer and erect

FLOWERS
The bright, sky-blue flowers can be added to the leaves to make a tea that aids digestion

LEAVES
The bitter leaves can be blanched and then sautéed with garlic and red peppers or anchovies and served with pasta

5 ft (1.5 m)

GROWTH HABIT
Tap-rooted, clump-forming perennial with a spread of 18–24 in (45–60 cm).

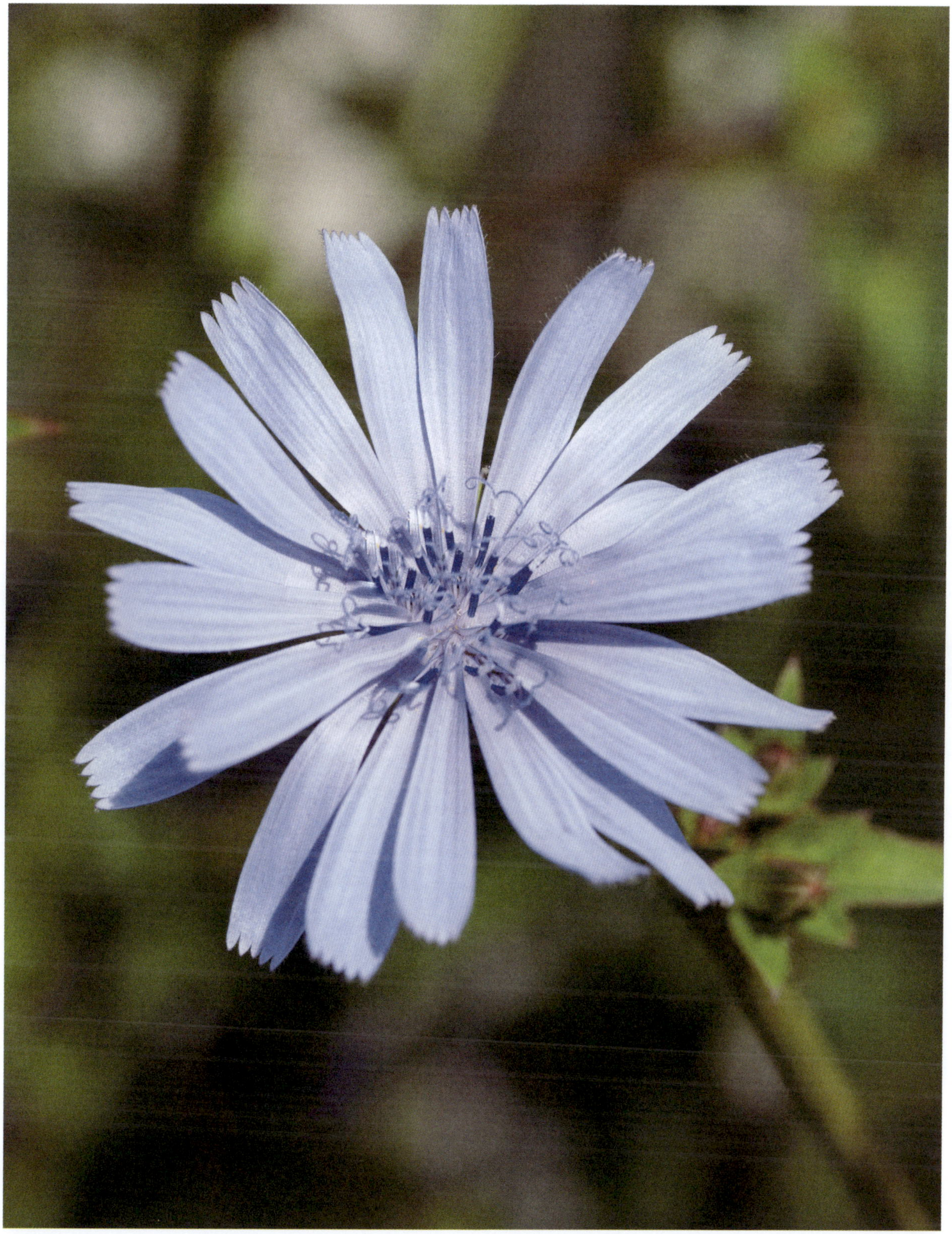

Crataegus laevigata
HAWTHORN

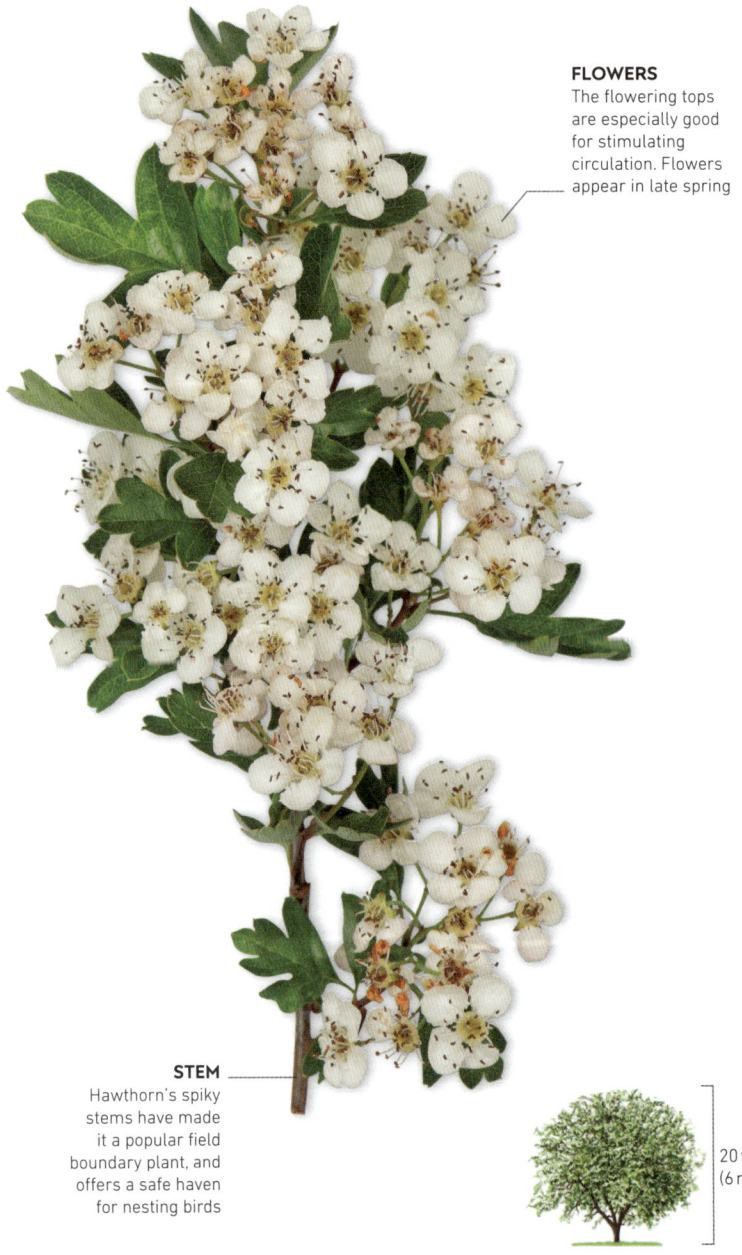

FLOWERS
The flowering tops are especially good for stimulating circulation. Flowers appear in late spring

STEM
Hawthorn's spiky stems have made it a popular field boundary plant, and offers a safe haven for nesting birds

GROWTH HABIT
Deciduous shrub or small tree; spread 15–25 ft (5–8 m).

20 ft (6 m)

Thorny shrubs and trees from various species of hawthorn are found throughout northern temperate zones. *Crataegus laevigata* is the European species, but *Crataegus pinnatifida* is native to northern China, and is also used as a medicinal herb. The berries were traditionally made into a savory jelly to eat with cheese, game, and cold meats.

PARTS USED Flowering tops, berries
MAIN CONSTITUENTS Bioflavonoid glycosides (incl. rutin and quercetin), triterpenoids, procyanidins, polyphenols, saponins, tannins, coumarins, minerals
ACTIONS Peripheral vasodilator, cardiac tonic, astringent, relaxant, antioxidant

HOW TO USE

INFUSION Drink 1 cup (2 tsp herb per cup boiling water) of the flowering tops 3 times daily to improve peripheral circulation or to support treatments for high blood pressure. Alternatively, drink ½ cup (2 tsp of the berries per cup boiling water) up to 6 times daily for acute diarrhea or digestive upsets. The same mixture can be used as a general tonic for the heart: drink 2 cups daily.
TINCTURE Take 20–40 drops (1–2 ml) of a standard tincture of either the berries or the flowering tops for high blood pressure; best combined with other herbs as appropriate.
JUICE Pulp the berries in a food processor, squeeze out the juice, and take in 2 tsp (10 ml) doses twice daily for sluggish digestion and diarrhea.

HOW TO SOURCE

GROW It can be grown from seed if planted in the fall and allowed to overwinter in a cold frame, but is more often propagated from cuttings in spring. Plant heeled cuttings in a small pot and, once rooted, pot into 8 in (20 cm) pots until sufficiently established to plant out. Will self-seed.
FORAGE Common hedge shrubs are found on field borders and roadsides in northern temperate zones. It is best to gather from shrubs within fields rather than those adjacent to roads. The flowering tops can be gathered in late spring/early summer for use in teas, and the berries in late fall to make into jelly.
HARVEST Gather flowering tops in spring, and the red berries in fall when ripe.

CAUTION Seek professional advice before self-medicating with hawthorn for heart disorders, or if using prescribed medication.

Curcuma longa
TURMERIC

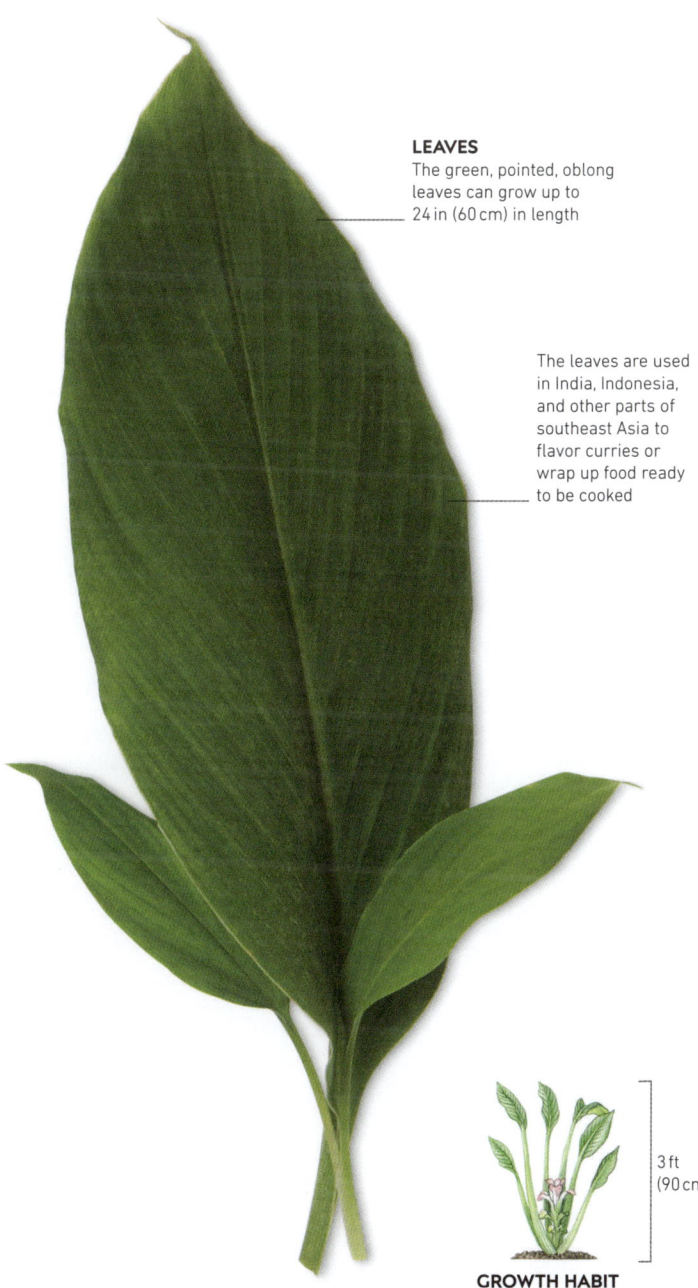

LEAVES
The green, pointed, oblong leaves can grow up to 24 in (60 cm) in length

The leaves are used in India, Indonesia, and other parts of southeast Asia to flavor curries or wrap up food ready to be cooked

3 ft (90 cm)

GROWTH HABIT
Aromatic perennial with shiny, pointed leaves and an indefinite spread.

Familiar to many people as a key ingredient in curry powder, turmeric originates in southern Asia, and has a long history of use in both Ayurveda and traditional Chinese medicine. It is largely used for digestive and liver disorders, although modern research also suggests that it has potent antioxidant properties and can reduce cholesterol levels.

PARTS USED Rhizome
MAIN CONSTITUENTS Volatile oil, curcumin (yellow pigment), resin, vitamins, minerals, bitter principle
ACTIONS Carminative, cholagogue, antioxidant, choleretic, detoxifier, antibacterial, anti-inflammatory, antitumor activity, hypolipidemic

HOW TO USE

DECOCTION Drink 1 cup (1 tsp herb per cup boiling water) up to 3 times daily for digestive problems including nausea, gastritis, excessive stomach acid, indigestion, and liver or gall bladder disorders. Can also be combined with remedies for arthritis such as angelica or devil's claw and taken 3 times daily.
TINCTURE Take 40–80 drops (2–4 ml) in a little water 3 times daily to help reduce blood cholesterol levels, or take 1 tsp (5 ml) up to 3 times daily for period pain.
POWDER Take ½–1 level tsp (1–2 g) stirred into a cup of water, fruit juice, or milk for arthritic problems or eczema.
OINTMENT Apply 2–3 times daily for athlete's foot, psoriasis, or ringworm.

HOW TO SOURCE

GROW Prefers moist, fertile soil with high humidity and partial shade. Will only grow in warm regions (minimum temperature 59–64°F/15–18°C), but can be cultivated under glass elsewhere. Sow seeds at 70°F (21°C) in fall. Alternatively, propagate by root division while the plant is dormant in winter or by root cuttings in fall.
FORAGE Unlikely to be found growing wild outside dry forest areas in India and some other parts of southern Asia.
HARVEST The rhizome is dug in fall and is boiled and steamed before drying.

CAUTION May occasionally cause skin rashes or increase photosensitivity. Avoid therapeutic doses in pregnancy, but culinary quantities are perfectly safe. Seek professional advice if you suffer from gallstones.

Cymbopogon citratus
LEMONGRASS

Originally native to grasslands in southeast Asia, lemongrass is now cultivated in many tropical regions, including Guatemala, the West Indies, and the Philippines, both as a culinary herb and for its essential oil. The herb is a popular digestive remedy in parts of Asia, and is used as a flavoring in perfumery and the food industry.

PARTS USED Leaves and stems, essential oil
MAIN CONSTITUENTS Volatile oil mostly citral (65–85 percent) as well as nerol, geraniol, citronellol, myrcene, and borneol
ACTIONS Antispasmodic, carminative, febrifuge, analgesic, antidepressant, antiseptic, astringent, antibacterial, antifungal, sedative, tonic

HOW TO USE

LOTION Dilute 30 drops of essential oil in 1 tbsp vodka, then add to ½ cup water and use in a spray bottle as an insect repellent (fleas, ticks, and lice), or as a deodorant and antiperspirant.
MASSAGE RUB Dilute 20 drops of essential oil in 2 fl oz (60 ml) of almond oil and massage into aching muscles, or use on the abdomen for stomach cramps.
INFUSION Drink 1 cup (1-2 tsp herb per cup boiling water) 3 times daily for gas, indigestion, or stomach cramps.
POULTICE Simmer a handful of chopped fresh lemongrass for 1–2 minutes in olive oil and use on arthritic or painful joints.

HOW TO SOURCE

GROW Grow in containers in cooler areas and over winter in a conservatory or heated greenhouse, as not frost hardy (minimum temperature 45°F/7°C). In frost-free areas plant in fertile, moist, well-drained soil in full sun, keeping 24 in (60 cm) between plants. Sow seeds (at 64°F/18°C) in early spring in seed trays and transplant to 3½ in (7 cm) pots when large enough. Alternatively, propagate by root division in late spring.
FORAGE Unlikely to be found growing wild other than in its native area of grassland in southeast Asia.
HARVEST Gather stems through the year.

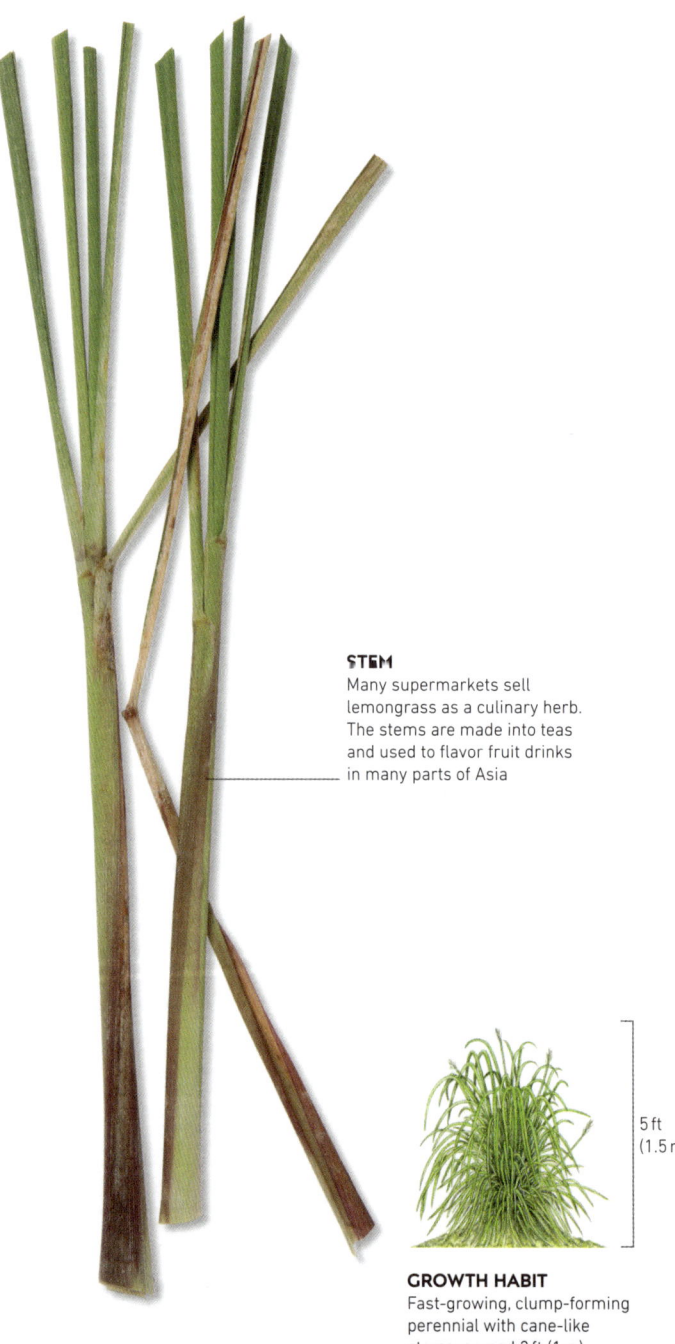

STEM
Many supermarkets sell lemongrass as a culinary herb. The stems are made into teas and used to flavor fruit drinks in many parts of Asia

5 ft
(1.5 m)

GROWTH HABIT
Fast-growing, clump-forming perennial with cane-like stems; spread 3 ft (1 m).

CAUTION Do not take the essential oil internally without professional advice. Avoid therapeutic doses during pregnancy, but culinary quantities are safe.

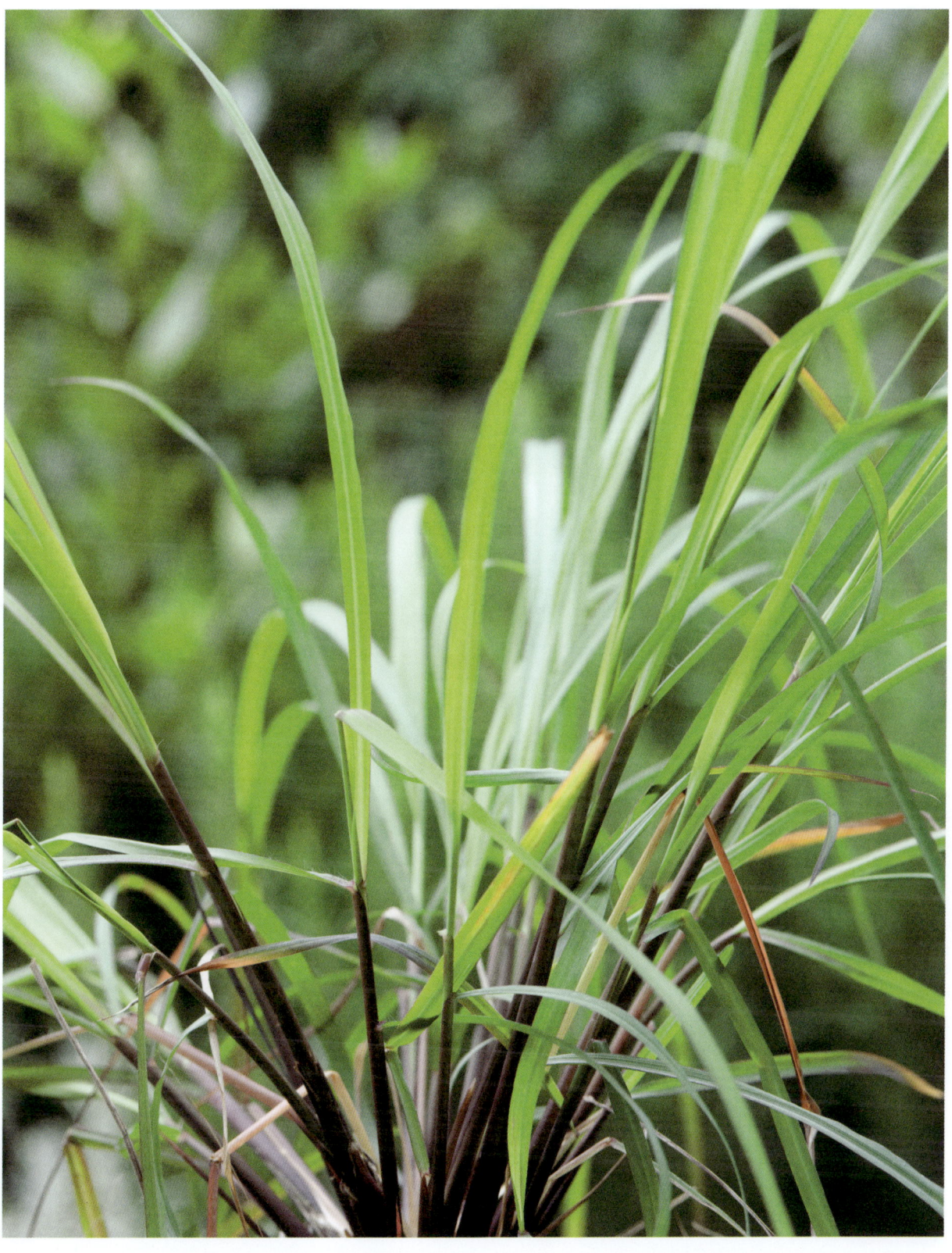

Cynara cardunculus var. scolymus
GLOBE ARTICHOKE

FLOWER HEADS
The flower heads are harvested before opening, boiled as a vegetable, and generally served with melted butter

HEARTS
Artichoke hearts, found at the center of the flowerheads, can be added to salads

GROWTH HABIT
Large perennial with a spread of 4 ft (1.2 m) and thistle-like flowers.

6 ft (1.8 m)

Originating in the Mediterranean region, the globe artichoke was probably developed from *Cynara cardunculus* in ancient times. The ball-like flower heads, which are picked before they open, are valued as a vegetable, while the hearts can be used in salads. Medicinally, the plant is used as a liver remedy that helps protect against toxins and infection and improve function.

PARTS USED Flower heads, leaves, root
MAIN CONSTITUENTS Sesquiterpene lactone (cynaropicrin), cynarin, inulin
ACTIONS Cholagogue, choleretic, liver restorative, hypoglycemic, diuretic, hypolipidemic

HOW TO USE

JUICE Mix an equal amount of juice from the leaves and flower heads with water and drink 1 cup daily as a liver tonic.
INFUSION Drink 1 cup (1 tsp dry leaves per cup of boiling water) 3 times daily for liver and gall bladder disorders, including liver damage or jaundice, or for indigestion, nausea, or abdominal bloating. Also helps reduce blood cholesterol levels and can be useful in the control of late-onset diabetes where treatment is focused on diet rather than medication.
DIET Eating artichoke hearts regularly can be helpful in the management of late-onset diabetes.
CAPSULES Take 3 x 250 mg capsules containing powdered leaf before meals morning and evening to improve liver function.

HOW TO SOURCE

GROW Prefers an open but sheltered site in full sun in well-drained soil; add well-rotted manure to the soil before planting. Sow seeds in a cold frame in spring and transplant to their final growing positions when large enough to handle. Alternatively, propagate from suckers in spring or take root cuttings in winter.
FORAGE Unknown in the wild.
HARVEST Cut the leaves before flowering. Gather the flower heads before the bracts open from the second year onward to eat as a vegetable.

Dioscorea villosa
WILD YAM

Perhaps best known as the herb that gave rise to the first oral contraceptive pill, wild yam is native to the southern and eastern US and central America, although it is now naturalized in many semitropical areas worldwide. The chemical from the yam, diosgenin, was identified in the 1930s, and by 1960 was being used to manufacture the hormone progesterone.

PARTS USED Root and tuber
MAIN CONSTITUENTS Alkaloids, steroidal saponins (mainly dioscin, which breaks down to diosgenin), tannins, phytosterols, starch
ACTIONS Relaxant for smooth muscle, antispasmodic, cholagogue, anti-inflammatory, diaphoretic, antirheumatic, diuretic

HOW TO USE

DECOCTION Take ½–1 cup 3 times daily of a decoction made by simmering ¼oz (10 g) in 1 pint (600 ml) of water for 20 minutes for colicky pains associated with IBS or diverticulosis. Drink ½ cup every 3–4 hours for period pains, or sip cups constantly during labor to relieve pain.
TINCTURE Take 40–60 drops (2–3 ml) 3 times daily for menopausal problems.
FLUID EXTRACT Take 20–40 drops (1–2 ml) in a little water 3 times daily for arthritis: usually combined with other herbs such as black cohosh, crampbark, meadowsweet, or white willow for rheumatoid arthritis. Also useful to stimulate liver function.

HOW TO SOURCE

GROW Prefers light to medium (sandy to loamy) soil that is moist but well drained, and requires partial shade. Usually grown from root cuttings, or from pea-sized tubers found growing in the leaf axils in late summer that can be collected and planted immediately. The plants are dioecious (have separate sexes), so both male and female plants are needed to set seeds, which can be sown in a cold frame in early spring and transplanted when large enough to handle.
FORAGE Generally found in damp woods, swamps, thickets, and hedges in central and southern US and parts of central America.
HARVEST Dig tubers and roots in fall, and wash and dry them.

CAUTION Saponin content may cause nausea in sensitive individuals.

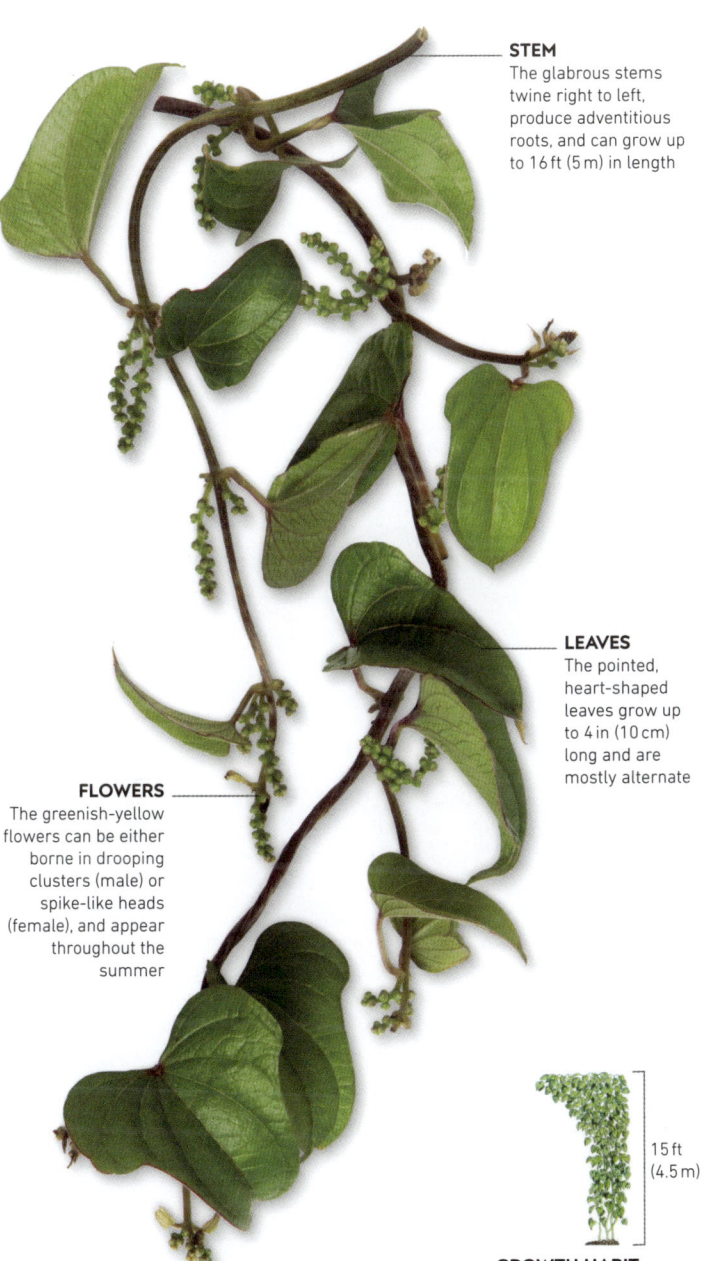

STEM
The glabrous stems twine right to left, produce adventitious roots, and can grow up to 16 ft (5 m) in length

LEAVES
The pointed, heart-shaped leaves grow up to 4 in (10 cm) long and are mostly alternate

FLOWERS
The greenish-yellow flowers can be either borne in drooping clusters (male) or spike-like heads (female), and appear throughout the summer

15 ft (4.5 m)

GROWTH HABIT
Trailing vine with heart-shaped leaves and reddish-brown stems.

Echinacea purpurea
ECHINACEA

Native to the eastern part of the US, echinacea was once known as "Missouri snakeroot" and was traditionally used by Native Americans for fevers and poorly healing wounds. It was introduced into Europe in the 19th century and has been extensively researched since, largely as an antibiotic remedy for treating a broad range of infections.

PARTS USED Root, leaves
MAIN CONSTITUENTS Volatile oil (incl. humulene), glycosides, alkamides, inulin, polysaccharides, antibiotic polyacetylenes
ACTIONS Immune stimulant, anti-allergenic, lymphatic tonic, antimicrobial, anti-inflammatory

HOW TO USE
INFUSION Drink 1 cup (1–2 tsp fresh leaves per cup of boiling water) 3 times daily for common colds, chills, or influenza.
DECOCTION Take 2 tsp of a decoction (1–2 tsp root per cup boiling water) every 2–4 hours for acute stages of infections. Combines well with hemp agrimony.
GARGLE/MOUTHWASH Use 1 cup of above root decoction or 2 tsp of tincture in a cup of warm water 2–3 times daily for sore throats, mouth ulcers, and tonsillitis.
TINCTURE Take 1 tsp of tincture 3 times daily for urinary infections; combine with an equal amount of cleavers tincture for enlarged lymphatic nodes or glandular fever. For colds and influenza, take 2 tsp of tincture as symptoms occur and repeat up to 4 times daily for 48 hours.
CREAM/OINTMENT Use on infected cuts, boils, acne, and skin sores.

HOW TO SOURCE
GROW Prefers fertile, moist, well-drained soil in full sun. Sow seeds in containers in spring and pot; when well established, plant in permanent positions. Alternatively, divide established plants in fall or spring or take root cuttings in late fall or early winter.
FORAGE Unlikely to be found growing wild outside the US. Over-cropping has endangered this plant, so avoid foraging for it in its native habitat.
HARVEST The leaves can be gathered throughout the growing season, and the roots of four-year-old plants are lifted in fall after flowering is over.

CAUTION Avoid if taking immunosuppressant medication. High doses can occasionally cause nausea and dizziness.

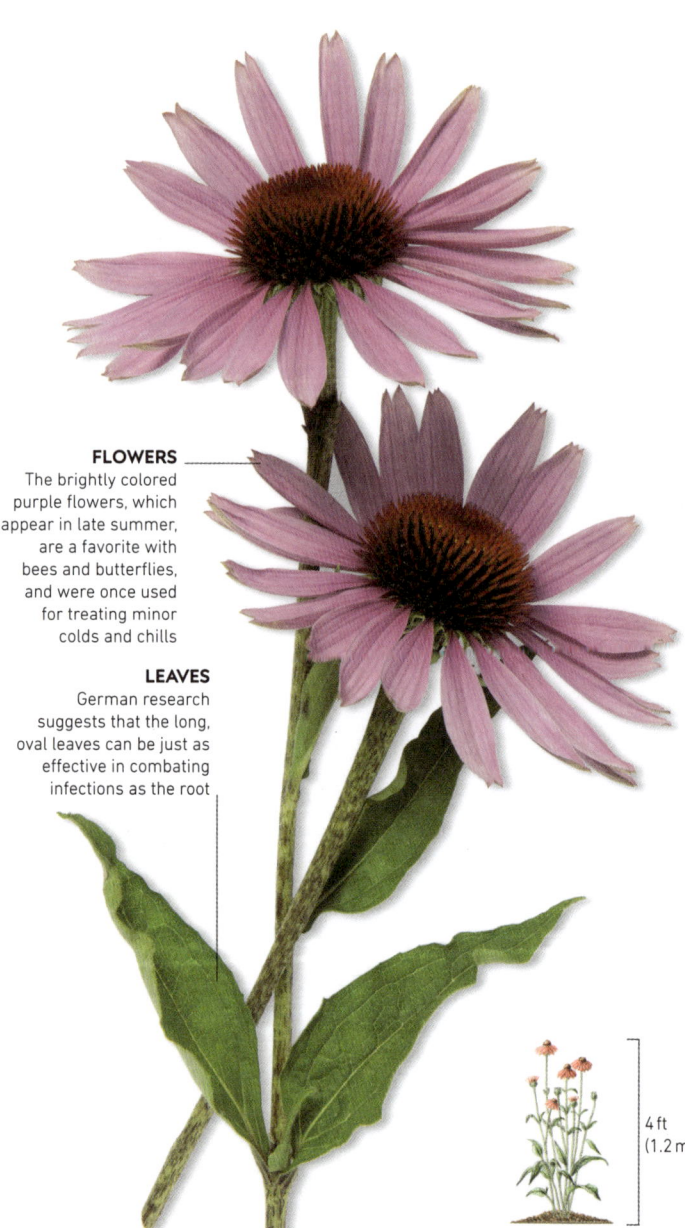

FLOWERS
The brightly colored purple flowers, which appear in late summer, are a favorite with bees and butterflies, and were once used for treating minor colds and chills

LEAVES
German research suggests that the long, oval leaves can be just as effective in combating infections as the root

4 ft (1.2 m)

GROWTH HABIT
Upright, rhizomatous perennial with daisy-like flowers; spread 18 in (35 cm).

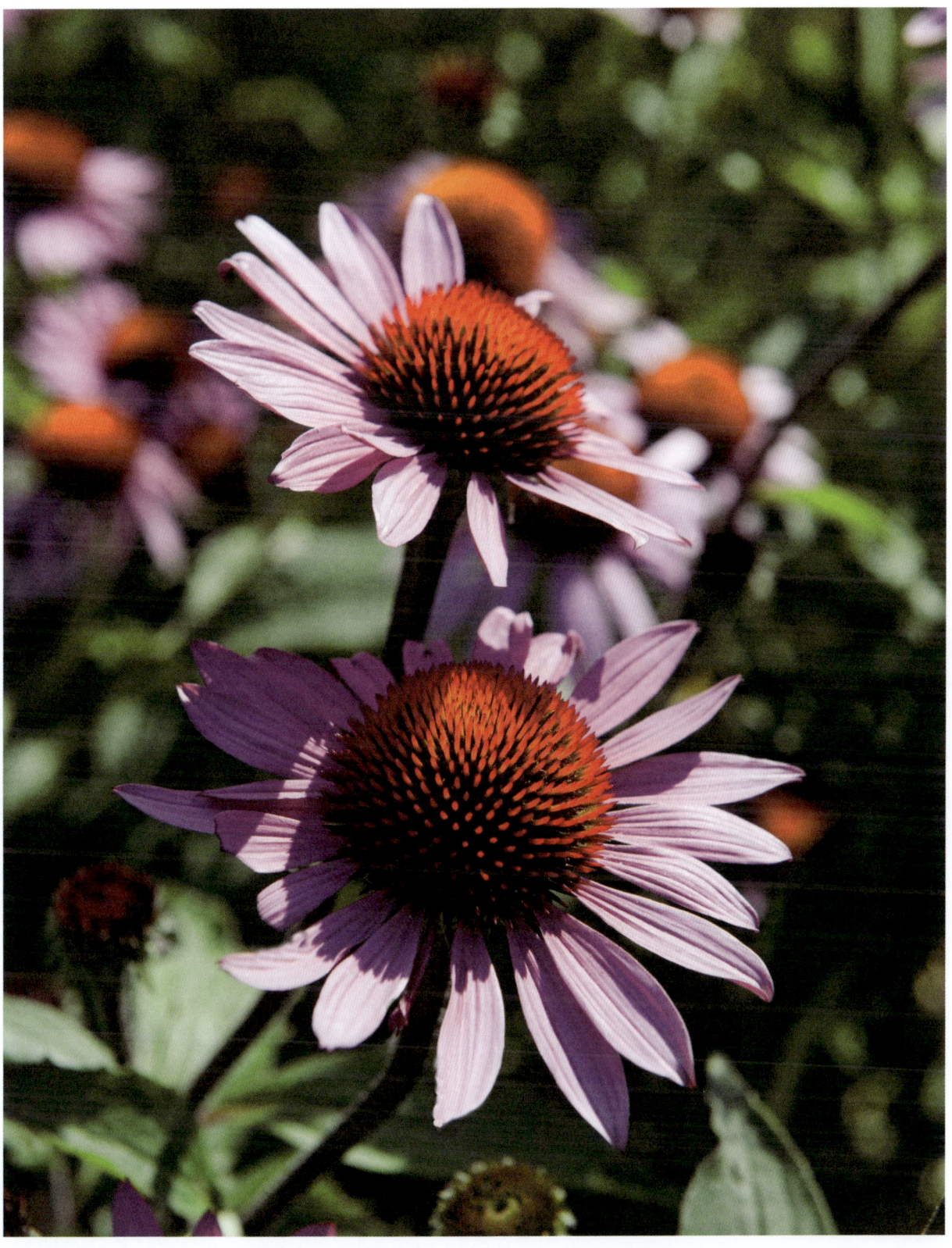

Equisetum arvense
HORSETAIL

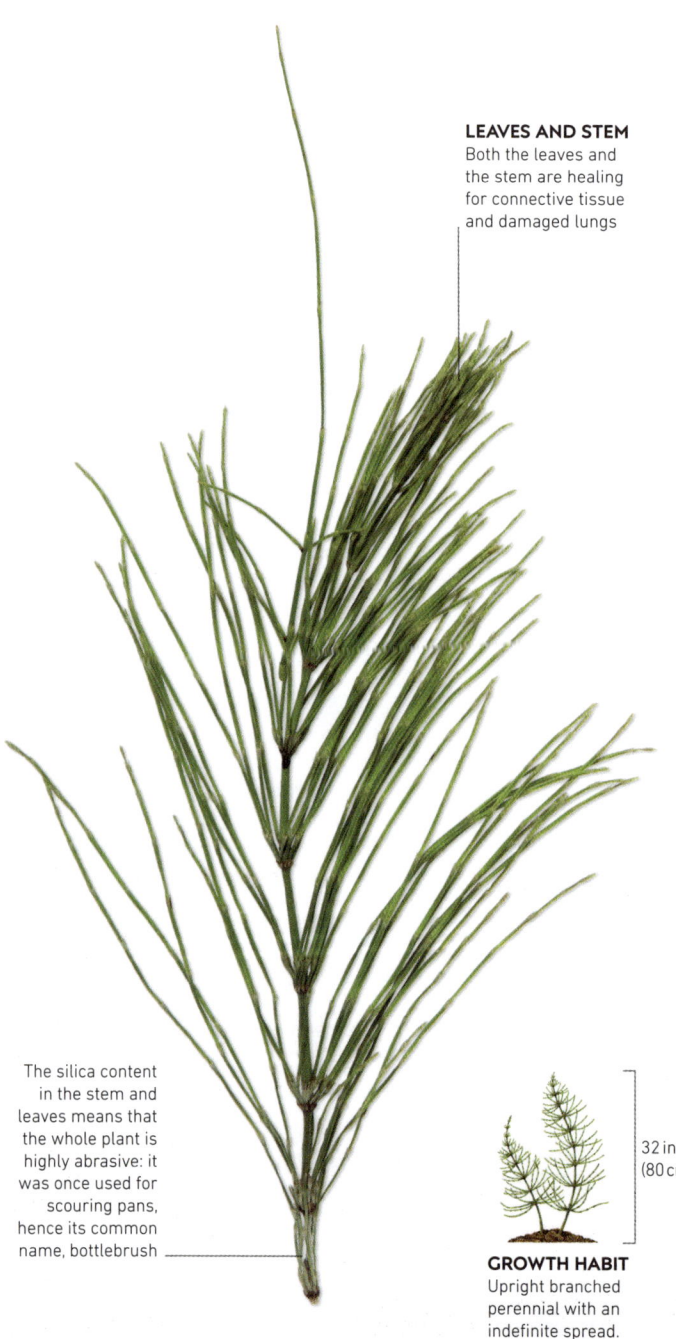

LEAVES AND STEM
Both the leaves and
the stem are healing
for connective tissue
and damaged lungs

The silica content
in the stem and
leaves means that
the whole plant is
highly abrasive: it
was once used for
scouring pans,
hence its common
name, bottlebrush

GROWTH HABIT
Upright branched
perennial with an
indefinite spread.

32 in
(80 cm)

Native to Europe, Asia, and North America,
horsetail is a survivor from prehistoric times.
This early plant has been unchanged for
millennia and once formed the vegetation
that decomposed to produce coal seams. It
encourages the healing of connective tissue,
and has been used as a wound herb to stop
bleeding since ancient times.

PARTS USED Aerial parts
MAIN CONSTITUENTS Silicic acid and silicates,
alkaloids (incl. nicotine), tannins, saponins, flavonoids,
bitter principles, other minerals (incl. potassium,
manganese, magnesium), phytosterols
ACTIONS Astringent, hemostatic, diuretic, anti-
inflammatory, tissue healer, increases coagulation

HOW TO USE

DECOCTION Take ½–1 cup of a decoction (p.176)
made from ½oz (15 g) of the herb to 1 pint (600 ml)
water 3 times daily for excessive menstruation,
inflammation of the urinary tract, prostate problems,
or chronic lung disorders.
JUICE Take 1–2 tsp (5–10 ml) 3 times daily for
damaged lungs or urinary disorders.
BATH Add 1 cup of the decoction to bath water for
sprains, fractures, or irritable skin conditions
including eczema.
POULTICE Use 1 tsp of powder made into a paste
with a little water, or a handful of the fresh aerial parts
sweated in a bowl over a saucepan of simmering
water (bain-marie); spread on gauze and use for leg
ulcers, wounds, sores, or chilblains.
MOUTHWASH/GARGLE Use ½ cup of a decoction
with an equal amount of water for mouth or gum
infections or sore throats.
NAIL SOAK Soak a few leaves in apple cider vinegar
for two weeks, then strain and use the liquid as a nail
soak twice a week to strengthen brittle nails.

HOW TO SOURCE

GROW Prefers moist soil in sun or partial shade. Usually
propagated by root division in early spring. Under statutory
control as an invasive weed in some countries.
FORAGE Found in meadows, hedgerows, and waste
ground. Don't confuse with marsh horsetail (*Equisetum
palustre*), a larger plant that contains toxic alkaloids.
HARVEST Cut stems in the growing season.

CAUTION Seek professional guidance in all cases
of blood in the urine, or for sudden changes in
menstrual flow leading to heavy bleeding. Do not
use for more than four weeks continuously without
professional guidance.

Eucalyptus globulus
EUCALYPTUS

Native to Australia and Tasmania, the eucalyptus, or "blue gum," tree is now cultivated worldwide both as a commercial crop and for its ability to absorb water and dry up marshes. It is an important remedy among Australian Aboriginals, although in medicine the essential oil is more commonly used, largely as an antiseptic.

PARTS USED Leaves, essential oil
MAIN CONSTITUENTS Volatile oil (incl. cineole), tannins, aldehydes, bitter resin
ACTIONS Antiseptic, decongestant, antibiotic, antispasmodic, stimulant, febrifuge, hypoglycemic, anthelmintic

HOW TO USE

DECOCTION Simmer 3–4 leaves per cup of water for 10 minutes in a covered pan and take ½–1 cup 3 times daily for the early stages of colds, chills, nasal catarrh, influenza, asthma, sinusitis, sore throats, and other respiratory disorders.
CHEST RUB Use 10 drops (½ml) of eucalyptus oil in 1 fl oz (30ml) of almond oil as a chest rub for colds, bronchitis, asthma, and respiratory problems.
STEAM INHALATION Use 10 drops (½ml) of essential oil or 6 leaves in a bowl of boiling water as a steam inhalation for colds and chest infections.
COMPRESS Soak a pad in a mixture of 10 drops of essential oil and 4 fl oz (120ml) of water and apply to inflammations, painful joints, or minor burns.

HOW TO SOURCE

GROW Prefers moisture-retentive soil that is neutral-to-slightly acid in a sunny site that is also sheltered from cold, dry winds. Sow the seeds at 70°F (21°C) in spring and grow until large enough to transplant into final positions, although buying young trees from a nursery is a quicker process. As the plant absorbs so much water, it can deplete the soil over a significant area.
FORAGE Now found—often in commercial plantations—in many tropical, subtropical, and temperate areas worldwide, although it can also be found growing wild in marshy areas. Collect the leaves as required.
HARVEST Gather the leaves as required throughout the year.

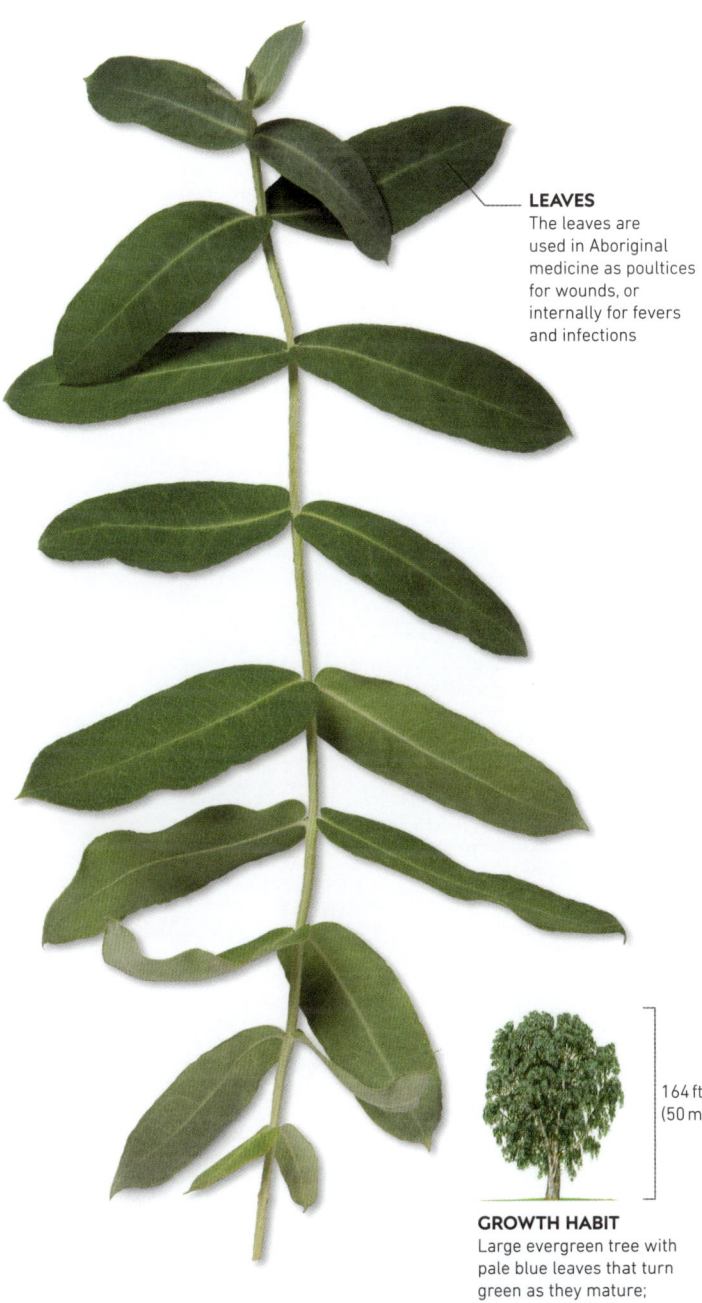

LEAVES
The leaves are used in Aboriginal medicine as poultices for wounds, or internally for fevers and infections

164 ft
(50 m)

GROWTH HABIT
Large evergreen tree with pale blue leaves that turn green as they mature; spread 80 ft (25 m).

CAUTION Do not take the essential oil internally; fatalities have been reported from comparatively low doses.

Eupatorium cannabinum
HEMP AGRIMONY

Native to Europe, hemp agrimony was traditionally used for feverish colds or as a poultice for skin sores. A bitter compound called eupatoriopicrin has now been identified in the plant and is believed to have an antitumor action. The plant also appears to be immunostimulant—increasing resistance in viral infections. However, it also contains toxic alkaloids, so must be used with caution.

PARTS USED Aerial parts, root
MAIN CONSTITUENTS Volatile oil (incl. thymol, azulenes, alpha-terpinene), flavonoids, sesquiterpene lactones (incl. eupatoriopicrin), pyrrolizidine alkaloids
ACTIONS Febrifuge, diuretic, antiscorbutic, laxative, cholagogue, expectorant, immune stimulant, antirheumatic, diaphoretic, tonic

HOW TO USE

NB: Take for short periods and only under professional guidance
INFUSION Traditionally used in the treatment of certain skin conditions, rheumatism, and arthritis, but use only under guidance from a qualified herbalist.
POULTICE Pulp a handful of fresh leaves in a blender, spread on gauze, and use on suppurating skin sores or ulcers.

HOW TO SOURCE

GROW Tolerates a range of soil conditions and grows in sun or partial shade, although prefers moist soil. Sow seeds in a cold frame in early spring and lightly cover with topsoil. Transplant to 3½ in (7 cm) pots and plant in early summer or when well established; allow 24 in (60 cm) between plants. Alternatively, sow seeds where you want them to grow in spring or fall.
FORAGE Found in damp woods, ditches, waste ground, or marshy areas. Naturalized in parts of western Asia and North Africa.
HARVEST Cut flowering aerial parts in late summer/early fall. Dig roots in fall.

FLOWER HEADS
The pink flower heads, which appear from summer to early fall, are a favorite with butterflies and bees

The leaves were traditionally used to wrap up bread to prevent mold

LEAVES
The leaves can be pulped and the juice extracted to use as an insect repellent to rub into the coats of dogs and horses

5 ft (1.5 m)

GROWTH HABIT
Herbaceous perennial with cannabis-like leaves; spread 4 ft (1.2 m).

CAUTION Contains pyrrolizidine alkaloids, which are carcinogenic, so only use under professional guidance. High doses may cause nausea and vomiting. Avoid during pregnancy.

Eupatorium purpureum
GRAVEL ROOT

Originally found in damp thickets in the eastern US, gravel root is grown as a statuesque garden ornamental in many parts of the world. Its other common name, Joe Pye weed, is reputedly named after a Native American medicine man who used it to treat typhus. The herb is used for clearing gravel and kidney stones and for other problems affecting the urinary tract.

PARTS USED Rhizome and root
MAIN CONSTITUENTS Eupatorin, volatile oil, flavonoids, resin
ACTIONS Soothing diuretic, anti-lithic, tonic, antirheumatic, astringent

HOW TO USE

DECOCTION Take ½ cup of a decoction made of 1 tsp dried root to 1 cup water and simmered for 20 minutes for kidney stones, gravel, or painful urination. This mixture was traditionally used to ease the pain of childbirth. Gravel root is believed to enhance the removal of waste products by the kidneys, so the decoction is also useful in rheumatism and gout to improve the excretion of uric acid.
TINCTURE Use 40–80 drops (2–4 ml) 3 times daily for urinary disorders including cystitis and gravel, or discharges associated with infection. It combines well with white dead-nettle (*Lamium album*) for prostate problems and with parsley piert (*Aphanes arvensis*), pellitory-of-the-wall (*Parietaria judaica*), or hydrangea (*Hydrangea* spp.) for kidney stones.

HOW TO SOURCE

GROW Prefers moist, fertile soil in sun or partial shade. Sow seeds in spring in a cold frame and when the seedlings are large enough to handle, transplant them to final positions. Allow at least 36 in (90 cm) between plants. Best grown at the back of a border, but is popular in planting schemes as it flowers late in the season.
FORAGE Unlikely to be found growing wild beyond the eastern part of the US, although it might occur as a garden escapee. As the root is used, it is best not to collect from the wild. In Europe, the related species *Eupatorium cannabinum* (hemp agrimony, see opposite) is more likely to be found growing as a hedge plant.
HARVEST The roots of two-year-old, or older, plants are dug in fall.

CAUTION Avoid during pregnancy.

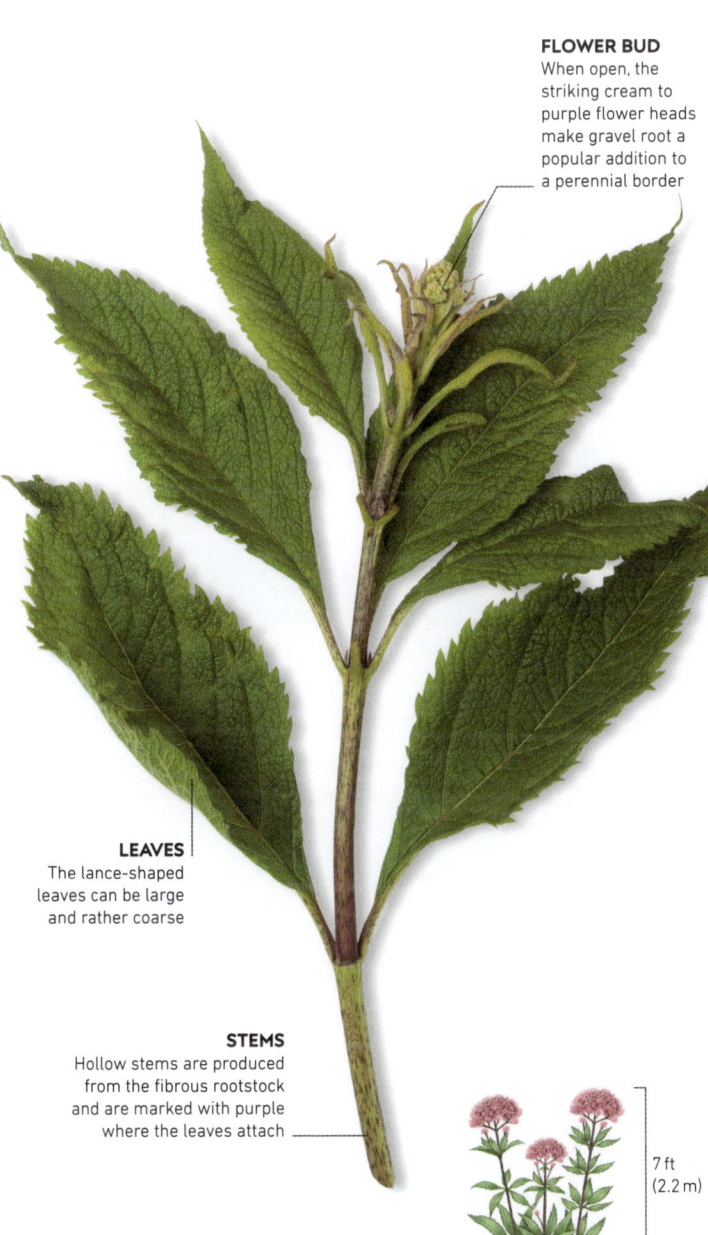

FLOWER BUD
When open, the striking cream to purple flower heads make gravel root a popular addition to a perennial border

LEAVES
The lance-shaped leaves can be large and rather coarse

STEMS
Hollow stems are produced from the fibrous rootstock and are marked with purple where the leaves attach

7 ft (2.2 m)

GROWTH HABIT
Robust, clump-forming perennial with erect stems; spread 3 ft (1 m).

Filipendula ulmaria
MEADOWSWEET

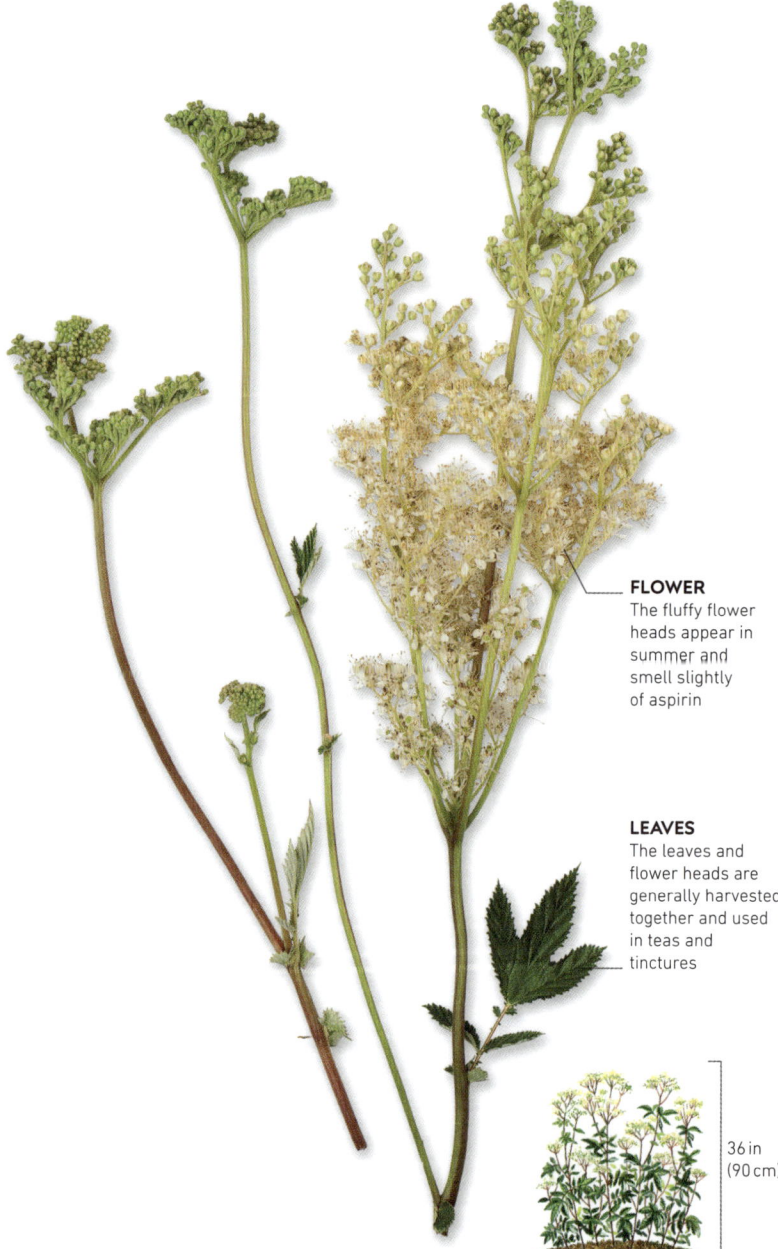

FLOWER
The fluffy flower heads appear in summer and smell slightly of aspirin

LEAVES
The leaves and flower heads are generally harvested together and used in teas and tinctures

36 in
(90 cm)

GROWTH HABIT
Clump-forming perennial; spread 24 ft (60 cm).

Growing in damp ditches throughout Europe and western Asia, meadowsweet takes its name from its original use of flavoring mead, or honey wine. Today it is highly regarded as an antacid herb, helping both to combat excess stomach acid leading to indigestion and gastritis and to reduce the body's acidity generally, so helping with arthritic conditions.

PARTS USED Aerial parts, flowers
MAIN CONSTITUENTS Salicylates, flavonoids (incl. rutin and hyperin), volatile oil (incl. salicylaldehyde), citric acid, mucilage, tannins
ACTIONS Antacid, anti-inflammatory, antirheumatic, soothing digestive remedy, diuretic, diaphoretic, anticoagulant

HOW TO USE

INFUSION Drink 1 cup (1–2 tsp herb per cup boiling water) of leaves and flowers 3 times daily for feverish colds or mild rheumatic pains. Drink ½ cup every 2 hours for acid reflux or indigestion. Can be given to children for stomach upsets; consult an herbalist for advice on dosage.
FLUID EXTRACT Take 40 drops–1 tsp (2–5 ml) 3 times daily for gastritis, gastric ulceration, or chronic rheumatism. Combine with angelica, bogbean (*Menyanthes trifoliata*), or willow for arthritis.
COMPRESS Soak a pad in dilute tincture and apply to painful arthritic joints or for rheumatism or neuralgia.

HOW TO SOURCE

GROW Prefers fertile, non-acid, moist-to-boggy soil in a sunny or lightly shaded position. Sow seeds in fall in a cold frame and transplant the following spring when the seedlings are established. Allow 24 in (60 cm) between plants. Alternatively, propagate by division in fall or spring, or by root cuttings in winter.
FORAGE Found in damp meadows and hedge ditches throughout Europe and western Asia. The aerial parts can be collected as flowering begins, or the flowers harvested separately when in full bloom.
HARVEST Collect in summer just before, or at, flowering.

CAUTION Avoid meadowsweet during pregnancy. Avoid in cases of salicylate (or aspirin) sensitivity.

Foeniculum vulgare
FENNEL

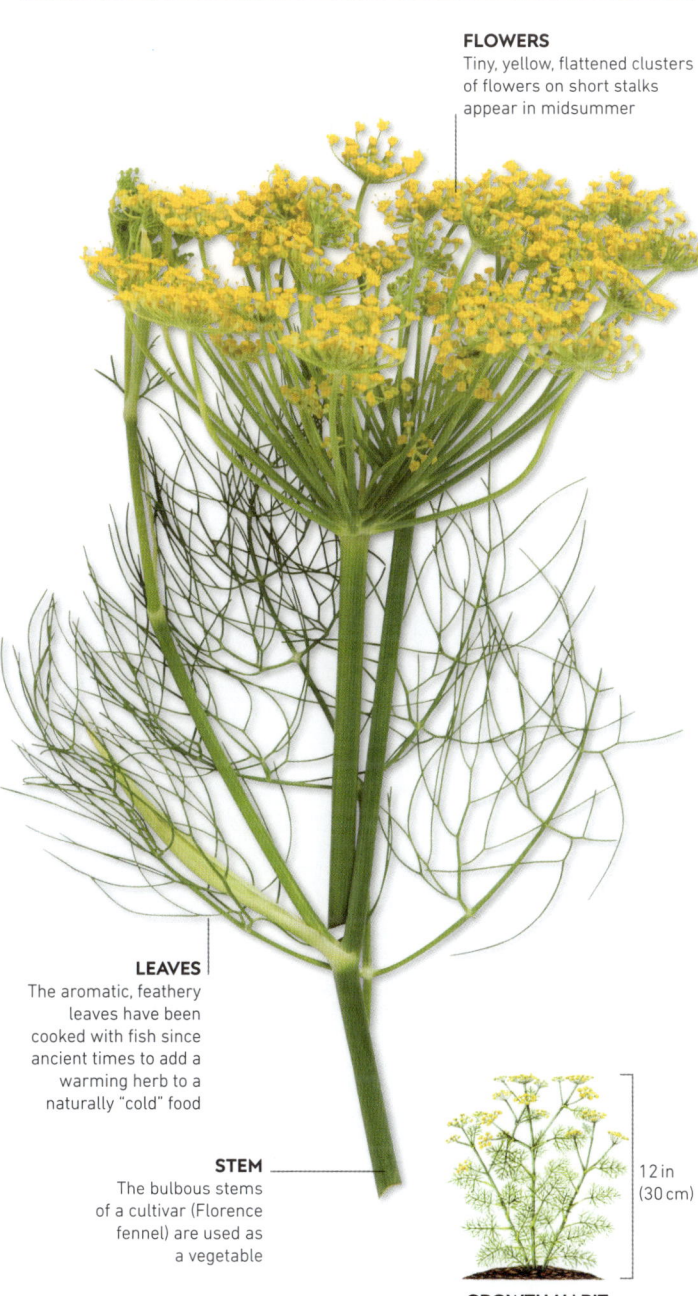

FLOWERS
Tiny, yellow, flattened clusters of flowers on short stalks appear in midsummer

LEAVES
The aromatic, feathery leaves have been cooked with fish since ancient times to add a warming herb to a naturally "cold" food

STEM
The bulbous stems of a cultivar (Florence fennel) are used as a vegetable

12 in (30 cm)

GROWTH HABIT
Deep-rooted perennial with a spread of 18 in (50 cm) and tiny flowers and feathery leaves.

Cultivated as both an herb and a vegetable since Roman times, fennel originated in Mediterranean areas, but by the 8th century CE had spread to northern Europe. It is widely available as an after-dinner herbal drink in tea bags to improve digestion, and has been used as a culinary herb with fish for centuries.

PARTS USED Seeds, root, leaves, essential oil
MAIN CONSTITUENTS Volatile oil (incl. estragole, anethole), essential fatty acids, flavonoids (incl. rutin), vitamins, minerals
ACTIONS Carminative, circulatory stimulant, anti-inflammatory, encourages milk flow, mild expectorant, diuretic

HOW TO USE

INFUSION ½–1 tsp of seeds to 1 cup of boiling water as an after-dinner tea to combat gas and indigestion. A standard infusion (p.176) taken 3 times daily can increase milk flow when breastfeeding.
MOUTHWASH/GARGLE Use 1 cup of above infusion of seeds as a wash for gum disorders or a gargle for sore throats.
TINCTURE 5–10 drops (¼–½ml) as a remedy for constipation to combat griping pains.
DECOCTION Drink 1 cup (1 tsp dry root per cup boiling water) 3 times daily for disorders linked to high uric acid levels.
CHEST RUB Add 5–10 drops (¼–½ml) each of fennel, thyme, and eucalyptus essential oil to 4 tsp (20 ml) of almond oil and massage into the chest for coughs and bronchitis.

HOW TO SOURCE

GROW Sow fennel seeds where you want them to grow in spring and thin to 12 in (30 cm), or transplant self-sown seedlings. Generally fairly hardy, but may suffer in severe winters. Can be treated as a biennial. The dulce variety is grown as a vegetable.
FORAGE Generally grows on waste ground and in coastal areas, but self-seeded plants growing outside gardens can be found in many places. Gather the leaves in summer for culinary use and the seeds in fall for teas and medicinal use.
HARVEST Collect the leaves in summer and the seeds in fall. Lift the root, if using, once the leaves have died down.

CAUTION Essential oils should not be taken internally except under professional advice.

Fragaria vesca
WILD STRAWBERRY

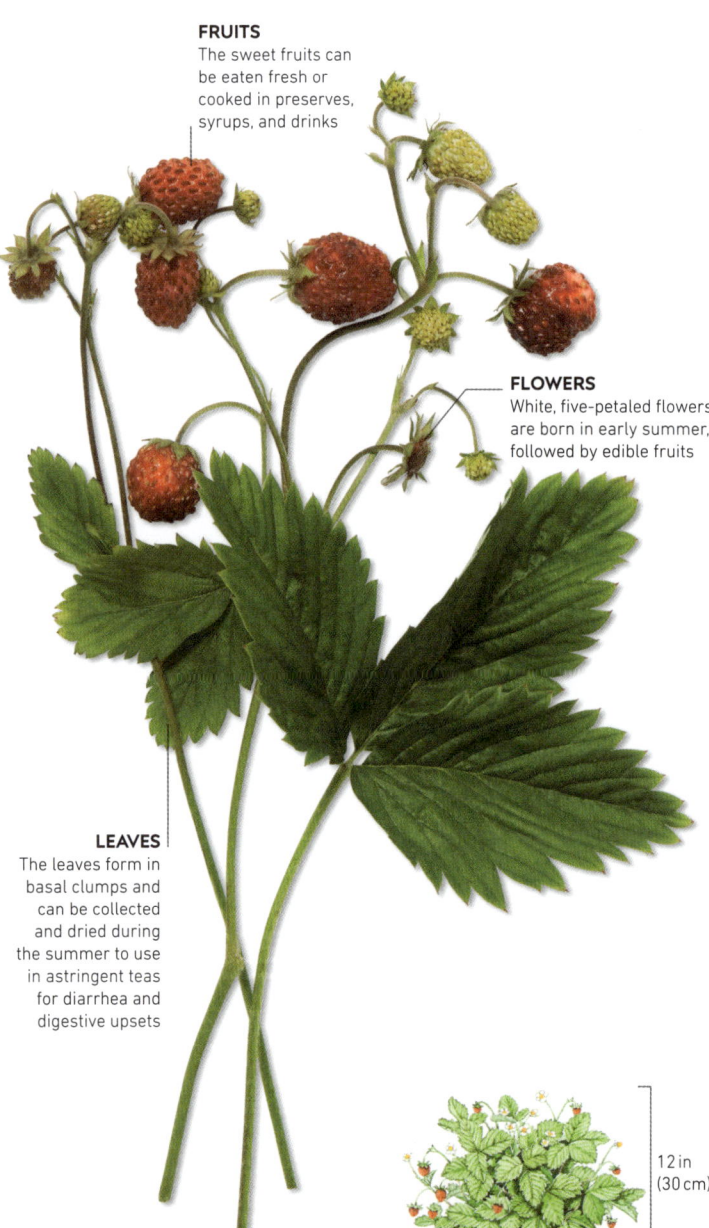

FRUITS
The sweet fruits can be eaten fresh or cooked in preserves, syrups, and drinks

FLOWERS
White, five-petaled flowers are born in early summer, followed by edible fruits

LEAVES
The leaves form in basal clumps and can be collected and dried during the summer to use in astringent teas for diarrhea and digestive upsets

12 in
(30 cm)

GROWTH HABIT
Low-growing perennial with edible fruits in summer that spreads by stolons; indefinite spread.

Alpine strawberries, now grown worldwide, originated from this wild strawberry and have smaller, more aromatic fruits than "cultivated" strawberries (which were developed in the 18th century from an American hybrid). Wild strawberry is found in woodlands and grassy areas of Europe, western Asia, and North America. Its leaves and fruits are used medicinally—mainly in astringent teas.

PARTS USED Leaves, fruit
MAIN CONSTITUENTS
Leaf: Volatile oil, flavonoids, tannins
Fruit: Fruit acids, salicylates, sugar, vitamins B, C, and E
ACTIONS Astringent, anti-inflammatory, wound herb, diuretic, laxative, liver tonic, cleansing

HOW TO USE

INFUSION Drink 1 cup (2 tsp herb per cup of boiled water) of the leaves 3 times daily for diarrhea.
MOUTHWASH/GARGLE Use 1 cup of the above infusion of the leaves for sore throats and gum disease.
LOTION Use the above infusion of the leaves as a lotion to bathe minor burns, cuts, and grazes.
FRESH BERRIES Traditionally regarded as cooling, strawberries have, in the past, been prescribed for gout, arthritis, rheumatism, and tuberculosis. They can also be soothing for gastritis and in convalescence.
JUICE Juice some fresh berries and take in 2 tsp (10 ml) doses 3 times daily to combat infections and as a mild, cleansing laxative in constipation and arthritic disorders.
POULTICE The crushed fresh berries can be used as a poultice to soothe sunburn and skin inflammations.

HOW TO SOURCE

GROW Prefers moist but well-drained fertile soil that is rich in organic matter, in sun or partial shade. Propagate by sowing seeds in trays in spring or fall and lightly covering them with soil. Keep moist and transplant to 3 in (7.5 cm) pots when large enough to handle. Alternatively, grow from rooted stolons (horizontal shoots) separated from the mother plant in late summer. It can be grown as an edging plant in an herb garden.
FORAGE Can be found in hedges, grassy areas, and woodlands in many parts of the world. Gather the berries when ripe and the leaves throughout the summer.
HARVEST Collect the fruit as it ripens in the summer and gather the leaves throughout the growing period.

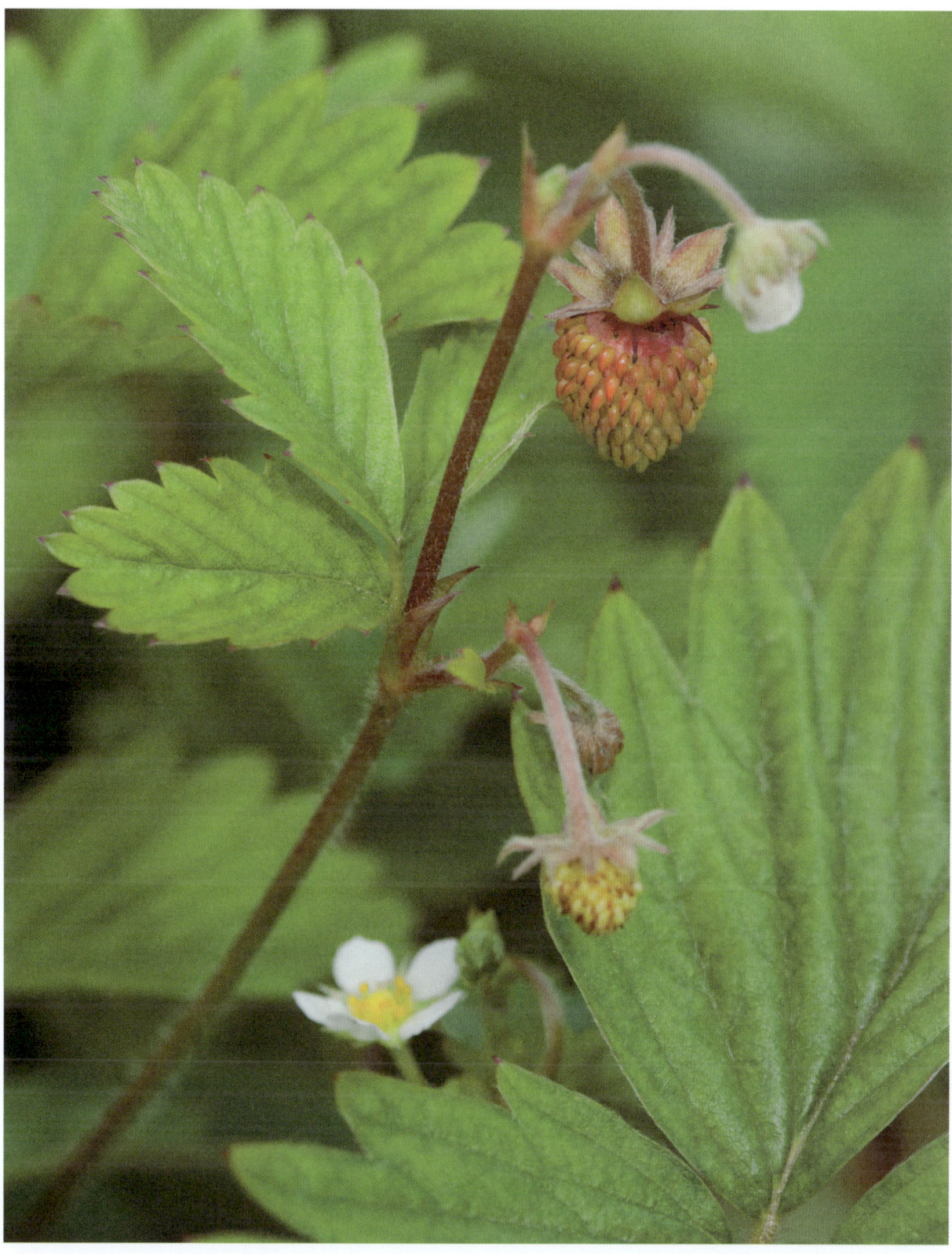

Galium aparine
CLEAVERS

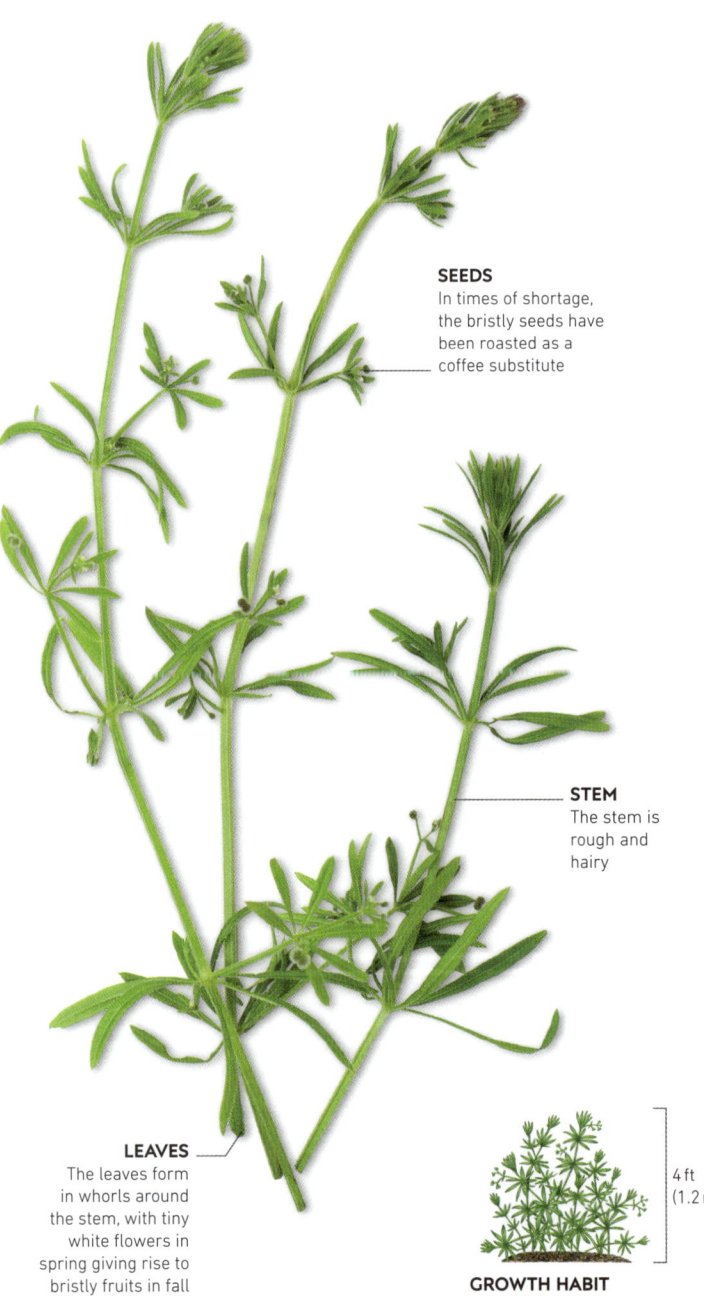

SEEDS
In times of shortage, the bristly seeds have been roasted as a coffee substitute

STEM
The stem is rough and hairy

LEAVES
The leaves form in whorls around the stem, with tiny white flowers in spring giving rise to bristly fruits in fall

GROWTH HABIT
Scrambling annual that climbs by hooked bristles; spread to 10 ft (3 m).

4 ft
(1.2 m)

A familiar garden weed, cleavers is found throughout Europe and northern and western Asia. In China, the whole plant is sometimes eaten as a vegetable. It has been used in cancer treatments since ancient times, although its efficacy has not been confirmed by modern research. It is, however, highly regarded as a cleanser for the lymphatic system.

PARTS USED Whole plant
MAIN CONSTITUENTS Flavonoids, anthraquinone derivatives (in the root), iridoids, coumarins, tannins, polyphenolic acids
ACTIONS Diuretic, lymphatic cleanser and detoxifier, astringent tonic, anti-inflammatory

HOW TO USE

JUICE Take 2 tsp (10 ml) of freshly made juice up to 3 times daily as a lymphatic cleanser and diuretic for conditions such as glandular fever, tonsillitis, and prostate disorders.
CREAM Use frequently for psoriasis; it is most effective if treatment begins early when the skin patches are still small.
INFUSION Drink 1 cup (2–3 tsp herb per cup boiling water) of the fresh herb 3 times daily for urinary problems such as cystitis and stones in the urinary tract. Usually combined with other urinary remedies such as yarrow, marshmallow, or buchu (*Agathosma* spp.).
TINCTURE Take up to 1 tsp (5 ml) 3 times daily as a lymphatic cleanser and detoxifier for any enlargement of the lymph nodes.
COMPRESS Apply a pad soaked in a standard infusion to scrapes, skin ulcers, and inflammations.

HOW TO SOURCE

GROW Regarded by most gardeners as an irritating annual weed, cleavers climbs by means of hooked bristles through shrubs to reach heights of 4 ft (1.2 m), and spreads to 10 ft (3 m). It is not a plant many would choose to cultivate, as it usually grows anywhere and everywhere, but the bristly fruits that appear in fall can be collected and immediately scattered where the plant is to grow the following year.
FORAGE From spring to fall, cleavers can be found scrambling through banks, hedgerows, and garden borders. The whole plant can be gathered, and is best used fresh.
HARVEST The whole plant is best gathered in the spring just before flowering.

Ginkgo biloba
GINKGO

A survivor of the fossil age, the ginkgo or maidenhair tree is the sole member of its genus and dates back at least 200 million years. The trees are either male or female and only flower when in close proximity. The edible seeds are used in traditional Chinese medicine for some types of asthma, while the leaves have become popular in the West for circulatory disorders.

PARTS USED Leaves, seeds
MAIN CONSTITUENTS Leaves: flavone glycosides, bioflavones, beta-sitosterol, lactones, anthocyanin Seeds: fatty acids, minerals, bioflavones
ACTIONS Leaves: vasodilator, circulatory stimulant Seeds: astringent, antifungal, antibacterial

HOW TO USE

FLUID EXTRACT Take 20–60 drops (1–3 ml) up to 3 times daily for diseases involving the peripheral circulation, or for cerebral arteriosclerosis in the elderly.
TINCTURE Take 60 drops–1 tsp (3–5 ml) 3 times daily for cardiovascular system disorders. It is generally combined with periwinkle (*Vinca* spp.) and lime flowers for circulatory problems, or melilot for venous disorders.
INFUSION Drink 1 cup of tea made from 3–4 seeds to 1 pint (600ml) of water 3 times daily for wheeziness, persistent coughs, or asthmatic conditions. Ginkgo can be combined with coltsfoot and mulberry leaves (*Morus* spp.).
TABLETS Widely available and generally recommended for poor circulation, erectile dysfunction, headaches, varicose veins, or memory loss.

HOW TO SOURCE

GROW Most commercially available trees are grown from cuttings from male trees; so female trees can be hard to find. Prefers fertile, moist, but well-drained soil in full sun. Grow from ripe seeds collected from a female tree in fall and plant in a cold frame, or take semi-ripe cuttings in summer. Avoid pruning.
FORAGE Rarely found in the wild, but widely cultivated as a specimen tree in parks and gardens.
HARVEST Collect leaves and fruits in fall.

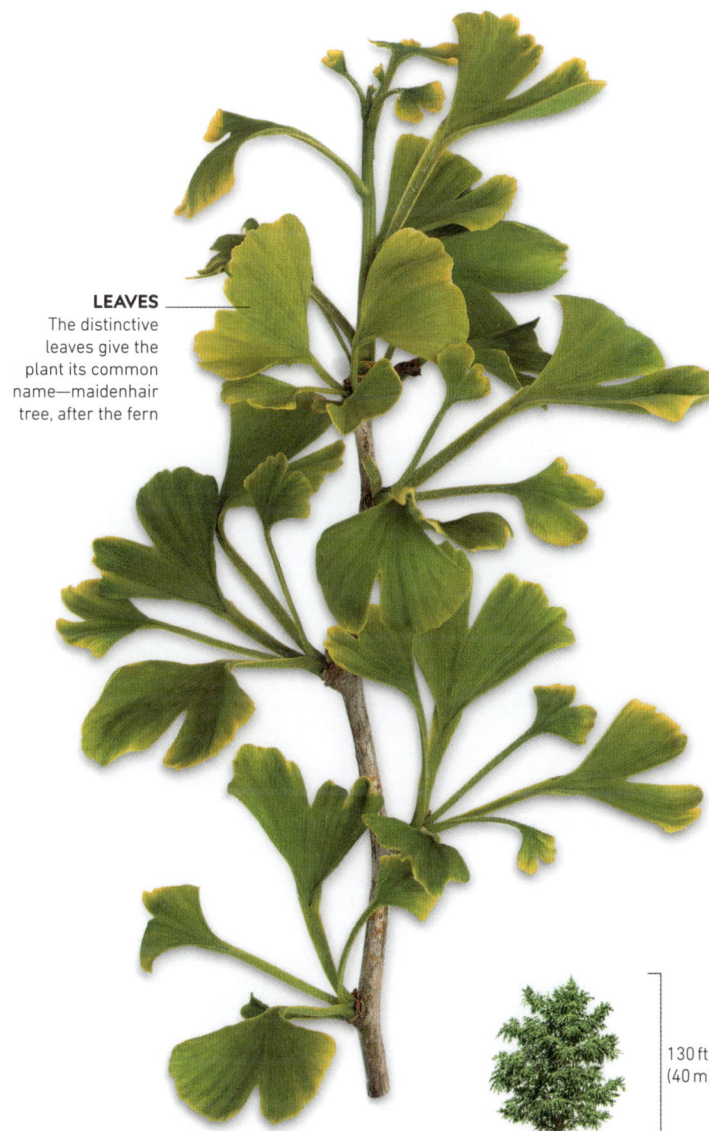

LEAVES
The distinctive leaves give the plant its common name—maidenhair tree, after the fern

130 ft
(40 m)

GROWTH HABIT
Upright, tall, spreading deciduous tree; spread 65 ft (20 m).

CAUTION Avoid if taking aspirin or warfarin. High doses of the seeds can lead to skin disorders and headaches. Restricted in some countries.

Glycyrrhiza glabra
LICORICE

A native of the Mediterranean region and southwest Asia, licorice has been valued for its sweet taste since ancient times. The Romans also used it as a remedy for asthma and coughs. Its cultivation spread to northern Europe in the 15th century. A related Asian species (*Glycyrrhiza uralensis*) is known as "the grandfather of herbs," and is widely used in Chinese medicine.

PARTS USED Root

MAIN CONSTITUENTS Saponins, glycyrrhizin, estrogenous substances, coumarins, flavonoids, sterols, asparagine

ACTIONS Anti-inflammatory, demulcent, tonic stimulant for adrenal cortex, mild laxative, expectorant, lowers cholesterol levels, soothing for gastric mucosa

HOW TO USE

TINCTURE Take 40 drops–1 tsp (2–5 ml) 3 times daily for gastritis, peptic ulceration, mouth ulcers, or excessive stomach acid. Add a similar amount to cough syrups.

FLUID EXTRACT Take 20–40 drops (1–2 ml) 3 times a day to strengthen the adrenal glands, especially after steroidal therapy, or as a digestive tonic.

DECOCTION Drink 1 cup (½–1 tsp dry root per cup boiling water) up to 3 times daily to reduce stomach acid and ease any inflammation or ulceration. Take 1 cup last thing at night for mild constipation.

SYRUP Combine the decoction with an equal amount of honey to make a cough syrup. Combines well with thyme, hyssop, or elecampane for a sore throat and chest problems including bronchitis, asthma, and chest infections.

WASH Add 1 tsp (5 ml) of tincture to 1¾ fl oz (50 ml) of warm water to bathe skin inflammations and irritant skin rashes.

HOW TO SOURCE

GROW Prefers deep, neutral to alkaline, well-drained soil in full sun. Sow seeds in fall or spring and transplant into 3 in (7.5 cm) pots when large enough. Grow in containers until sturdy enough to plant.

FORAGE Grows wild in southern Europe. Collecting wild roots is not recommended. Gather the seed pods to cultivate at home.

HARVEST Gather the roots of three- or four-year-old plants in fall.

CAUTION Do not take therapeutic doses if pregnant. Avoid if you have high blood pressure or take digoxin-based drugs. Do not take for prolonged periods except under professional advice.

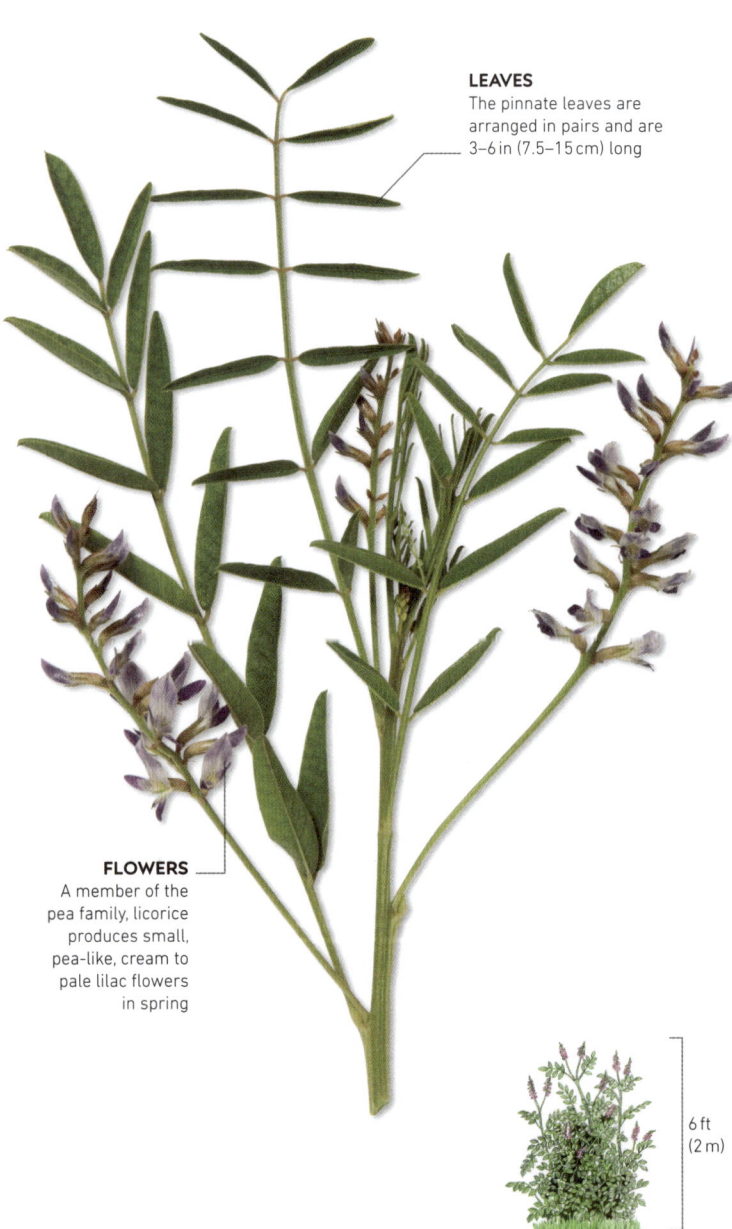

LEAVES
The pinnate leaves are arranged in pairs and are 3–6 in (7.5–15 cm) long

FLOWERS
A member of the pea family, licorice produces small, pea-like, cream to pale lilac flowers in spring

6 ft (2 m)

GROWTH HABIT
Tap-rooted perennial with oblong pods; spread 3 ft (1 m).

Hamamelis virginiana
WITCH HAZEL

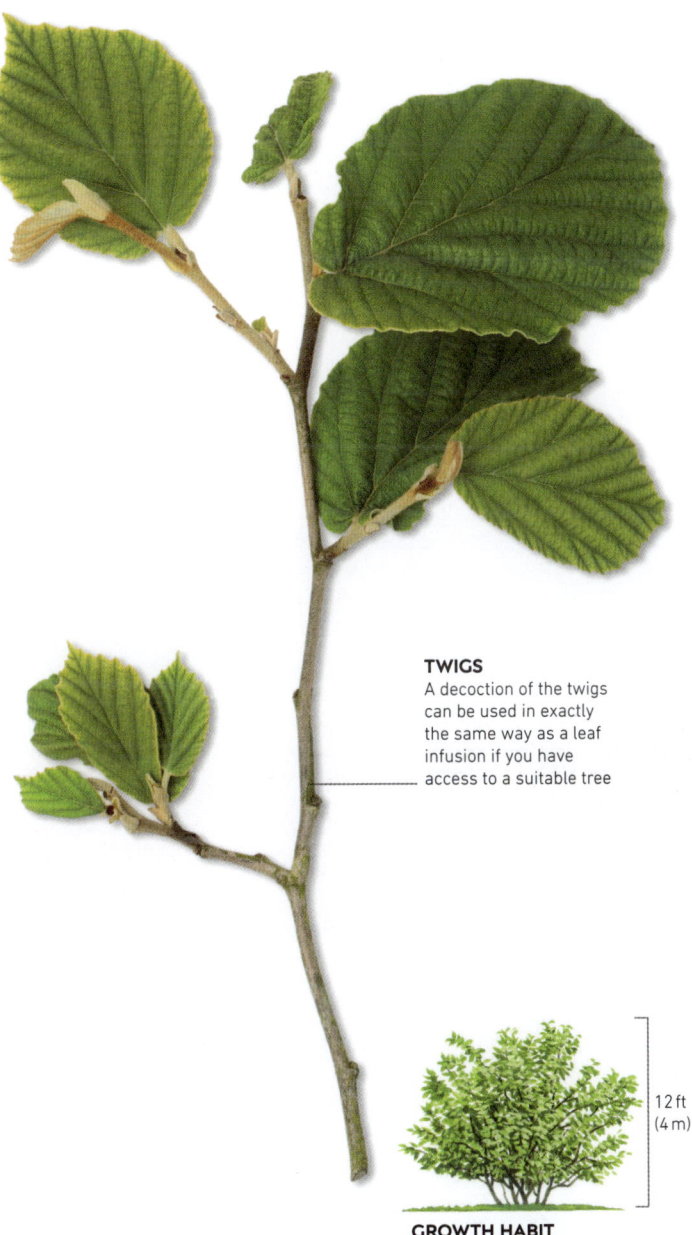

TWIGS
A decoction of the twigs can be used in exactly the same way as a leaf infusion if you have access to a suitable tree

12 ft
(4 m)

GROWTH HABIT
A small deciduous single- or multi-stemmed tree or shrub with a spread of 12 ft (4 m).

Used by Native Americans for traumatic injuries and aching muscles, Virginian witch hazel was originally found in North America's moist woodland areas, from Nova Scotia to Florida. Today it is widely cultivated for its medicinal properties, and as an attractive garden ornamental with heavily scented fall flowers. Distilled Virginian witch hazel is a familiar first-aid remedy.

PARTS USED Leaves, twigs
MAIN CONSTITUENTS Tannins, flavonoids (incl. kaempferol and quercetin), saponins, bitters, volatile oil (incl. eugenol and safrole), choline, gallic acid
ACTIONS Astringent, stops internal and external bleeding, anti-inflammatory

HOW TO USE

DISTILLATE/HYDROSOL The leaves and twigs are distilled commercially to produce a mixture of water and essential oil (sometimes preserved with alcohol). It can be used to stop bleeding from cuts, scrapes, or nosebleeds, to bathe varicose veins and irritant skin rashes, and in compresses for sprains or sore eyes.
INFUSION Pour 1 cup boiling water over 1 tsp leaves and drink 1 cup 3 times daily for diarrhea, hemorrhoids, or capillary fragility.
MOUTHWASH/GARGLE Use 1 cup of above infusion of the leaves for sore throats, mouth ulcers, tonsillitis, pharyngitis, and spongy or bleeding gums.
TINCTURE Add 1 tsp (5 ml) of the bark tincture to 1¾ fl oz (50 ml) of water and use as an alternative to distilled witch hazel.
CREAM/OINTMENT Use the bark for minor cuts, scrapes, bruises, hemorrhoids, or varicose veins.

HOW TO SOURCE

GROW Prefers moist, rich, sandy, or peaty soil with partial shade, but can tolerate poorer soil and full sun. Sow ripe seeds in a cold frame in fall. The seeds can be slow to germinate, but grow in larger pots until the young tree is large enough to plant out. Alternatively, take softwood cuttings in summer or hardwood cuttings in fall.
FORAGE Virginian witch hazel may be found growing wild in woodlands on the eastern side of North America. Gathering bark from wild trees is not recommended, as it can damage the tree, although leaves and a few twigs can be harvested in summer and early fall before flowering.
HARVEST The leaves are gathered in summer and the bark in fall. The twigs can be cropped when the tree is dormant.

Houttuynia cordata
DOKUDAMI

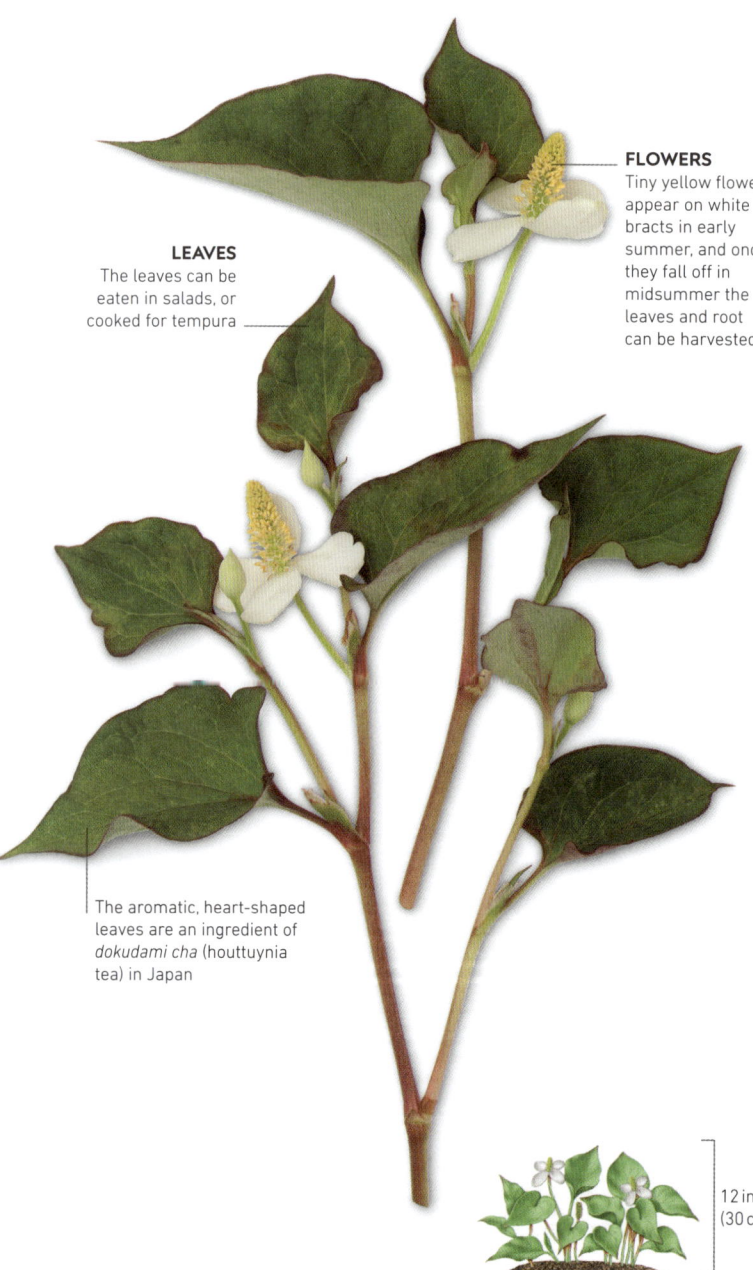

FLOWERS
Tiny yellow flowers appear on white bracts in early summer, and once they fall off in midsummer the leaves and root can be harvested

LEAVES
The leaves can be eaten in salads, or cooked for tempura

The aromatic, heart-shaped leaves are an ingredient of *dokudami cha* (houttuynia tea) in Japan

12 in (30 cm)

GROWTH HABIT
Vigorous spreading rhizomatous perennial; spread indefinite.

This plant was once used as an antidote to poisons and its common name, dokudami, translates as "poison blocking" in Japanese. While its Chinese name, *yu xing cao*, means "fish-smelling plant." Dokudami is a common addition to savory dishes. One of the most popular medicinal herbs in Japan, it is used widely as a cleanser and detoxifier.

PARTS USED Leaves, root
MAIN CONSTITUENTS Flavonoids (incl. quercetin and hyperin), terpenes (incl. limonene and camphene), linalool, sitosterols, potassium salts, volatile oil (incl. decanoyl-acetaldehyde)
ACTIONS Astringent, diuretic, antibacterial, laxative, urinary antiseptic, anti-inflammatory, antitussive, wound herb

HOW TO USE

TINCTURE Take up to 2 tsp (10 ml) 3 times daily for urinary infections or pain on urination; also said to improve capillary integrity when taken long term, so use for thread veins and broken capillaries.
INFUSION Make an infusion (p.176) of 2–3 tsp fresh herb per cup of boiling water. Drink on 1 day each month as a general detoxifier.
SYRUP Add 1 lb (450 g) of honey to 1 pint (600 ml) of above infusion containing equal amounts of dokudami and Chinese balloon flower and take in 1 tsp (5 ml) doses 4–5 times daily for coughs with thick, yellow-green sputum.
DECOCTION Drink 1–2 cups (2–3 tsp whole plant per cup boiling water) daily for boils and abscesses, although abscesses will not improve unless drained.
LOTION/OINTMENT Use on cuts, scrapes, acne, boils, athlete's foot, or insect bites.

HOW TO SOURCE

GROW Prefers damp, fertile soil in full sun or dappled shade, but will grow in dry conditions, and may require protection in cold areas in winter. Sow seeds in trays in the summer, pot on, and transplant to their final growing positions in spring when well established. Can be invasive.
FORAGE Native to marginal aquatic and marshy areas in China, Japan, Laos, and Vietnam. It is classified as an alien invasive species in North America and Australia.
HARVEST Cut after flowering in summer.

CAUTION A cooling herb, so avoid in cold syndromes.

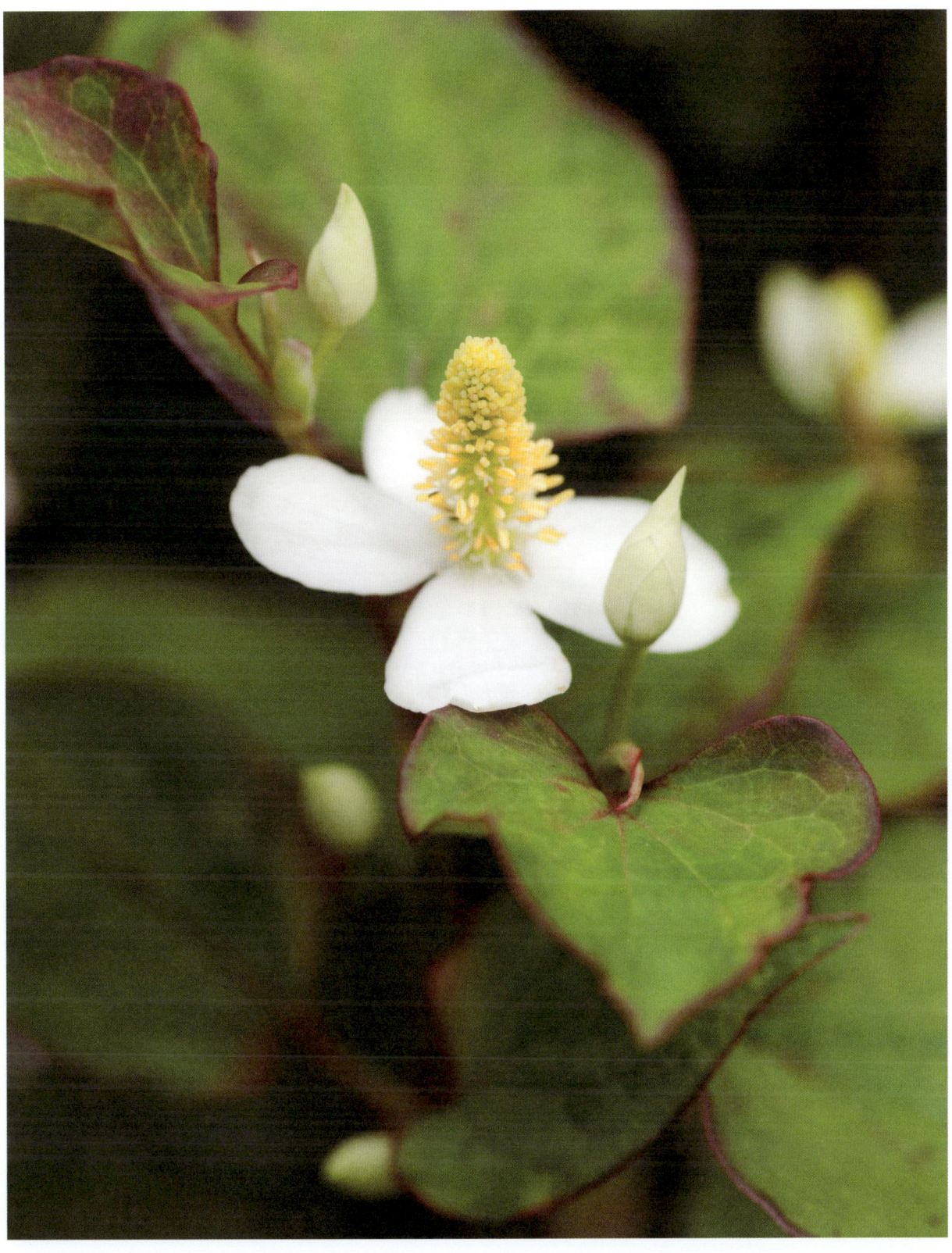

Humulus lupulus
HOPS

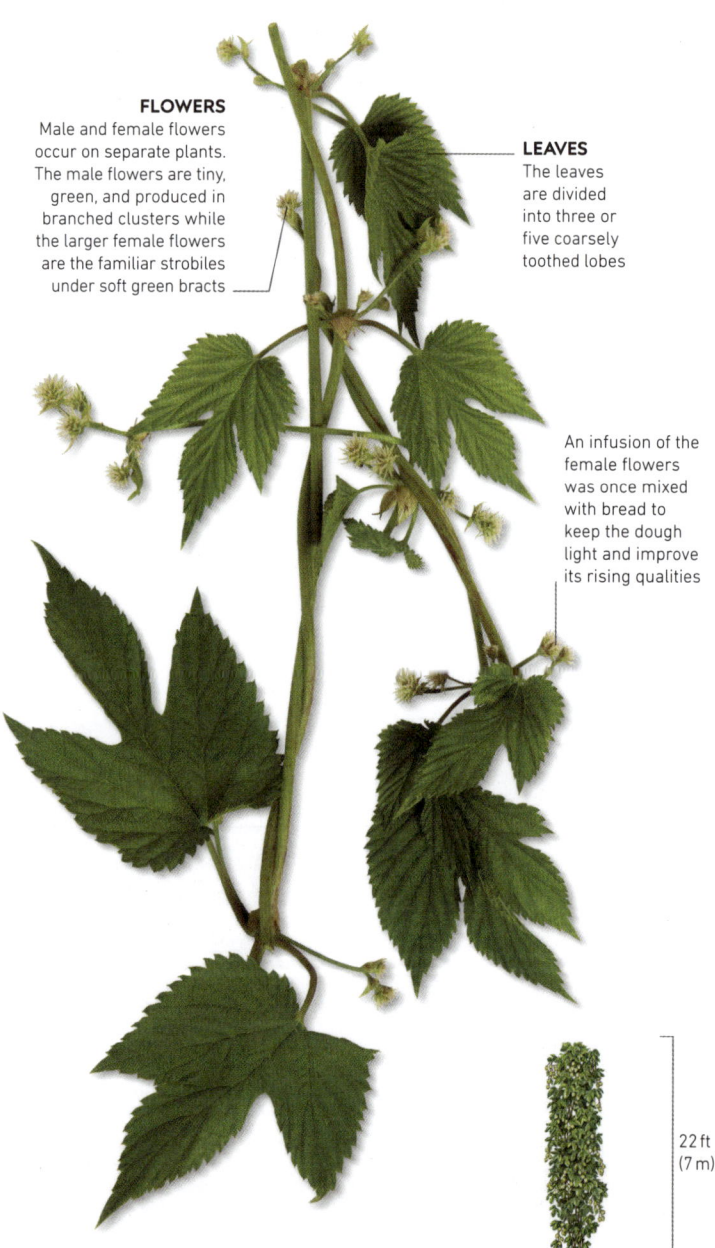

FLOWERS
Male and female flowers occur on separate plants. The male flowers are tiny, green, and produced in branched clusters while the larger female flowers are the familiar strobiles under soft green bracts

LEAVES
The leaves are divided into three or five coarsely toothed lobes

An infusion of the female flowers was once mixed with bread to keep the dough light and improve its rising qualities

22 ft
(7 m)

GROWTH HABIT
A vigorous, deciduous perennial climber with bristly stems.

The strobiles, or female flowers, of the hop plant have been used since the 11th century for brewing beer, while the Romans used the leaves as a salad herb. The plant, which is native to Europe, is sedative and bitter, so it is used medicinally both for nervous disorders and digestive problems. It is also estrogenic, leading to a loss of libido in men who regularly drink large amounts of beer.

PARTS USED Strobiles (female flowers)
MAIN CONSTITUENTS Bitter principles (incl. humulone and valeric acid), tannins, volatile oil (incl. humulene), estrogenic substances, asparagine, flavonoids
ACTIONS Sedative, anaphrodisiac, restoring tonic for the nervous system, bitter digestive stimulant, diuretic, soporific, astringent.

HOW TO USE

TINCTURE Take 20–40 drops (1–2 ml) in water 3 times a day as a sedative for nervous tension and anxiety, to stimulate the digestion in poor appetite, and to ease gut spasms and colic.
INFUSION For insomnia, use 2–4 fresh strobiles per cup of boiling water, infuse for 5 minutes, and drink 30 minutes before bedtime. Freshly dried hops can also be used (older plant material is less effective).
WASH Use a standard infusion of fresh or freshly dried hops (above) as a wash for chronic ulcers, skin eruptions, or wounds.
COMPRESS Add 2 tsp (10 ml) of tincture to 4 fl oz (120 ml) of water, soak a pad in the mixture, and use as a compress on varicose ulcers.

HOW TO SOURCE

GROW Prefers fertile, well-drained soil in sun or partial shade, and must be supported on canes or trellises. Sow the seeds in spring in trays in a propagator at 59°F (15°C) and transplant to their final growing positions when established. Alternatively, propagate by softwood cuttings in spring or early summer. Cut down old growth in winter.
FORAGE Likely to be found in hedges or waste ground, especially if plants have self-seeded outside commercial hop-growing areas. Collect the female flowers.
HARVEST Collect the strobiles in summer.

CAUTION Do not take if suffering from depression. The growing plant can cause contact dermatitis. Harvesting large amounts can disrupt a menstrual cycle.

Hydrastis canadensis
GOLDENSEAL

Used by Native American tribes for a wide range of ailments including whooping cough, liver disorders, and heart problems, goldenseal originated in North America's mountain woodlands. Today its used mainly for ulceration and inflammations affecting the mucous membranes. By the 20th century, over-harvesting caused the plant to become endangered.

PARTS USED Rhizome

MAIN CONSTITUENTS Alkaloids (incl. hydrastine, canadine, and berberine), volatile oil, resin

ACTIONS Astringent, tonic, digestive, bile stimulant, anti-inflammatory, antibacterial, anticatarrhal, laxative, healing to gastric mucosa, uterine stimulant, stops internal bleeding

HOW TO USE

TINCTURE Take 10–40 drops (0.5–2 ml) 3 times a day for catarrhal conditions, mucous colitis, gastroenteritis, or vaginal discharge, as a liver tonic for sluggish digestion, or to help control heavy menstrual and postpartum bleeding.

MOUTHWASH/GARGLE Use 40–60 drops (2–3 ml) of tincture in 3½ fl oz (100 ml) of warm water for mouth ulcers, gum disease, sore throats, and catarrhal conditions.

CAPSULES Use 1 x 300 mg capsule 3 times daily for catarrh, infections, or with powdered eyebright to relieve hay fever symptoms.

HOW TO SOURCE

GROW Prefers moist, well-drained, slightly acid to neutral soil in shade. Plant seeds in a cold frame in small pots when ripe. Pot and plant when large enough, or propagate by root division in fall.

FORAGE The plant is designated as "vulnerable" on the IUCN Red List of endangered species and should not be harvested from the wild.

HARVEST Roots of mature plants are lifted in the fall and dried.

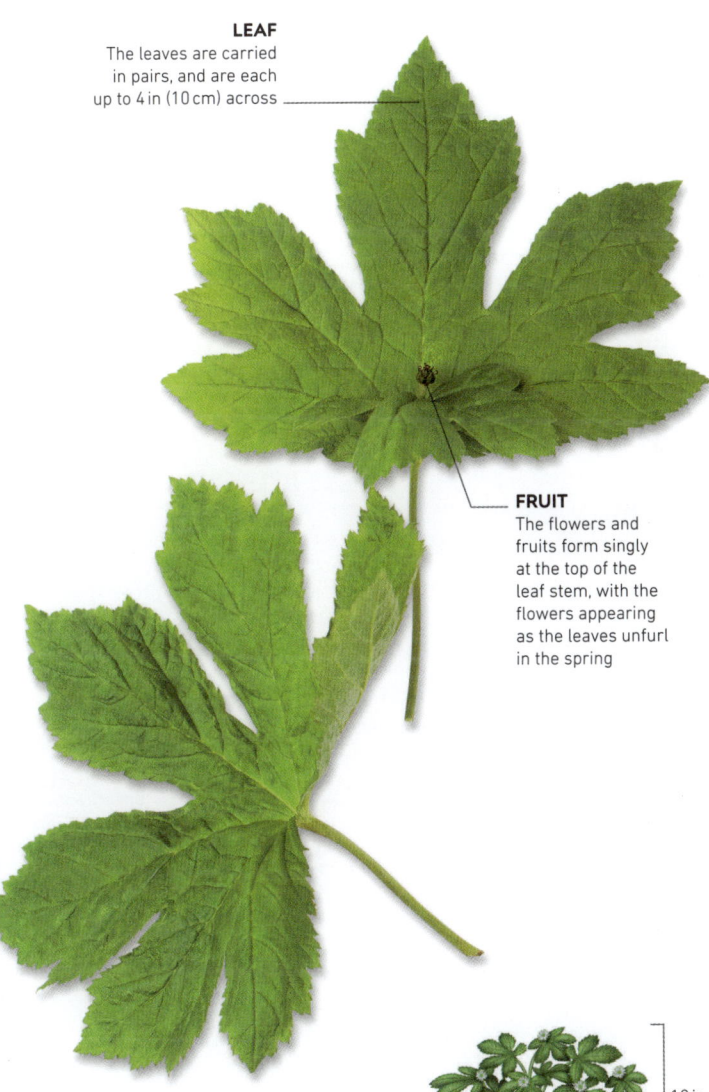

LEAF
The leaves are carried in pairs, and are each up to 4 in (10 cm) across

FRUIT
The flowers and fruits form singly at the top of the leaf stem, with the flowers appearing as the leaves unfurl in the spring

12 in (30 cm)

GROWTH HABIT
A rhizomatous, deciduous perennial; spread 6–12 in (15–30 cm) or more.

CAUTION A uterine stimulant, so avoid during pregnancy and lactation. Avoid if you have high blood pressure. Prolonged use can reduce absorption of B vitamins.

Hypericum perforatum
ST. JOHN'S WORT

Native to temperate zones in Europe and Asia, St. John's wort has been used as a wound herb since the Crusades, and was widely regarded as a cure-all in earlier centuries. It was also used for treating hysteria and mental illness. Today it is widely prescribed in parts of Europe for depression; the quality of commercial preparations, readily available to purchase, can vary.

PARTS USED Aerial parts, flowering tops
MAIN CONSTITUENTS Hypericin, pseudohypericin, flavonoids (incl. rutin), volatile oil, tannins, resins
ACTIONS Astringent, analgesic, antiviral, anti-inflammatory, sedative, restoring tonic for the nervous system, and vulnerary

HOW TO USE

INFUSION Make an infusion of 1 cup boiling water over 1–2 tsp (5–10 ml) of the aerial parts. Drink 1 cup 3 times daily for anxiety, irritability, or emotional upsets associated with menopause or PMS.
TINCTURE Take 40 drops–1 tsp (2–5 ml) 3 times daily for nervous tension leading to exhaustion and depression. 5–10 drops of tincture at night can be useful for childhood bed-wetting.
WASH Use 1 cup of above infusion of aerial parts to bathe wounds, skin sores, or bruises.
MACERATED OIL Apply a little oil 2–3 times daily to minor burns, sunburn, cold sores, cuts, or scrapes. Massage gently to relieve inflamed joints and tendonitis, and
to ease nerve pains. Up to 10 drops of lavender or yarrow essential oil with 1 tsp (5 ml) of the oil increases efficacy.

HOW TO SOURCE

GROW Prefers a sunny position and well-drained, alkaline soil. Sow seeds in seed trays in fall or spring and pot when large enough to handle. Harden off before planting in final positions. Established clumps can be divided by root division in spring or fall.
FORAGE Found growing wild, often in hedges, in many parts of the world.
HARVEST Gather the whole plant just before flowering, or just the flowering tops in midsummer.

CAUTION Avoid during pregnancy. May cause gastrointestinal disturbances and allergic reactions. Interacts with many prescription drugs and oral contraceptives. Photosensitive: do not apply topically before sun exposure.

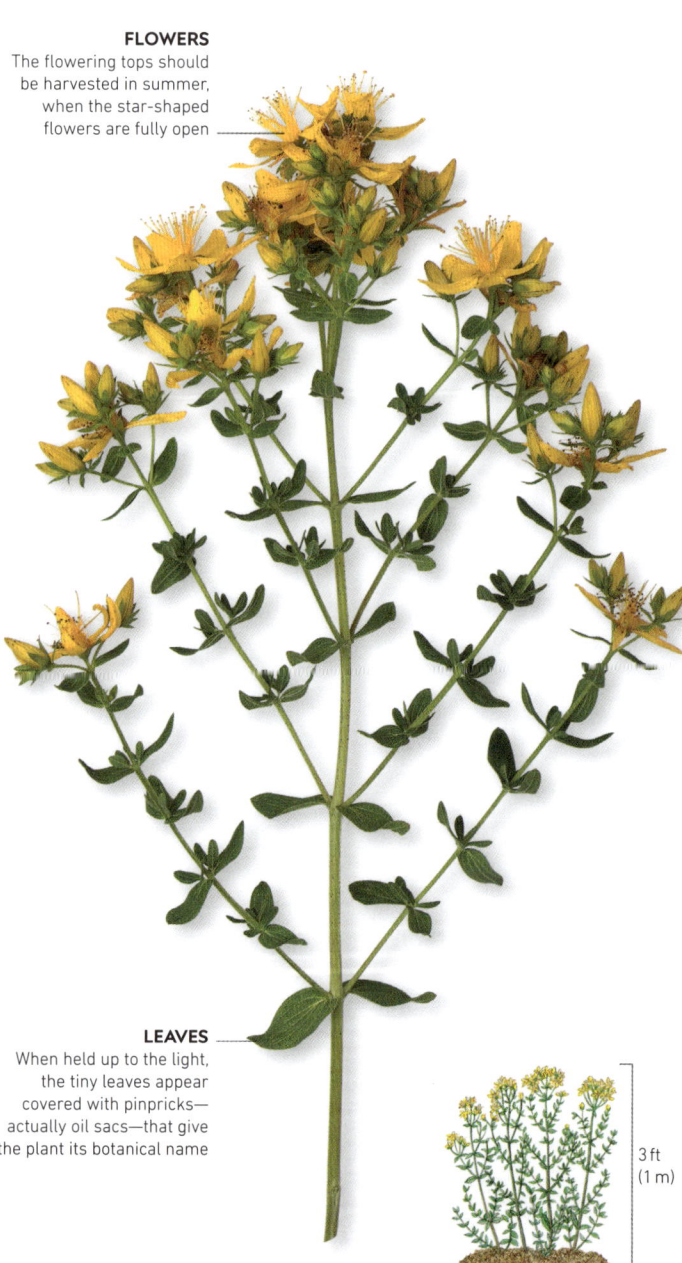

FLOWERS
The flowering tops should be harvested in summer, when the star-shaped flowers are fully open

LEAVES
When held up to the light, the tiny leaves appear covered with pinpricks—actually oil sacs—that give the plant its botanical name

GROWTH HABIT
Compact, erect perennial with a spread of 3 ft (1 m).

3 ft (1 m)

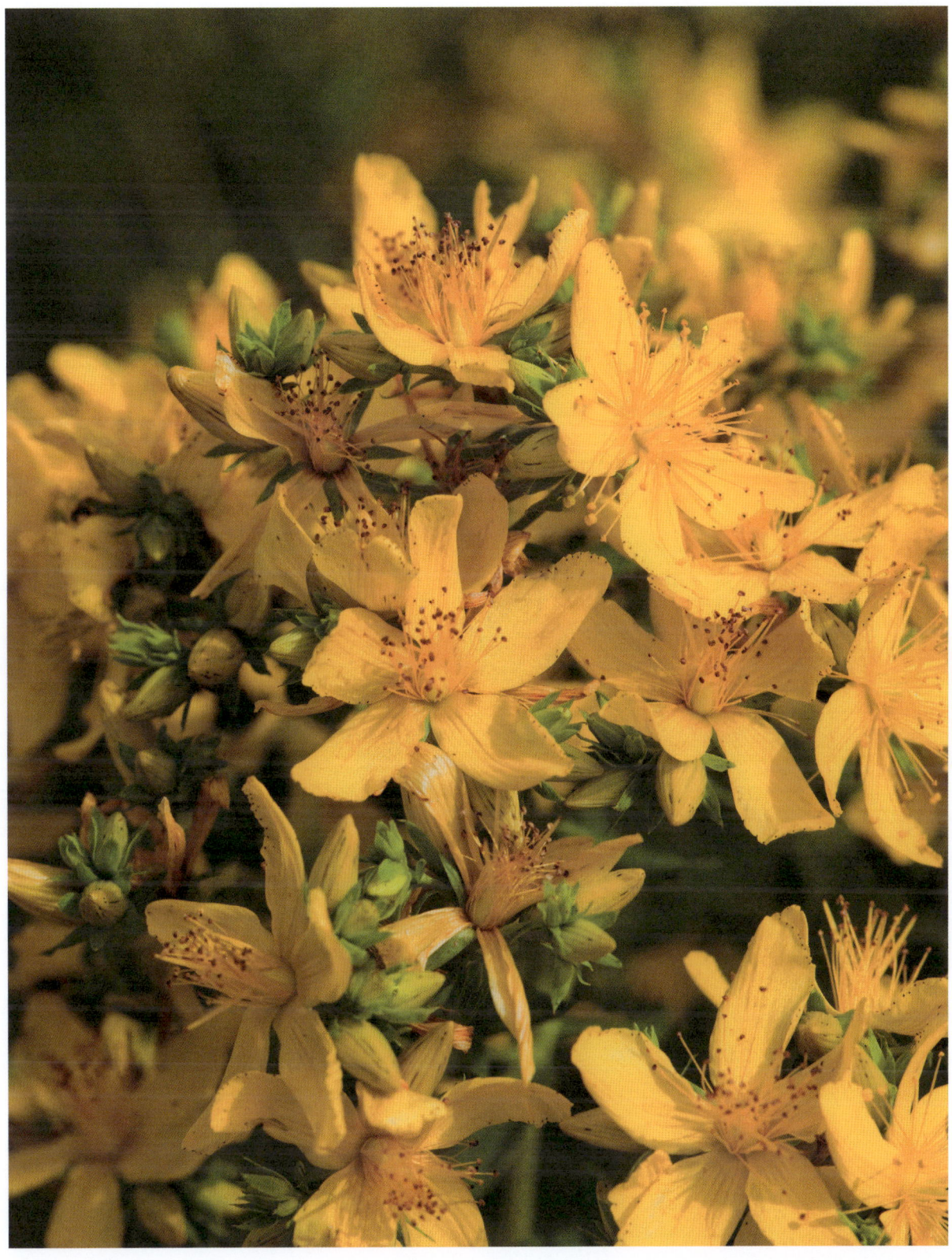

Hyssopus officinalis
HYSSOP

Originally found in rocky areas around the Mediterranean, hyssop is now cultivated in many parts of the world and is often grown as low edging in knot gardens or as a companion plant to keep butterflies from brassicas. It can be used both as a culinary herb to flavor stews and in remedies for coughs and feverish chills.

PARTS USED Aerial parts, flowers, essential oil
MAIN CONSTITUENTS Volatile oil (incl. camphor and pinocamphone), flavonoids, terpenes (incl. marrubiin), hyssopin, tannins
ACTIONS Expectorant, carminative, diaphoretic, anticatarrhal, antispasmodic, hypertensive, emmenagogue, some antiviral action reported (to *Herpes simplex*)

HOW TO USE

INFUSION Drink ½ cup of a hot infusion (1–2 tsp herb per cup of boiling water) every 2 hours to encourage sweating in the early stages of colds or flu.
TINCTURE Take 40–80 drops (2–4 ml) 3 times daily for gas, indigestion, bloating, or colic, especially if anxious.
SYRUP Combine 1 pint (600 ml) of an infusion of the whole herb (or the flowers only, if you have them) with 1 lb (450 g) honey to make a syrup for productive coughs and catarrh. Take in 1 tsp (5 ml) doses as required. Combines well with coltsfoot, thyme, or mullein flowers.
CHEST RUB Combine 1 tbsp (15 ml) macerated oil of hyssop with 2 drops (1 ml) each of essential oils of thyme and eucalyptus as a chest rub for bronchitis and chesty colds.

HOW TO SOURCE

GROW Prefers fertile, neutral to alkaline soil, and full sun. Grow from seeds in trays in fall or spring and transplant to final positions when established; allow up to 36 in (90 cm) between plants. Alternatively, take softwood cuttings in summer. Prune lightly after flowering, and harder in spring.
FORAGE Unlikely to be found growing in the wild beyond the Mediterranean region.
HARVEST Gather leaves and flower buds in summer and sprigs in the growing season.

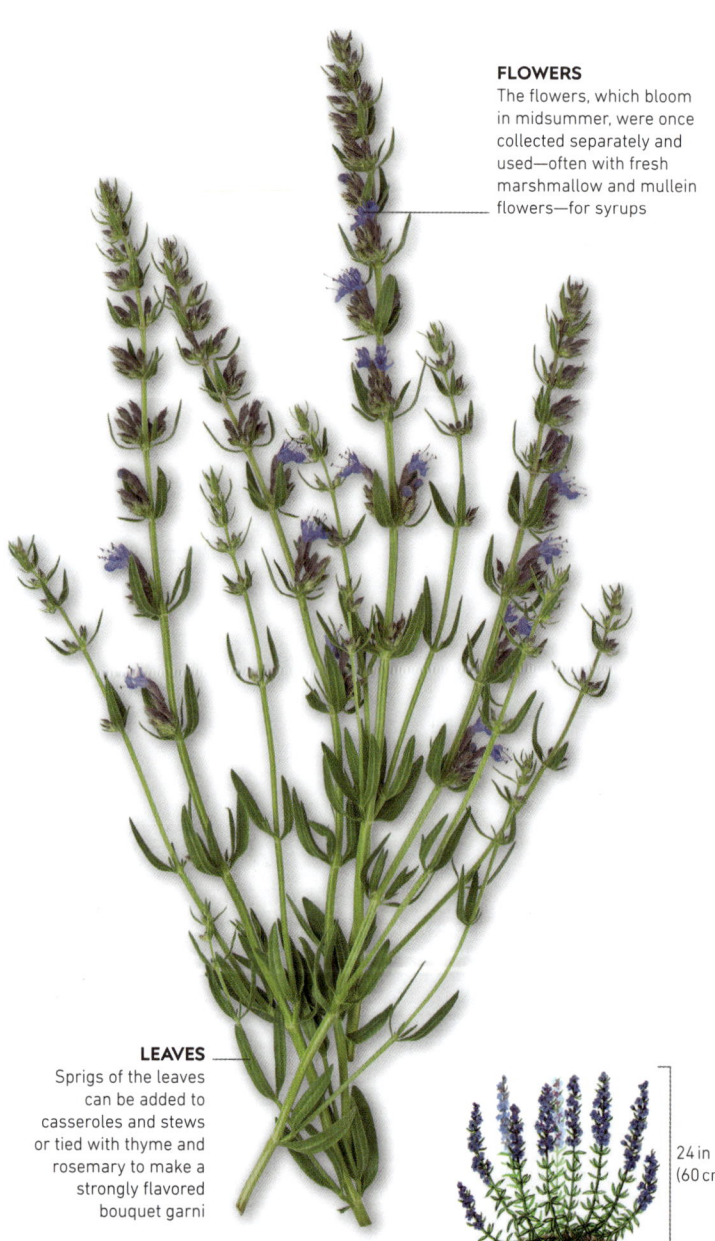

FLOWERS
The flowers, which bloom in midsummer, were once collected separately and used—often with fresh marshmallow and mullein flowers—for syrups

LEAVES
Sprigs of the leaves can be added to casseroles and stews or tied with thyme and rosemary to make a strongly flavored bouquet garni

24 in (60 cm)

GROWTH HABIT
A semi-evergreen shrub with whorled flower spikes and a spread of 24–36 in (60–90 cm).

CAUTION In high doses the essential oil can trigger epileptic seizures; use only under professional guidance. Avoid during pregnancy.

Inula helenium
ELECAMPANE

FLOWER
The flowers of a related species (*Inula japonica*) are used in cough remedies in China

LEAVES
The large, bright green leaves can be up to 28 in (70 cm) in length and have a soft, downy underside

GROWTH HABIT
Tall, upright, rhizomatous perennial; spread 5 ft (1.5 m).

6 ft
(2 m)

Native to woods and grassy areas across Europe and western Asia, elecampane is largely used today as a cough remedy and respiratory tonic. In earlier ages, it was regarded much more as a cure-all: the Romans prescribed the herb for digestive upsets and sciatica; while the Anglo-Saxons used it for skin diseases, leprosy, and for sudden onset disorders or "elf-shot."

PARTS USED Root and rhizome
MAIN CONSTITUENTS Inulin, helenin, volatile oil (incl. azulenes and sesquiterpene lactones), sterols, possible alkaloids, mucilage
ACTIONS Tonic, stimulating expectorant, diaphoretic, antibacterial, antifungal, antiparasitic

HOW TO USE

DECOCTION Make an infusion (p.176) of 1–2 tsp herb per cup of boiling water (best made with fresh root). Drink 1 cup 3 times daily for bronchitis, asthma, and upper respiratory catarrh. This can also ease hay fever symptoms, and is valuable as a respiratory tonic. Sweeten with 1 teaspoon of honey if desired.
TINCTURE Take 60 drops–1 tsp (3–5 ml) 3 times daily for chronic respiratory complaints such as bronchitis.
SYRUP Combine 10 fl oz (300 ml) of a decoction (ideally from fresh root) with 8 oz (225 g) of honey to make a cough syrup and take in 1 tsp (5 ml) doses as required for productive coughs or to ease hay fever symptoms.

HOW TO SOURCE

GROW Prefers moist but well-drained soil in a sunny position. Sow the seeds in a cold frame in fall and transplant to their final position when established; allow 36 in (90 cm) between plants. Alternatively, propagate by division in spring or fall. The plant has a deep-rooted rhizome and, once established, can be difficult to eradicate. Flowers appear in summer.
FORAGE The root is generally used, which can make foraging difficult, although the plant is commonly found in hedges and grassy places. The flowers can be easily harvested in summer and used to make a mild cough syrup.
HARVEST The root is dug in fall, chopped, and dried quickly at a high heat.

CAUTION Avoid during pregnancy and if breastfeeding.

Jasminum officinale
JASMINE

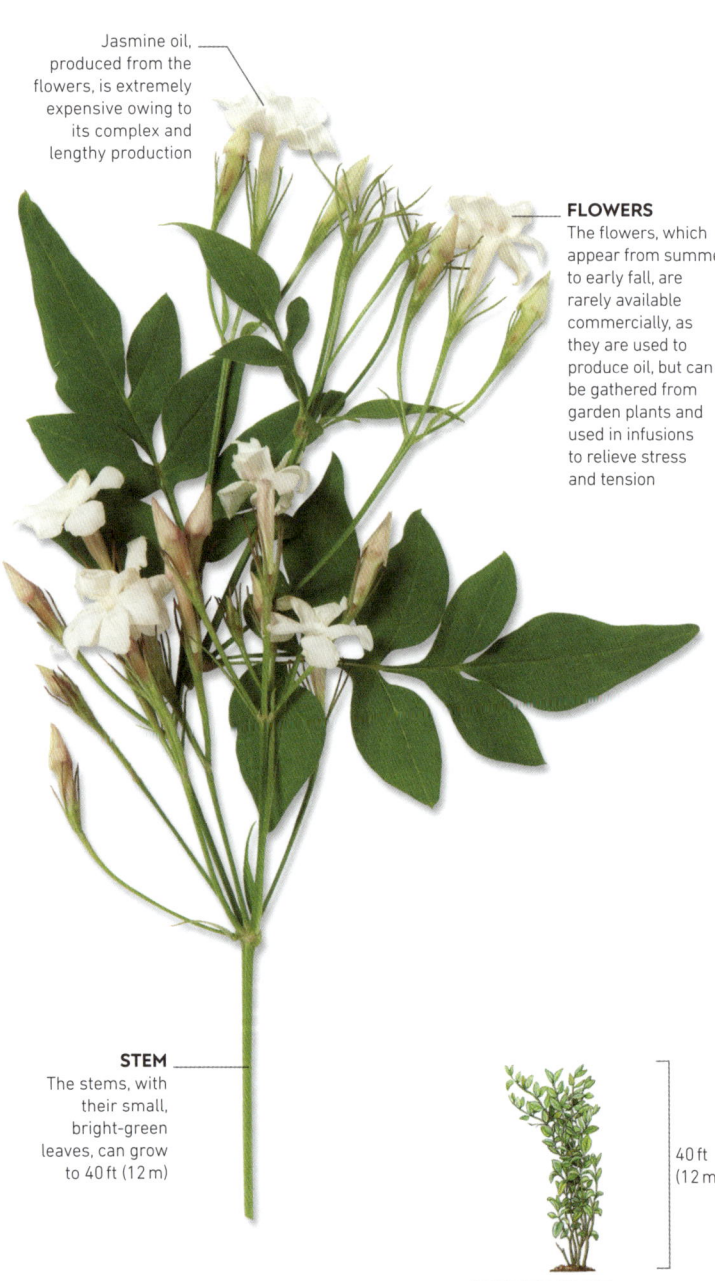

Jasmine oil, produced from the flowers, is extremely expensive owing to its complex and lengthy production

FLOWERS
The flowers, which appear from summer to early fall, are rarely available commercially, as they are used to produce oil, but can be gathered from garden plants and used in infusions to relieve stress and tension

STEM
The stems, with their small, bright-green leaves, can grow to 40 ft (12 m)

40 ft (12 m)

GROWTH HABIT
Woody stemmed deciduous climber with fragrant, white, star-shaped flowers.

Native to Himalayan regions, India, Pakistan, and parts of China, jasmine is widely grown as a garden ornamental and is also extensively cultivated for its essential oil, which is used mainly as a sedative and antidepressant. Its close relation, *Jasminum grandiflorum*, is known as *jati* in India and is considered an important spiritual tonic to emphasize love and compassion.

PARTS USED Flowers, essential oil
MAIN CONSTITUENTS Alkaloids (incl. jasminine), volatile oil (incl. benzyl alcohol, linalool, and linyl acetate), salicylic acid
ACTIONS Aphrodisiac, astringent, bitter, relaxing nervine, sedative, mild analgesic, galactagogue, antidepressant, antiseptic, antispasmodic, uterine tonic, encourages parturition

HOW TO USE

INFUSION Use 4–6 fresh flowers in 1 cup of boiling water, infuse for 5 minutes, and drink 2–3 times a day to relieve stress and tension, or for mild depression.
MASSAGE OIL Add 1–2 drops of essential oil to 1 tsp (5 ml) of almond oil for massage rubs to relieve anxiety, insomnia, or depression. Use 20 drops of essential oil in 1 fl oz (30ml) of almond oil to massage the abdomen during the first stages of labor. The same mixture can be used for period pains.
DIFFUSER Use 2–3 drops of essential oil in a diffuser to scent a bedroom for problems with impotence; a mutual massage between partners using 1–2 drops of jasmine oil in 1 tsp (5 ml) of almond oil before lovemaking can help.

HOW TO SOURCE

GROW Prefers fertile, well-drained soil in a sun or partial shade. Prune after flowering if necessary. Usually grown from semi-ripe cuttings in summer, although established plants will frequently self-seed.
FORAGE Rarely found in the wild outside its native area, although cultivated commercially worldwide.
HARVEST The flowers are traditionally gathered in the evening when their scent is greatest while in full bloom.

CAUTION Avoid during pregnancy or while breastfeeding.

Juniperus communis
JUNIPER

Native to Europe, North America, and many parts of Asia, juniper has long been associated with ritual cleansing and has been burned in various temples throughout history. Today the herb is mainly used as remedy for urinary disorders, while its essential oil is included in various massage rubs for muscle and joint pains.

PARTS USED Fruits, essential oil, cade oil
MAIN CONSTITUENTS Volatile oil (incl. myrcene and cineole), flavonoids, sugars, glycosides, tannins, vitamin C
ACTIONS Urinary antiseptic, diuretic, carminative, digestive tonic, emmenagogue, antirheumatic

HOW TO USE

TINCTURE Take 20–40 drops (1–2 ml) in a little water 3 times daily for urinary tract problems including cystitis, or to stimulate the digestion and ease flatulence.
INFUSION Infuse ½ oz (15 g) of crushed berries in 1 pint (600 ml) of boiling water for 30 minutes and take ½–1 cup 3 times daily for gastric upsets, stomach chills, or period pains. The infusion can also be sipped during the first stages of labor.
MASSAGE OIL Use 10 drops of juniper essential oil in 2 tsp (10 ml) of almond oil as a massage for arthritic pains.
HAIR RINSE Use 10 drops of cade oil in 1 tbsp almond oil, add to 1 pint (600 ml) of hot water, mix well, and apply for psoriasis affecting the scalp. Leave for 15 minutes or longer, and rinse thoroughly.

HOW TO SOURCE

GROW Tolerates almost all conditions including both acid and alkaline soils, sun and partial shade or exposed positions, but dislikes water-logged soil. Usually grown from seed sown in a propagator in fall or spring or by heeled cuttings in fall. Grow until the plants are well established and can be moved to their final positions.
FORAGE Found on moors, heaths, conifer woods, and shrubland in temperate regions throughout the northern hemisphere.
HARVEST Collect the "berries"—actually small cones—by shaking the branches over a ground cloth to dislodge them.

CAUTION Avoid during pregnancy. May irritate the kidneys after long-term use, so do not take for more than six weeks internally without a break or if there is already kidney damage.

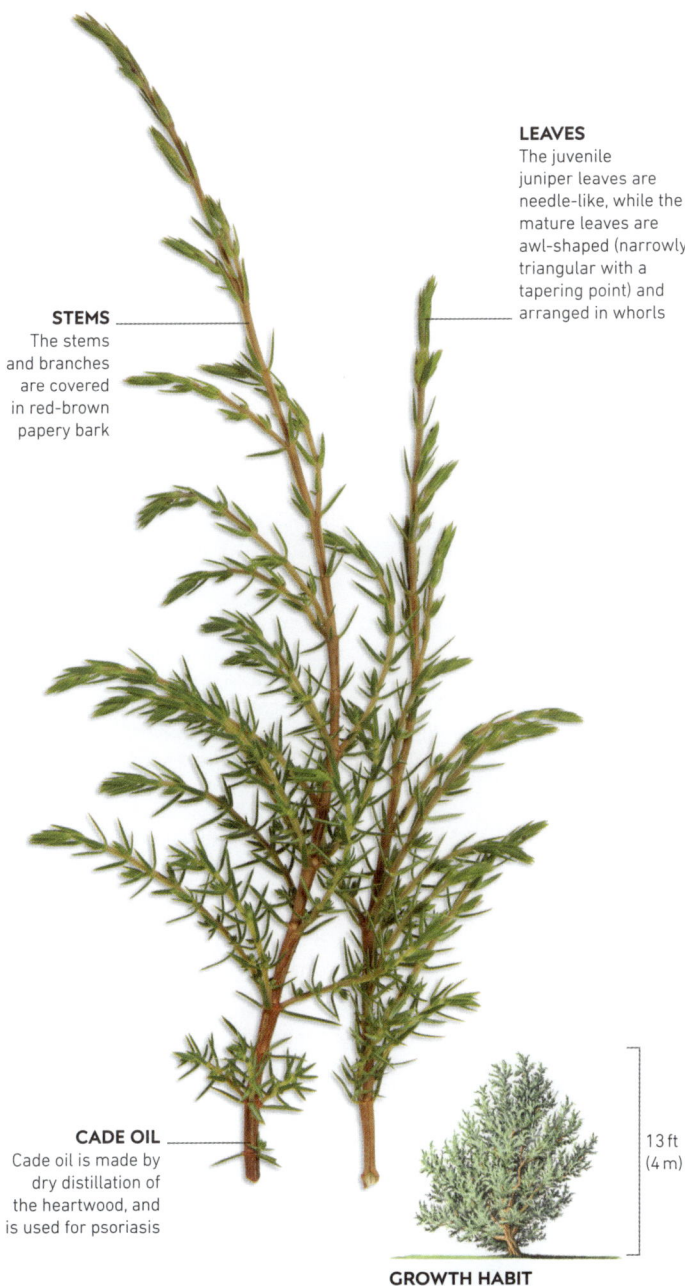

LEAVES
The juvenile juniper leaves are needle-like, while the mature leaves are awl-shaped (narrowly triangular with a tapering point) and arranged in whorls

STEMS
The stems and branches are covered in red-brown papery bark

CADE OIL
Cade oil is made by dry distillation of the heartwood, and is used for psoriasis

GROWTH HABIT
An upright shrub with a spread of 5 ft (1.5 m). Its fruits take two years to ripen.

13 ft (4 m)

Lavandula angustifolia
LAVENDER

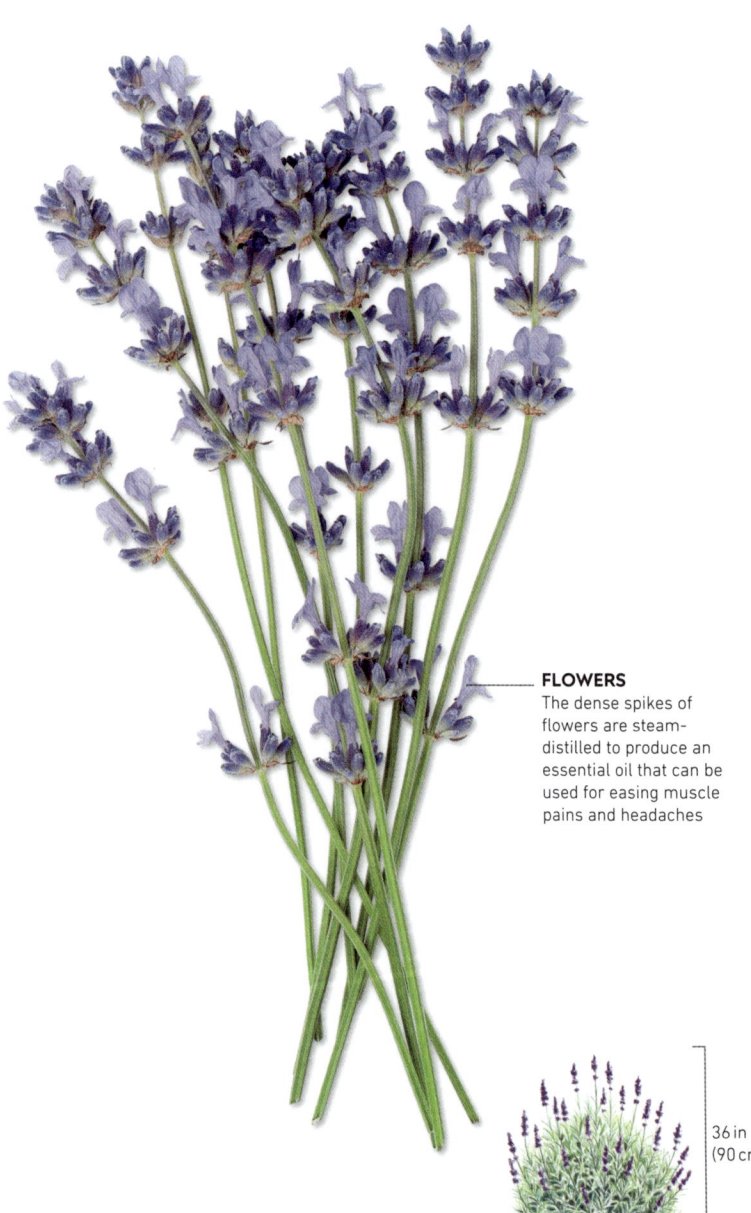

FLOWERS
The dense spikes of flowers are steam-distilled to produce an essential oil that can be used for easing muscle pains and headaches

36 in (90 cm)

GROWTH HABIT
Compact, bushy evergreen shrub with a spread of 36 in (90 cm).

Lavender takes it name from the Latin *lavare* (to wash), and has been used to scent bath oils and soaps for centuries. It originates in Mediterranean regions and is still closely associated with the perfume industry in southern France. The flowers are valued for their soothing and sedating properties, and the essential oil is used for muscle aches and respiratory problems.

PARTS USED Flowers, essential oil
MAIN CONSTITUENTS Volatile oil (mostly linalyl acetate and cineole), tannins, coumarins, flavonoids, triterpenoids
ACTIONS Relaxant, antispasmodic, tonic for the nervous system, circulatory stimulant, antibacterial, analgesic, carminative, cholagogue, antidepressant, anti-emetic

HOW TO USE

INFUSION Make an infusion of 1 cup of boiling water over 1–2 tsp flowers and drink 1 cup up to 3 times daily for nervous exhaustion or tension headaches. 1 cup before bedtime can also help with insomnia.
TINCTURE Take up to 1 tsp (5 ml) twice a day for headaches, depression, or nervous tension. Can also help ease asthma, especially where attacks are triggered by nervousness or stress.
MASSAGE OIL Dilute 40 drops (2 ml) of essential oil in 2 tsp (10 ml) carrier oil. Use for muscular pains, or rub into the temples and the nape of the neck for tension headaches or at the first sign of a migraine.
HAIR RINSE Dilute 20 drops (1 ml) of essential oil in a jug of water as a final hair rinse for head lice, and use a few drops of undiluted oil on a fine-toothed comb run through the hair to remove both lice and nits.
ESSENTIAL OIL Use undiluted on insect bites or stings, or add 10 drops to 1¾fl oz (50 ml) of water to use as a lotion for sunburn. Add 3–4 drops to a tissue and place on the pillow to aid sleep.

HOW TO SOURCE

GROW Prefers well-drained, moderately fertile soil in full sun. Germination from seed can be erratic; alternatively, take semi-ripe cuttings in summer.
FORAGE Native to dry, rocky regions in the Mediterranean and southwest Asia; may grow wild in other areas.
HARVEST Flowers are usually harvested in the mornings on sunny days in summer.

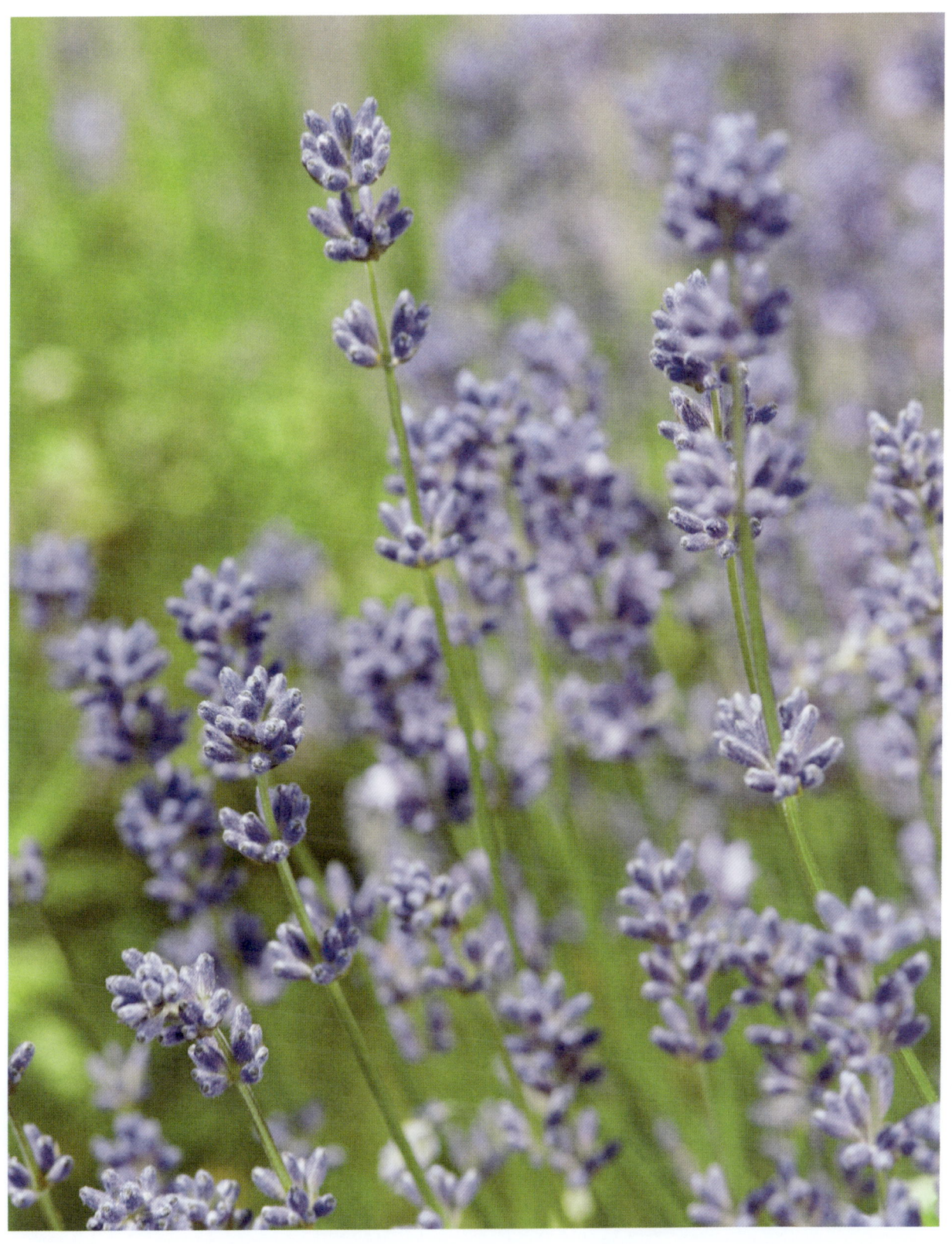

Leonurus cardiaca
MOTHERWORT

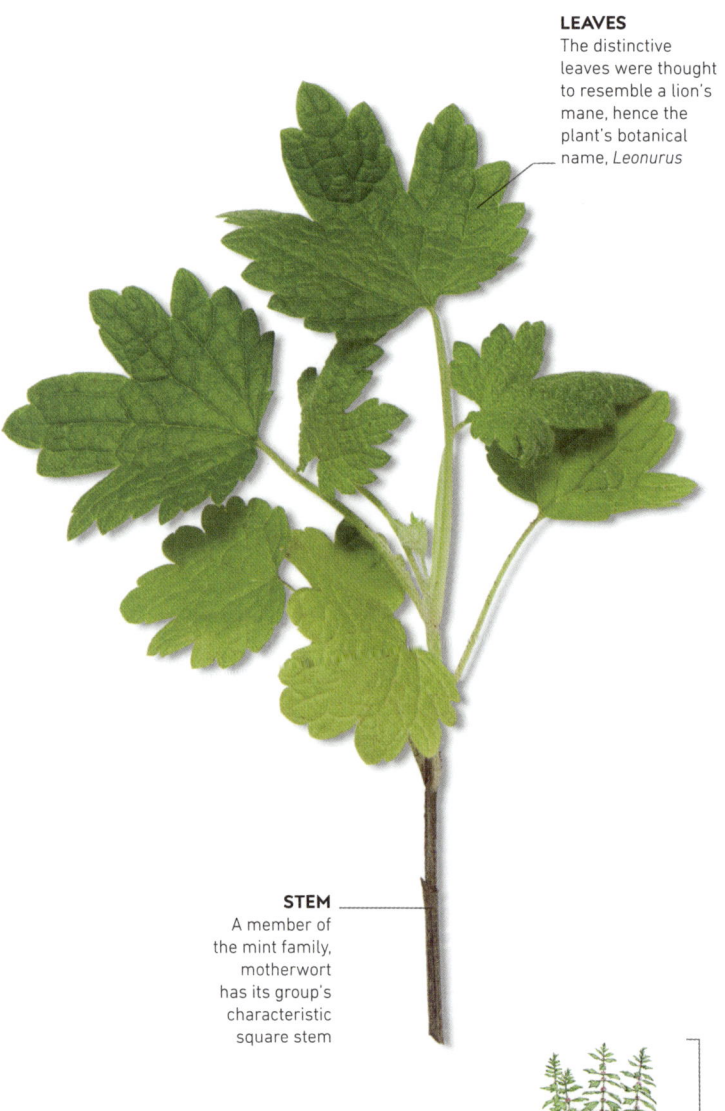

LEAVES
The distinctive leaves were thought to resemble a lion's mane, hence the plant's botanical name, *Leonurus*

STEM
A member of the mint family, motherwort has its group's characteristic square stem

GROWTH HABIT
Upright perennial with purple stems; spread 24 in (60 cm).

4 ft (1.2 m)

As its name suggests, motherwort has a long tradition as a woman's herb and was used both to calm the mother in childbirth and encourage contractions. Native to much of Europe, the plant has striking foliage and is sometimes grown as a garden ornamental. It is also used in treating heart conditions and it is commonly given for palpitations and to improve heart function.

PARTS USED Aerial parts
MAIN CONSTITUENTS Alkaloids (incl. stachydrine), iridoid (leonurine), flavonoids, diterpenes, volatile oil, tannins, vitamin A
ACTIONS Uterine stimulant, relaxant, cardiac tonic, carminative, antispasmodic, hypotensive, diaphoretic

HOW TO USE

INFUSION Drink 1 cup (1–2 tsp dry herb per cup boiling water) 3 times daily for anxiety, menopausal problems, or heart weakness. Sip the tea flavored with cloves (*Syzygium aromaticum*) during labor and after childbirth to help restore the womb and reduce the risk of bleeding. Combine with lemon balm and lime flowers and use 2–4 tsp per cup to relieve symptoms of angina pectoris.
TINCTURE Take 1 tsp (5 ml) 3 times daily for palpitations, menopausal problems such as hot flashes and emotional instability, rapid heartbeat, or PMS.
CAPSULES/POWDER Use as an alternative to the bitter infusion. Blend 1 level tsp of powdered herb with 1 tsp of honey, or take 2 x 500 mg capsules, 2–3 times daily.

HOW TO SOURCE

GROW Prefers moist but well-drained soil in sun or partial shade. Sow seeds in a cold frame in spring and transplant to their final position when the seedlings are well-established; allow 18 in (45 cm) between plants. Alternatively, propagate by division in spring or fall. It can self-seed enthusiastically and become invasive.
FORAGE May be found growing on waste ground, at woodland edges, or by roadsides across Europe. Avoid plants from busy roadsides to minimize pollutants.
HARVEST Gather in summer while the plant is flowering.

CAUTION A uterine stimulant, so avoid in pregnancy (except during labor) and heavy menstruation. Seek professional advice for all heart conditions.

Levisticum officinale
LOVAGE

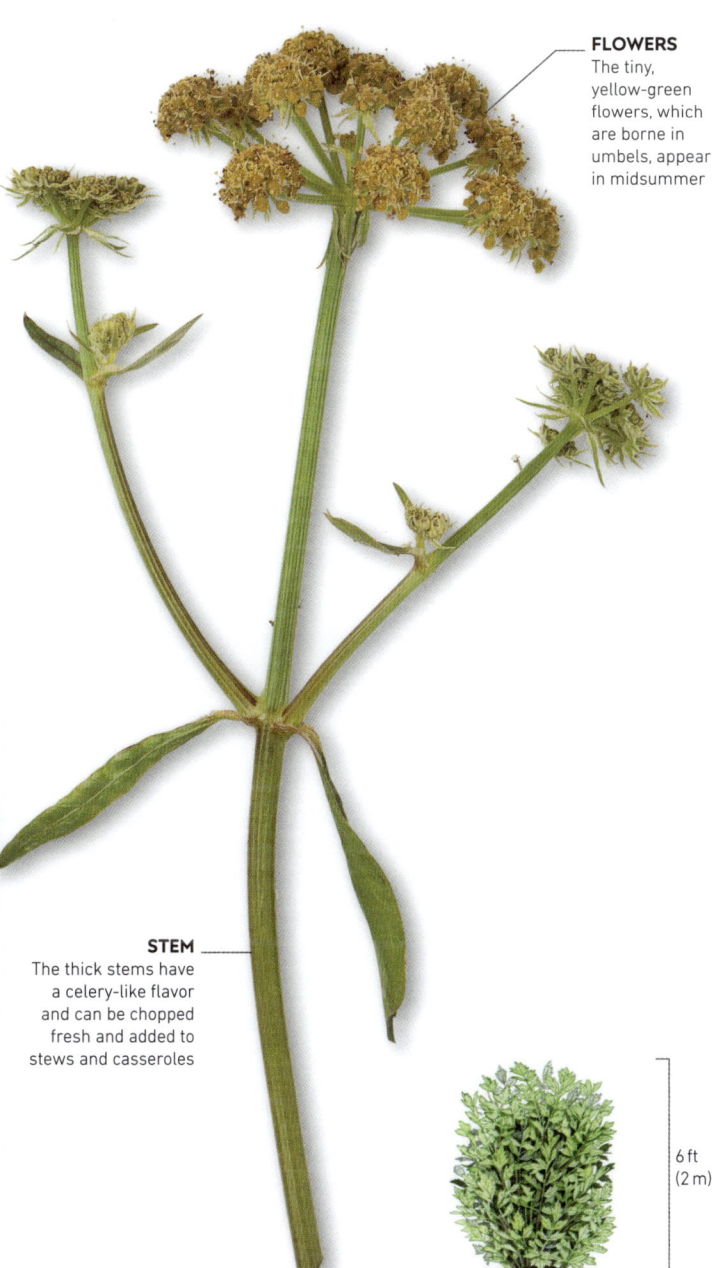

FLOWERS
The tiny, yellow-green flowers, which are borne in umbels, appear in midsummer

STEM
The thick stems have a celery-like flavor and can be chopped fresh and added to stews and casseroles

6 ft (2 m)

GROWTH HABIT
Perennial with triangular divided leaves and tiny yellow flowers; spread 36 in (90 cm).

Traditionally associated with love potions and aphrodisiacs, lovage was originally called *luveshe* (Old French) or "loveache." It originates in the eastern Mediterranean, although it is now widely naturalized. A culinary herb used in stock cubes, lovage is also used for treating various digestive, respiratory, and urinary problems, and is generally warming for the circulation.

PARTS USED Root, leaves, seeds
MAIN CONSTITUENTS Volatile oil (mostly phthalides), coumarins (incl. bergapten), beta-sitosterol, resins, and gums
ACTIONS Mild antibiotic, anticatarrhal, antispasmodic, diaphoretic, expectorant, sedative, carminative, mild diuretic, emmenagogue

HOW TO USE
DECOCTION Add ½oz (15 g) of the root to 1½ pints (900 ml) of water and simmer to reduce the volume by one third. Take ½–1 cup up to 3 times daily for indigestion, cystitis, rheumatism, gout, poor appetite, or painful menstruation. Combines well with an equal amount of agrimony infusion for indigestion.
TINCTURE Take 20–60 drops (1–3 ml) of the root tincture in warm water 3 times daily for indigestion, poor appetite, urinary tract problems, or period pain. Take every 2 hours for colic.
GARGLE Use 1 cup of the root decoction as a mouthwash for mouth ulcers or as a gargle for tonsillitis.
SEEDS Chew 2–3 seeds to relieve flatulence and indigestion.
FRESH LEAVES AND STEMS Chop and add to casseroles to flavor the stock.

HOW TO SOURCE
GROW Prefers fertile, moist, well-drained soil in full sun and an open position; tolerates other conditions. Sow seeds when ripe in early fall and transplant into position when large enough, or propagate by dividing established plants in spring.
FORAGE Sometimes found growing wild; harvest the leaves and seeds to use in cooking throughout the growing period. Lovage shoots appear early in the year, so can be useful when little else is available.
HARVEST Gather leaves through spring and early summer, seeds in late summer or fall, and the root in late fall.

CAUTION Avoid during pregnancy. The foliage can irritate skin.

Linum perenne
PERENNIAL FLAX

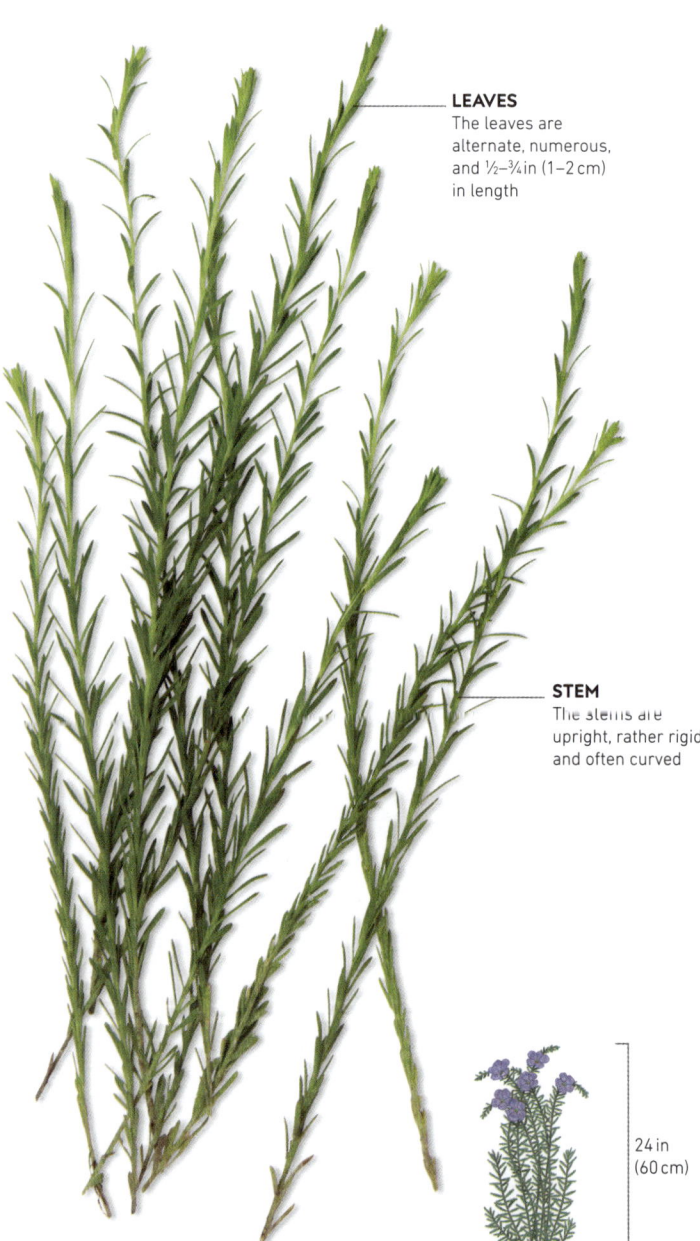

LEAVES
The leaves are alternate, numerous, and ½–¾ in (1–2 cm) in length

STEM
The stems are upright, rather rigid, and often curved

24 in (60 cm)

GROWTH HABIT
Herbaceous perennial with narrow, lance-shaped leaves and pale blue flowers.

Perennial flax is very similar to a related species, common flax or linseed (*Linum usitatissimum*), which is the more commonly cultivated form. Both are native to Europe, although linseed also grows from the Mediterranean to India. The seeds of perennial flax are used much like linseed, although—unlike common flax—the fresh aerial parts are also a traditional remedy.

PARTS USED Aerial parts, seeds, seed oil
MAIN CONSTITUENTS Mucilage; linoleic acid; cyanogenic glycosides; bitter principle; fixed oil incl. linolenic acid; vitamins A, B, D, and E; minerals; and amino acids
ACTIONS Antirheumatic, diuretic, anti-inflammatory, demulcent, soothing antitussive, antiseptic, laxative

HOW TO USE

INFUSION Add 2 oz (60 g) of fresh chopped aerial parts to 2 cups of boiling water and take 1 cup 3 times daily for colds.
POULTICE The seeds can be used as linseeds: crush or pulp in a blender or food processor, spread on gauze, and apply to boils, abscesses, or skin ulcers.
CRUSHED SEEDS Crush 1 oz (30 g) in a pestle and mortar or food processor and mix with yogurt as a dietary supplement providing essential fatty acids to support treatments for eczema, menstrual disorders, rheumatoid arthritis, or atherosclerosis.
SEEDS For constipation, mix 1–2 tsp of dried seeds with muesli, oatmeal, or yogurt and eat at breakfast. Then drink 1 cup of water or fruit juice.

HOW TO SOURCE

GROW Prefers well-drained light or sandy soil in full sun. Sow seeds in trays in early spring in a cold frame and transplant out after the last frosts; alternatively, sow seeds directly in spring after all danger of frost is past, or in late summer, and cover with a light dusting of topsoil. Transplant out, leaving 10 in (25 cm) between plants.
FORAGE Commonly found at higher altitudes (the Alps, for instance) and northern regions. Only collect seeds from sustainable populations. Collect the aerial parts while flowering in summer for use in infusions.
HARVEST Gather seeds in summer and aerial parts through the growing season.

CAUTION The seeds contain traces of prussic acid (which are potentially toxic in large quantities). Do not exceed stated dosages.

Lycium barbarum
GOJI

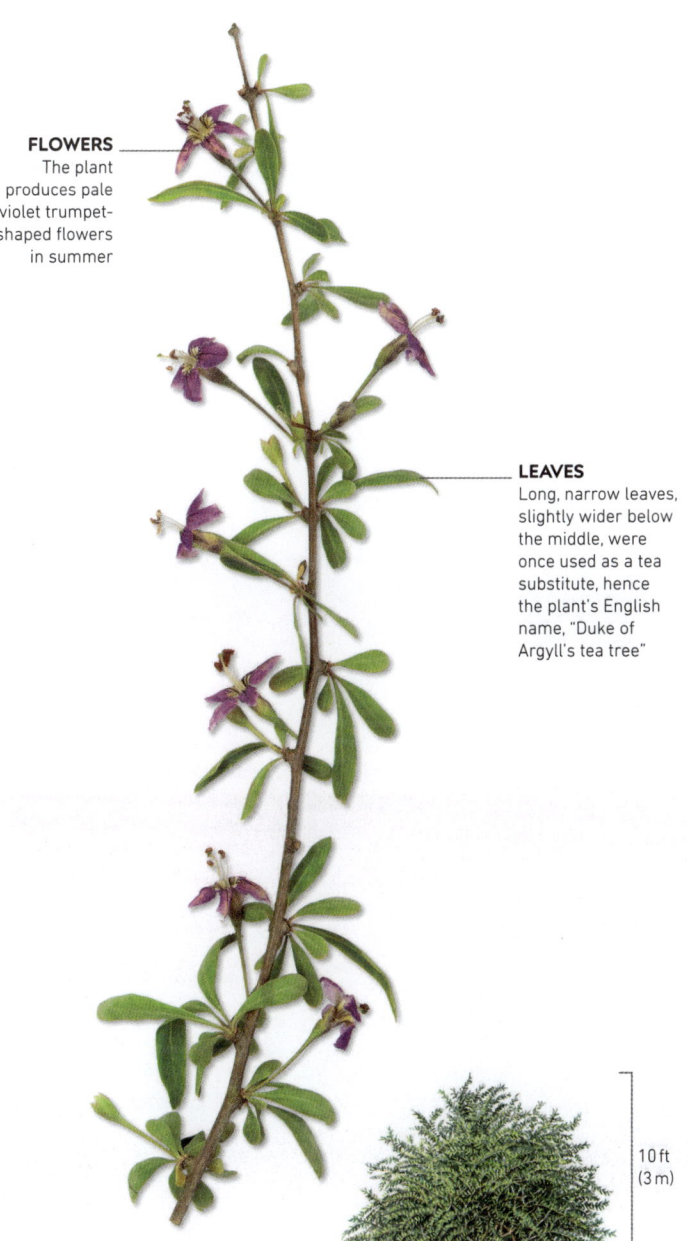

FLOWERS
The plant produces pale violet trumpet-shaped flowers in summer

LEAVES
Long, narrow leaves, slightly wider below the middle, were once used as a tea substitute, hence the plant's English name, "Duke of Argyll's tea tree"

10 ft (3 m)

GROWTH HABIT
Fast-growing deciduous woody shrub with thorny, arching stems, spread 6 ft (2 m); red berries in fall.

Native to China, goji—variously known as wolfberry, matrimony vine, or Chinese boxthorn—is used as a hedge shrub. Both the root bark and berries have been used in China for more than 2,000 years as remedies for various problems associated with weakened liver or kidney energy, including impotence and eye disorders.

PARTS USED Fruit
MAIN CONSTITUENTS Fruit: vitamins, minerals, amino acids, essential fatty acids. Bark: alkaloids, saponins, tannins
ACTIONS Hypotensive, hypoglycemic, hypolipidemic, immune stimulant, liver tonic and restorative

HOW TO USE

FRESH BERRIES Add up to 1 oz (30 g) to breakfast cereal or yogurt to increase vitamin and mineral intake, enhance energy and well-being, or stimulate the immune system.
DRIED BERRIES Add up to 1 oz (30 g) to soups and stews, or add to cakes and desserts as alternatives to blueberries.
TINCTURE Take 20–40 drops (1–2 ml) up to 3 times daily as a general energy tonic.
PATENT CHINESE REMEDIES Various products such as *qi ju di huang wan* (pills that include lycium and chrysanthemum) are used as a tonic for blood and yin energy, but are best prescribed by professional practitioners.

HOW TO SOURCE

GROW Prefers average soil in a sunny position and is drought tolerant. Sow fresh seeds ½ in (1 cm) deep in compost. Keep in a warm place until germinated, and pot when the leaves develop. Pinch out the tops when 4 in (10 cm) high to ensure bushy growth. Will produce fruit from the second year.
FORAGE Introduced into Europe in the 18th century, it can sometimes be found naturalized in hedges.
HARVEST Gather berries in fall. They discolor if touched by hand, so shake them into a cloth.

CAUTION Avoid therapeutic doses in pregnancy—small doses in cooking are perfectly safe. Avoid during colds or flu, if suffering from diarrhea, and/or if digestion is poor. Ensure that your supplies are of good quality.

Matricaria recutita
GERMAN CHAMOMILE

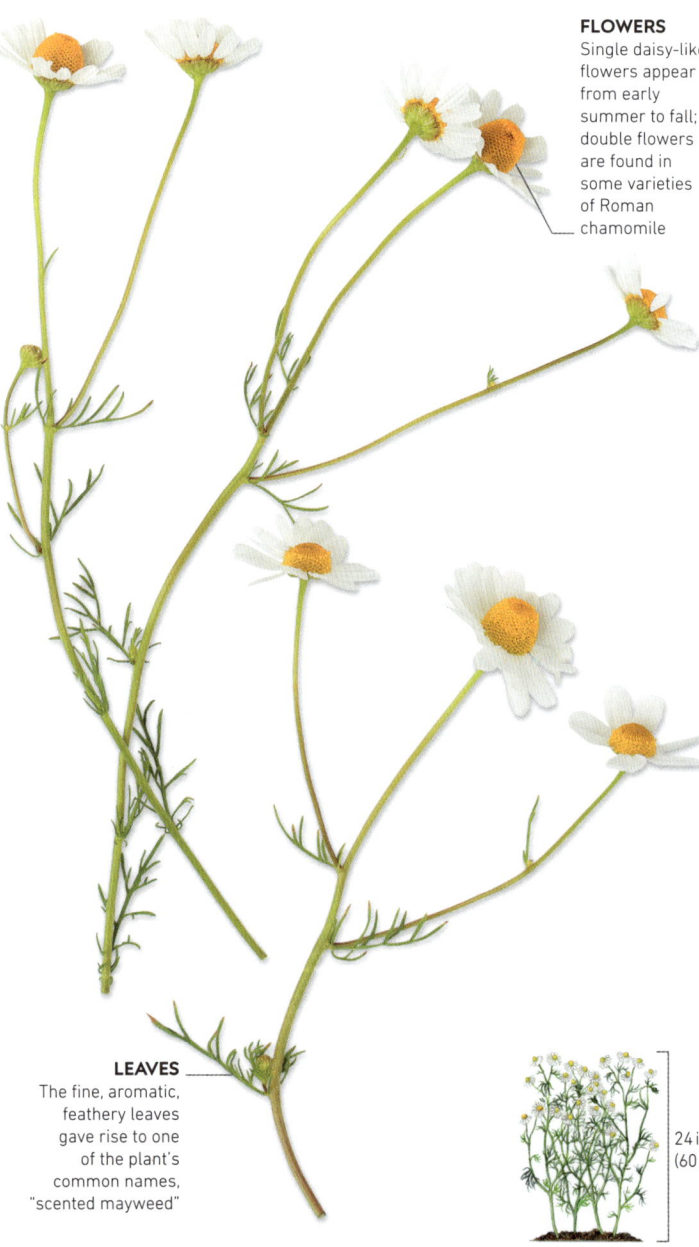

FLOWERS
Single daisy-like flowers appear from early summer to fall; double flowers are found in some varieties of Roman chamomile

LEAVES
The fine, aromatic, feathery leaves gave rise to one of the plant's common names, "scented mayweed"

GROWTH HABIT
Upright and branched; spread 4–15 in (10–38 cm).

24 in (60 cm)

Also known as scented mayweed, German chamomile's apple-scented fragrance is familiar to herbal tea drinkers, and is used both for digestive disorders and nervous problems and as an ingredient in anti-inflammatory creams and ointments. Its close relation, Roman chamomile (*Chamaemelum nobile*), is used in similar ways. It is native to Europe, western Asia, and India.

PARTS USED Flowers, essential oil
MAIN CONSTITUENTS Volatile oil (incl. proazulenes), flavonoids (incl. rutin), valeric acid, coumarins, tannins, salicylates, cyanogenic glycosides
ACTIONS Anti-inflammatory, nervine antispasmodic, bitter, sedative, tonic, anti-emetic, carminative, anti-allergenic

HOW TO USE

INFUSION Pour 1 cup boiling water over 2 tsp of flowers and leaves and take for mild digestive problems or insomnia. German chamomile is a gentle herb that is suitable for children at reduced doses.
STEAM INHALATION Add 2 tsp of flowers or 5 drops of essential oil to a basin of boiling water for hay fever or mild asthma.
TINCTURE Take 2 tsp (10 ml) of the flower tincture 3 times daily for irritable bowel syndrome or nervous tension.
BATHS Add 4–5 drops of essential oil to the bath to heal wounds or soothe the skin. Add 1 cup of strained infusion to a baby's bath at night to encourage sleep.
CREAM/OINTMENT/LOTION Use on insect bites, wounds, or eczema.
MOUTHWASH/GARGLE Use 2 tsp (10 ml) of tincture in a glass of warm water, or 1 cup of standard infusion for gum disease and mouth inflammations or as a gargle for sore throats.

HOW TO SOURCE

GROW Prefers well-drained, neutral to slightly acid soil, and a sunny site. Sow seeds where you want them to grow in fall or spring. It self-seeds freely.
FORAGE Found growing in Europe, western Asia, and India. Easily confused with other daisies, so be familiar with its distinctive smell before gathering.
HARVEST Gather flowers in summer.

CAUTION Can cause contact dermatitis. Avoid if you are allergic to the Compositae family.

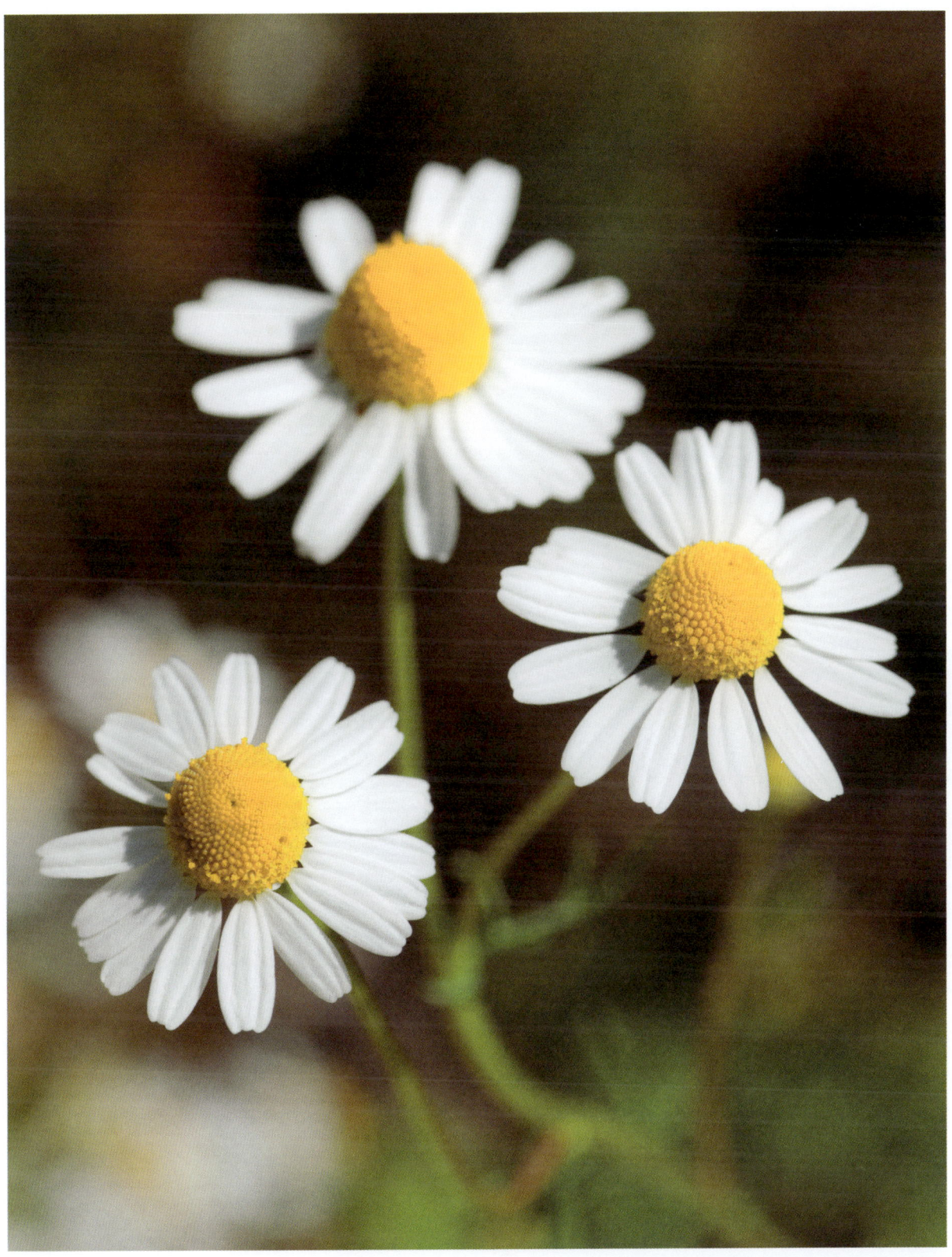

Medicago sativa
ALFALFA

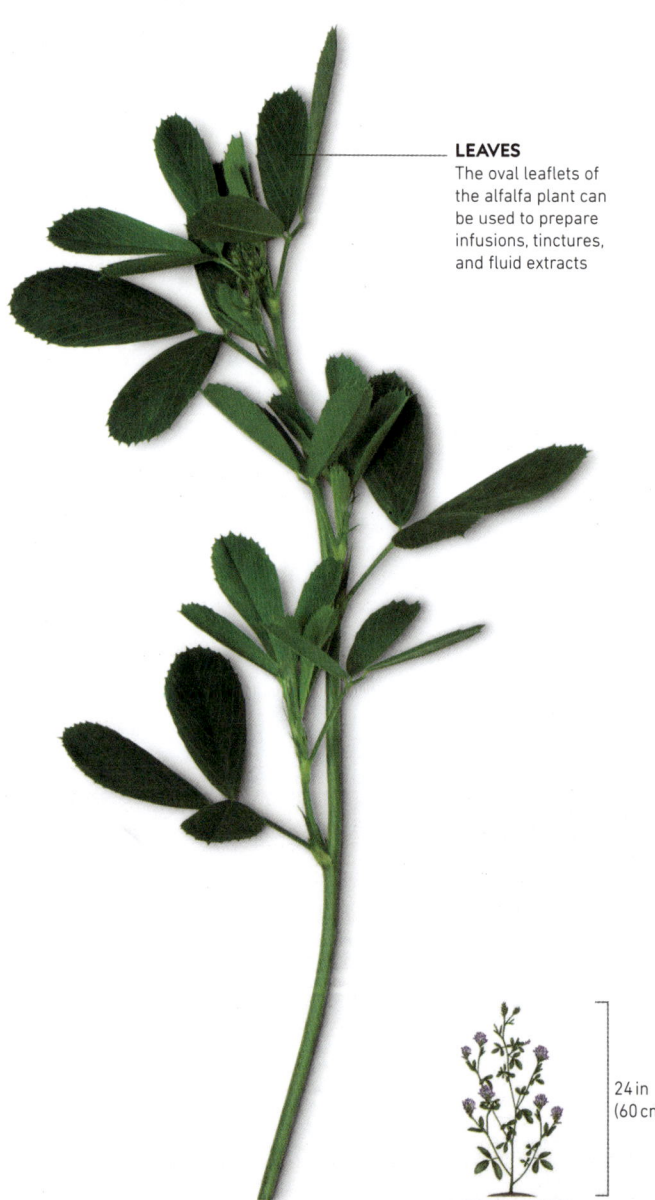

LEAVES
The oval leaflets of the alfalfa plant can be used to prepare infusions, tinctures, and fluid extracts

GROWTH HABIT
Hardy perennial with trifoliate leaves about ¾in (2 cm) wide with a folded margin; the blue flowers appear in dense racemes.

24 in
(60 cm)

Originating in South and Central Asia, alfalfa has long been grown as a feed for livestock. In Arabic, "alfalfa" means "father of all foods." High in vitamins and minerals, it has a reputation for increasing fertility, improving milk supply, and reducing menopausal symptoms. Alfalfa has also been shown to lower cholesterol and sugar levels, so can be helpful when treating type 2 diabetes.

PARTS USED Leaves, sprouted seeds
MAIN CONSTITUENTS Coumarins, saponins, isoflavonoids, phytosterols, phytoestrogens, alkaloids
ACTIONS Galactagogue, oestrogenic, hypolipidemic, hypoglycemic

HOW TO USE

INFUSION Take 1 cup of a standard infusion (p.176) of the leaves 3 times daily to increase milk production and strength in breastfeeding mothers.
TINCTURE Take 40 drops–1 tsp (2–5 ml) 3 times daily to improve menopausal symptoms.
FLUID EXTRACT Prepare a 1:1 fluid extract and take 1–2 tsp (5–10 ml) 3 times daily as a general energy tonic or as a preventative measure to reduce cholesterol levels. It can be useful in the control of late-onset diabetes where treatment is focused on diet rather than medication.
SPROUTED SEEDS Place 2 tbsp of alfalfa seeds in a jar, cover with water, and leave overnight. Drain the water and leave the seeds in a light place to sprout, washing them every day until they are the size you prefer. Fresh alfalfa sprouts are high in magnesium-rich chlorophyll, and can aid detoxification, gut health, and support the immune system. They make a crunchy addition to salads.

HOW TO SOURCE

GROW The plant is intensively grown as food for cattle and as green manure to improve soil, and it can also be grown as a houseplant. It will grow in all types of soil but prefers sandy, clay loam, or silt loam soil.
FORAGE Alfalfa can often be found near cultivated fields, where it is used to fix nitrogen in the soil. It recovers quickly from being cut back.
HARVEST The aerial parts of the plant are harvested in spring to late summer. As it grows back quickly, it can be harvested 4 times a year.

CAUTION Avoid during pregnancy, if you have an autoimmune disorder, or when taking blood-thinning medication.

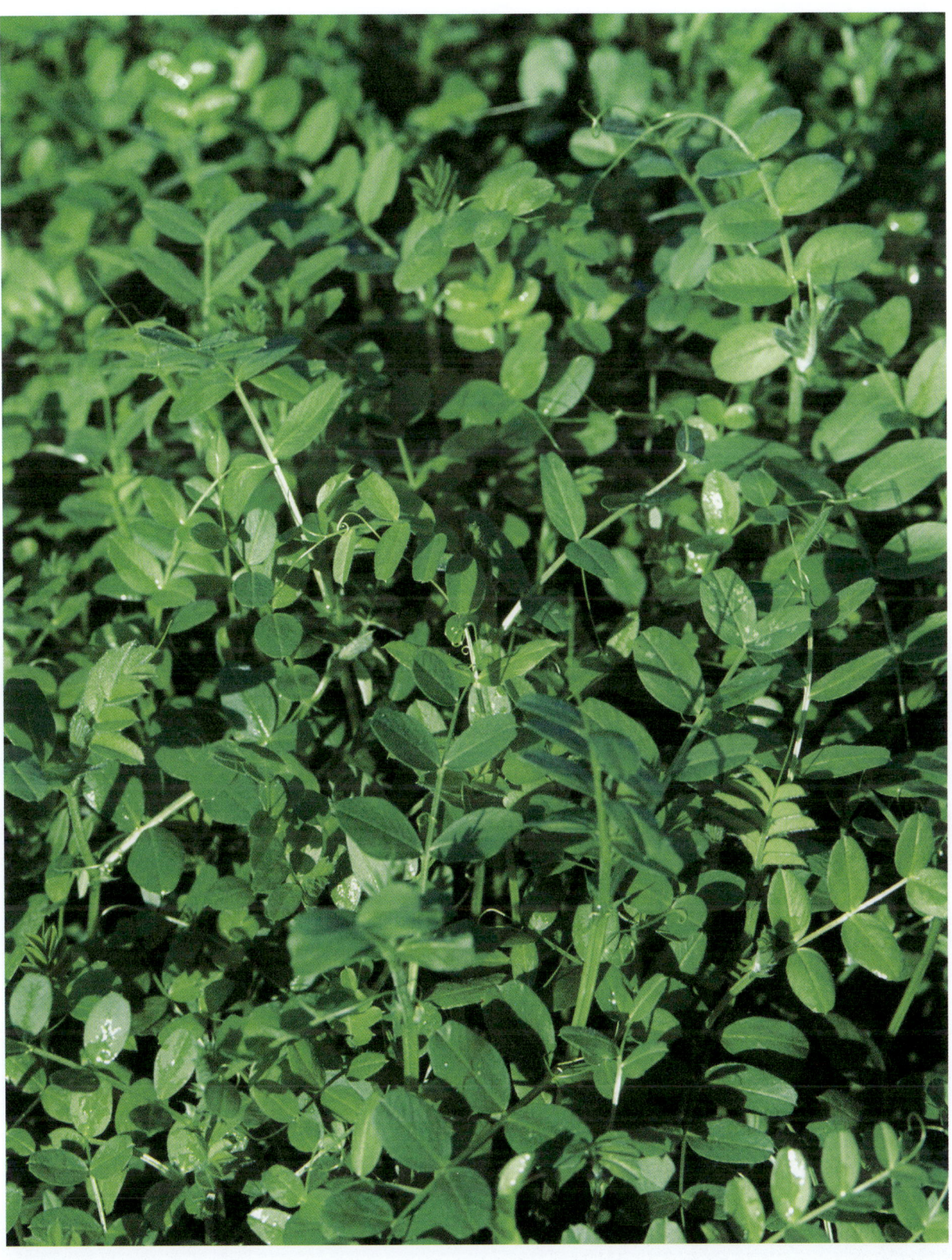

Melilotus officinalis
MELILOT

Also known as king's clover, melilot is native to Europe, north Africa, and temperate regions of Asia, and is widely cultivated as a fodder crop for silage. Today it is largely used for problems associated with venous circulation, including thrombosis and varicose veins, although in the past it was a popular remedy for indigestion, bronchitis, and insomnia in children.

PARTS USED Aerial parts
MAIN CONSTITUENTS Flavonoids, coumarins, resin, tannins, volatile oil; dicoumarol (an anti-coagulant) is produced as the plant ages and rots
ACTIONS Antispasmodic, anti-inflammatory, diuretic, expectorant, sedative, styptic, mild analgesic

HOW TO USE

INFUSION Drink ½–1 cup (1–2 tsp aerial parts per cup boiling water) up to 3 times daily for varicose veins, lymphatic swellings, hemorrhoids, anxiety, menopausal disorders, insomnia, or to reduce the risk of thrombosis. Can be used for insomnia in children; consult an herbalist for advice on children's dosage.
CREAM Combine with an equal amount of calendula cream and apply 3–4 times daily for varicose eczema.
OINTMENT Use several times daily for hemorrhoids.
COMPRESS Apply a pad soaked in 1 cup of infusion for facial or intercostal neuralgia.
EYE BATH Simmer 1 cup of well-strained infusion (above) gently for 2–3 minutes to sterilize the mix; allow to cool thoroughly, and use as an eye bath for conjunctivitis.

HOW TO SOURCE

GROW Prefers sun and well-drained neutral to alkaline soil; tolerates other conditions. Sow seeds in spring or summer where you want to grow them, then thin out to 24 in (60 cm) apart. Self-seeds in ideal conditions.
FORAGE Found in meadow borders, dry waste ground, and hedges. Collect the whole plant in late spring or early summer and use fresh, or dry immediately while still flowering. Collect the flowers separately to use in cold macerated oils.
HARVEST Gather while flowering in late spring or early summer.

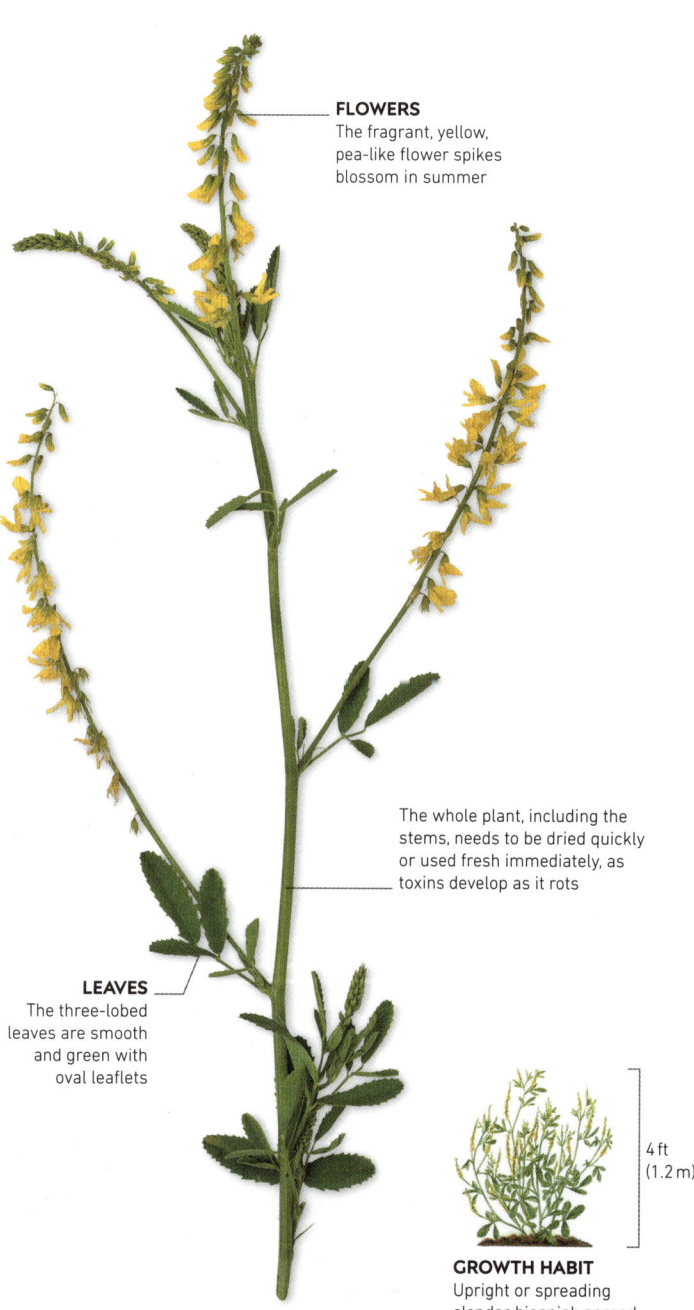

FLOWERS
The fragrant, yellow, pea-like flower spikes blossom in summer

The whole plant, including the stems, needs to be dried quickly or used fresh immediately, as toxins develop as it rots

LEAVES
The three-lobed leaves are smooth and green with oval leaflets

4 ft
(1.2 m)

GROWTH HABIT
Upright or spreading slender biennial; spread 8–36 in (20–90 cm).

CAUTION Do not take if on anticoagulant medication (such as warfarin or heparin); can be emetic in large doses.

Melissa officinalis
LEMON BALM

A European native, also known as "bee balm," this herb takes its botanical name from the Greek word for "honey bee" as it was regarded as being as healing and curative as honey. Both relaxing and toning for the nervous system, lemon balm is largely used today for anxiety, depression, nervous tension, and related digestive disorders.

PARTS USED Aerial parts, essential oil
MAIN CONSTITUENTS Volatile oil (incl. citronellal, linalool, and citral), polyphenols, tannins, bitter principle, flavonoids, rosmarinic acid
ACTIONS Sedative, antidepressant, digestive stimulant, peripheral vasodilator, diaphoretic, relaxing restorative for nervous system, carminative, antiviral, antibacterial

HOW TO USE

INFUSION Drink 1 cup (2–3 tsp fresh or dried leaves per cup boiling water) 3 times daily for depression, nervous exhaustion, indigestion or nausea; use a dilute infusion for children suffering from chicken pox.
CREAM/OINTMENT Use on sores, cold sores, poorly healing wounds, or insect bites.
LOTION Add 20 drops (1 ml) of essential oil to 3½ fl oz (100 ml) of water in a spray bottle and spray on skin to repel biting insects.
TINCTURE Take 10–20 drops in water 3–5 times daily for depression, tension headaches, and anxiety. Best made from fresh leaves.
MASSAGE OIL Add 5–6 drops of essential oil to 1 tbsp (15 ml) of almond oil and use as a massage for depression, tension, asthma, and bronchitis, or dab on cold sores at the first sign of symptoms.

HOW TO SOURCE

GROW Prefers moist, well-drained soil, but thrives in poor soil and tolerates full sun or shade. Sow seeds in a cold frame in spring and transplant when well established, or divide roots in spring when growth starts to appear in fall. Self-seeds, but can be invasive. Less vigorous variegated or golden cultivars are an alternative option.
FORAGE Grows in shrubby, partially shaded areas across Europe, or as cultivated plants that have self-seeded elsewhere.
HARVEST Gather the aerial parts just before the flowers open in summer, and the leaves throughout the growing period.

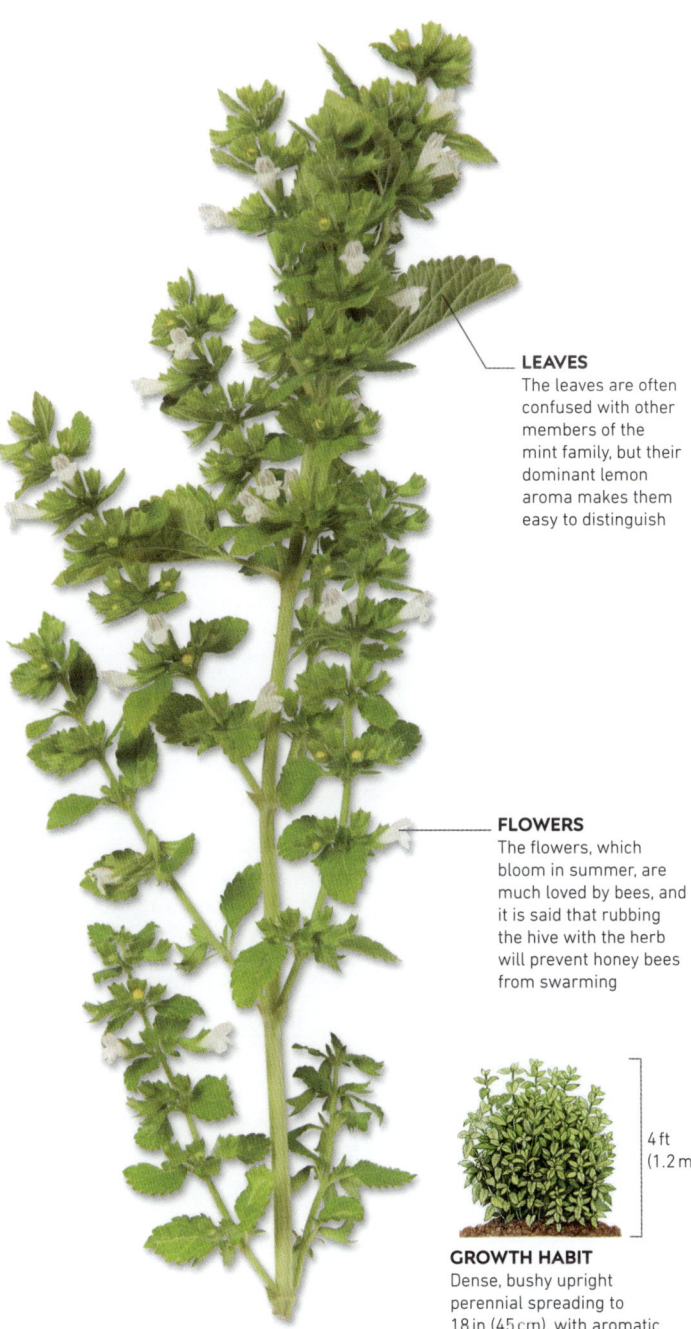

LEAVES
The leaves are often confused with other members of the mint family, but their dominant lemon aroma makes them easy to distinguish

FLOWERS
The flowers, which bloom in summer, are much loved by bees, and it is said that rubbing the hive with the herb will prevent honey bees from swarming

4 ft
(1.2 m)

GROWTH HABIT
Dense, bushy upright perennial spreading to 18 in (45 cm), with aromatic lemon-scented leaves.

Mentha x piperita
PEPPERMINT

There are more than 25 different types of mint, many of which cross-pollinate readily to produce variable hybrids. Peppermint, which originates in Europe, was the result of one such cross, possibly in ancient times, and is now naturalized worldwide. It is widely cultivated for its oil, which is used in flavorings and to scent perfumes and toiletries.

PARTS USED Aerial parts, essential oil
MAIN CONSTITUENTS Volatile oil (mainly menthol), tannins, flavonoids (incl. luteolin), tocopherols, choline, bitter principle, triterpenes
ACTIONS Antispasmodic, digestive tonic, anti-emetic, carminative, peripheral vasodilator, diaphoretic, cholagogue, analgesic, antiseptic

HOW TO USE

TEA Add 2–3 fresh leaves to 1 cup of boiling water and infuse for 5 minutes for everyday drinking; especially suitable after meals.
STEAM INHALATION Add a few fresh sprigs to a basin of boiling water and use as an inhalant to ease nasal congestion.
INFUSION Use ½oz (15 g) to 2 cups of boiling water and take ½–1 cup 2–3 times daily for nausea, indigestion, flatulence, or colic, or with other herbs for colds or catarrh.
LOTION Add 30 drops of essential oil to ½ cup vegetable oil and massage into aching muscles and joints, or use for scabies or ringworm. Use in a spray bottle as a mosquito repellent or foot deodorant.

HOW TO SOURCE

GROW Prefers fertile, moist soil in full sun or partial shade. Can be invasive if growing conditions are ideal. Propagated by division in spring or fall or by tip cuttings in spring or summer; easy to root if the sprigs are kept standing in water for a few days. As a hybrid, it is sterile and produces no seeds. In general, mints should not be grown from seed, as they cross-pollinate readily and may not come true.
FORAGE Generally found in moist areas. Native to Europe and the Mediterranean area; classified as invasive in parts of North America. Collect the leaves for tea throughout the growing season.
HARVEST Cut aerial parts before flowering.

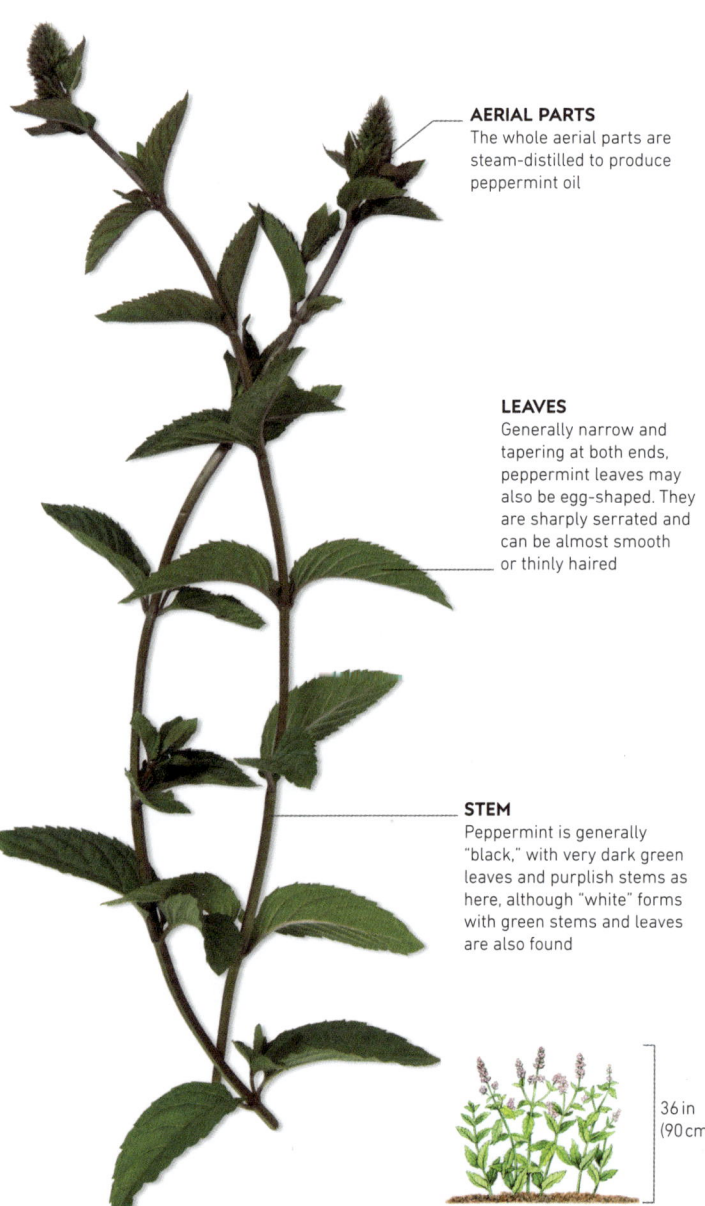

AERIAL PARTS
The whole aerial parts are steam-distilled to produce peppermint oil

LEAVES
Generally narrow and tapering at both ends, peppermint leaves may also be egg-shaped. They are sharply serrated and can be almost smooth or thinly haired

STEM
Peppermint is generally "black," with very dark green leaves and purplish stems as here, although "white" forms with green stems and leaves are also found

36 in (90 cm)

GROWTH HABIT
Herbaceous perennial with underground runners that can spread extensively.

CAUTION Do not use peppermint oil for children under the age of five.

Nepeta cataria
CATNIP

Also known as catmint, catnip—as the name implies—is much loved by cats, who will roll ecstatically in the young plants. Native to Europe and Mediterranean regions, but now naturalized in many parts of the world, the herb is used for digestive disorders or feverish chills. As a gentle remedy, it is also safe to use for many childhood disorders.

PARTS USED Aerial parts
MAIN CONSTITUENTS Volatile oil (incl. citronellol, geraniol, and nepetalactone), glycosides
ACTIONS Antispasmodic, antidiarrheal, emmenagogue, diaphoretic, carminative, nerve relaxant

HOW TO USE

INFUSION Drink 1 cup (2 tsp dry herb per cup boiling water) 3 times a day for colds, flu, stomach upsets, and indigestion. Reduce the dose, depending on age, for children and use for childhood illnesses, colic, or emotional upsets.
TINCTURE Take up to 1 tsp (5 ml) 3 times daily with the infusion for headaches associated with digestive disturbances. Use 1–2 tsp (5–10 ml) externally as a friction rub for rheumatism and arthritis.
ENEMA Use up to 1 quart (1 liter) of a well-strained standard infusion to clear toxic wastes from the colon.
OINTMENT Apply 2–3 times daily for hemorrhoids.

HOW TO SOURCE

GROW Prefers moist but well-drained soil in full sun. Sow the seeds in fall in trays of compost in a cold frame and transplant to 3 in (7.5 cm) pots when large enough to handle. Plant in early summer in their final growing positions. Alternatively, propagate by root division in fall or spring or take cuttings in spring or early summer. Self-seeds in favorable conditions, especially in gardens where there are no cats. Said to repel aphids, cucumber beetles, and other pests in companion planting.
FORAGE Found in shrubby, waste ground and wayside places in many parts of Europe and Asia, and now naturalized in North America. Collect the aerial parts in summer.
HARVEST Cut the aerial parts just as the plant is starting to flower.

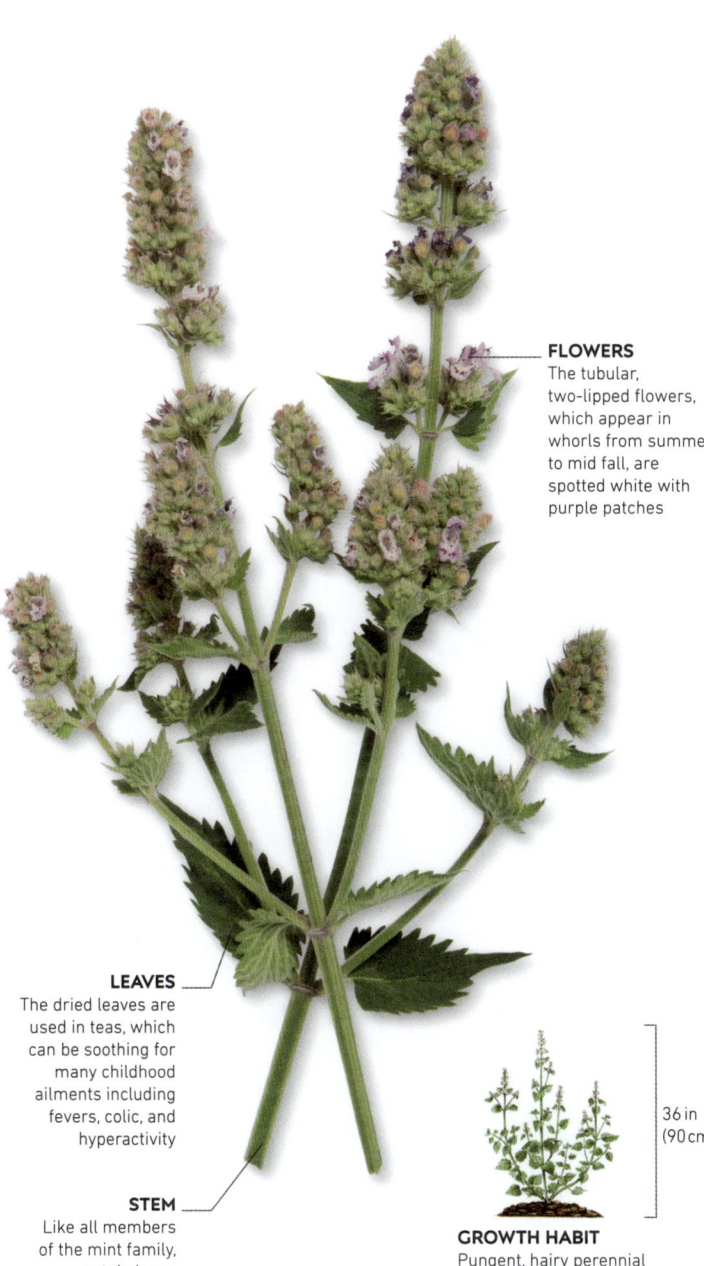

FLOWERS
The tubular, two-lipped flowers, which appear in whorls from summer to mid fall, are spotted white with purple patches

LEAVES
The dried leaves are used in teas, which can be soothing for many childhood ailments including fevers, colic, and hyperactivity

STEM
Like all members of the mint family, catnip has a square stem

36 in (90 cm)

GROWTH HABIT
Pungent, hairy perennial with gray-green oval leaves and a spread of 9–24 in (23–60 cm).

CAUTION Do not take in pregnancy.

Oenothera biennis
EVENING PRIMROSE

Native to North America, evening primrose is now grown worldwide both as a garden ornamental and as a commercial crop to supply a global trade in its seed oil, which is rich in essential fatty acids. The oil is marketed as a food supplement and remedy for a variety of ailments, including skin, arthritic, and menstrual disorders.

PARTS USED Seed oil, leaves, stems, flowers
MAIN CONSTITUENTS Seeds: rich in essential fatty acids, including gamma-linolenic acid—a precursor of prostaglandin E1
ACTIONS Whole plant: astringent, sedative.
Seed oil: hypotensive, anticoagulant, hypolipidemic

HOW TO USE

INFUSION Drink 1 cup (2–3 tsp leaves and stems per cup of boiling water) 3 times daily for digestive upsets including poor appetite and diarrhea.
SYRUP Combine 1 lb (450 g) of sugar or honey with 1 pint (600 ml) of above infusion of the leaves and stems, bring to a boil, and simmer gently for 10 minutes; take in 1–2 tsp (5–10 ml) doses as required for whooping cough.
CAPSULES Commercial capsules often contain vitamin E as a preservative; take 500 mg daily or follow the directions on the pack. Generally used for menopausal problems, skin disorders including psoriasis and eczema, and rheumatoid arthritis. The oil is also combined with fish oils as an anti-aging remedy. Follow the directions on the package.
CREAM/SEED OIL Use 2–3 times daily on dry, scaly skin.

HOW TO SOURCE

GROW Prefers poor to moderately fertile, light, well-drained soil in full sun; tolerates dry periods. Sow seeds in a cold frame in late spring and transplant when established in summer, or sow directly in late summer to fall.
FORAGE Naturalized in many parts of the world and often found in dry, stony, waste areas. Collect the leaves and stems in the second year when the flower stem appears.
HARVEST Collect the seeds when ripe.

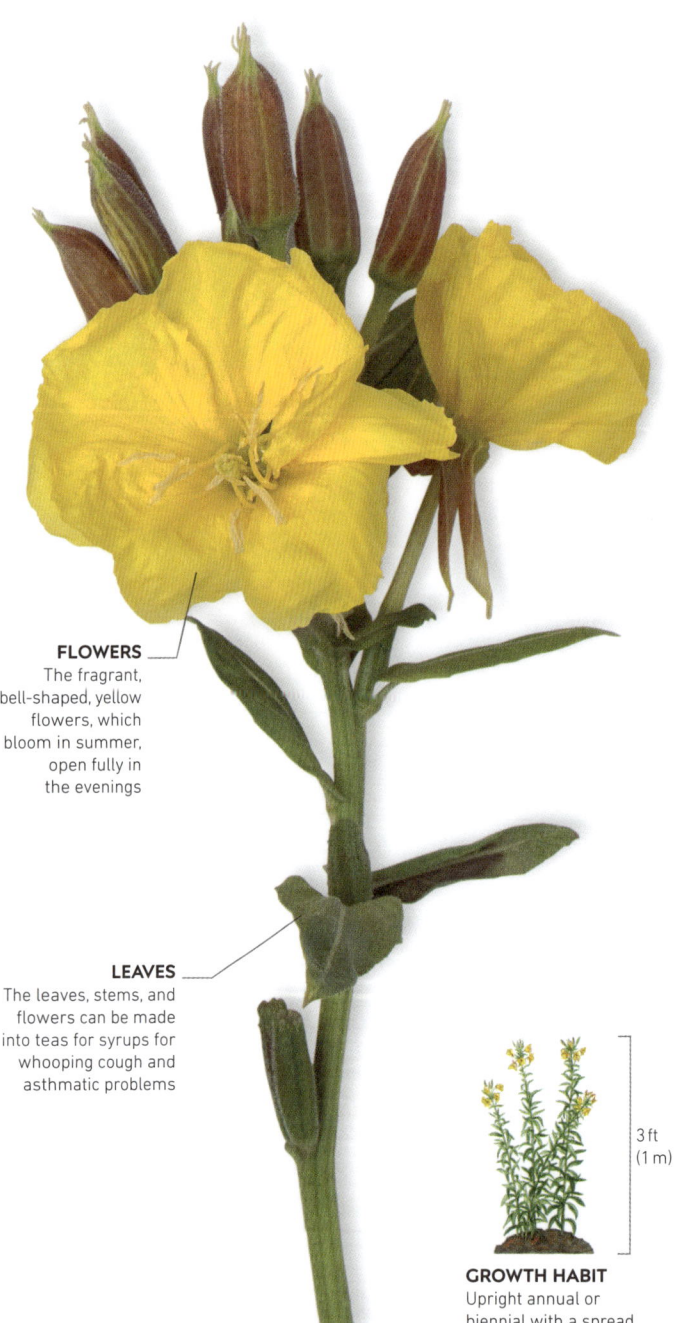

FLOWERS
The fragrant, bell-shaped, yellow flowers, which bloom in summer, open fully in the evenings

LEAVES
The leaves, stems, and flowers can be made into teas for syrups for whooping cough and asthmatic problems

GROWTH HABIT
Upright annual or biennial with a spread of 9–12 in (22–30 cm).

3 ft (1 m)

CAUTION Do not take the oil if suffering from epilepsy.

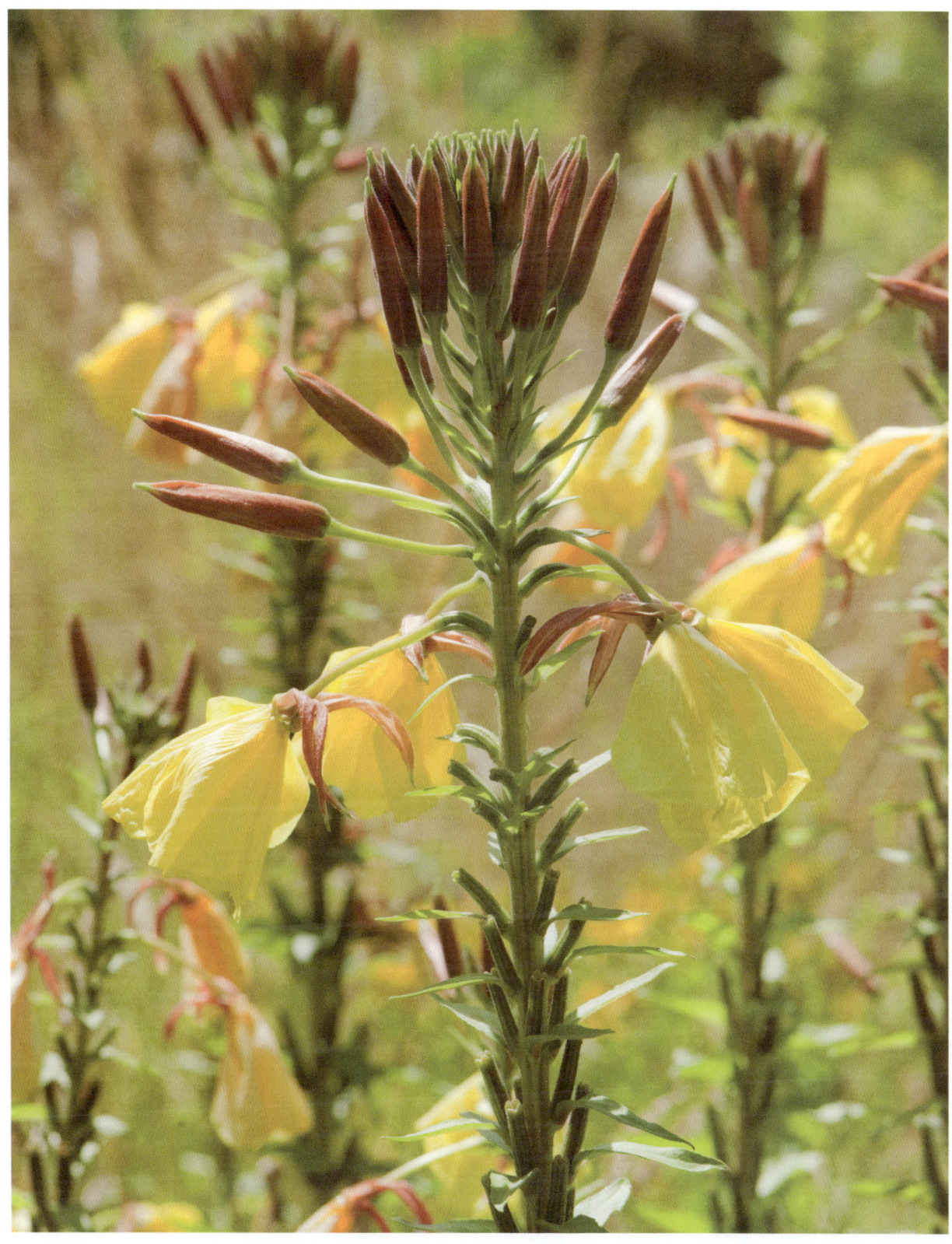

Olea europaea
OLIVE

The Ancient Greeks crowned the winners of the first Olympic Games with olive leaves, and historically the olive has been seen as the tree of life and a symbol of peace. Native to the Mediterranean, Middle East, and the south of Russia, olive trees were traditionally used as a liver and cardiac tonic, and have antimicrobial properties. They are now cultivated widely all over the world.

PARTS USED Fruit and leaves
MAIN CONSTITUENTS Phenolics (incl. flavonoids derived from luteolin and rutin), triterpenes (incl. oleanolic and betulinic acids), volatile oils (incl. aldehydes, sesquiterpenes, and monoterpenes)
ACTIONS Hypotensive, diuretic, antiseptic, spasmolytic, antifungal, antibacterial, antiviral

HOW TO USE

INFUSION Take 1 cup of a standard infusion (p.176) of the dried leaves 3 times daily to improve blood pressure.
TINCTURE Take 40 drops–1 tsp (2–5 ml) as an immune and cardiovascular tonic.
OIL Regular consumption of olive oil in cooking or salad dressings helps reduce cholesterol. Olive oil is also often used as a base oil for infusions of herbs such as comfrey leaves, calendula flowers, or horse chestnuts. Place the herbs in a jar of oil for 2 weeks, drain, and add to cosmetics, soaps, and creams to soften dry lesions, heal wounds, and soothe burns.
CAPSULES Take 500–1,000 mg per day of standardized leaf extract in capsule form to lower blood pressure and boost the immune system.

HOW TO SOURCE

GROW Can be grown either from seed or from cuttings; seed should be sown in fall, while cuttings should be taken and planted during summer. The tree needs full sun and well-drained soil. It grows very slowly and will take 5–12 years before it bears fruit.
FORAGE Branches are often pruned in the spring or summer on a sunny day and left on the ground. This is a good time to forage and harvest the leaves without doing damage to the tree or fruit.
HARVEST The fruit is harvested in fall by picking, or by beating the tree and collecting the dropped fruit on a ground sheet. The best-quality olive oil is from the first pressing and is usually labeled as such.

CAUTION High doses of olive oil (1–4 tbsp a day) can have a laxative effect.

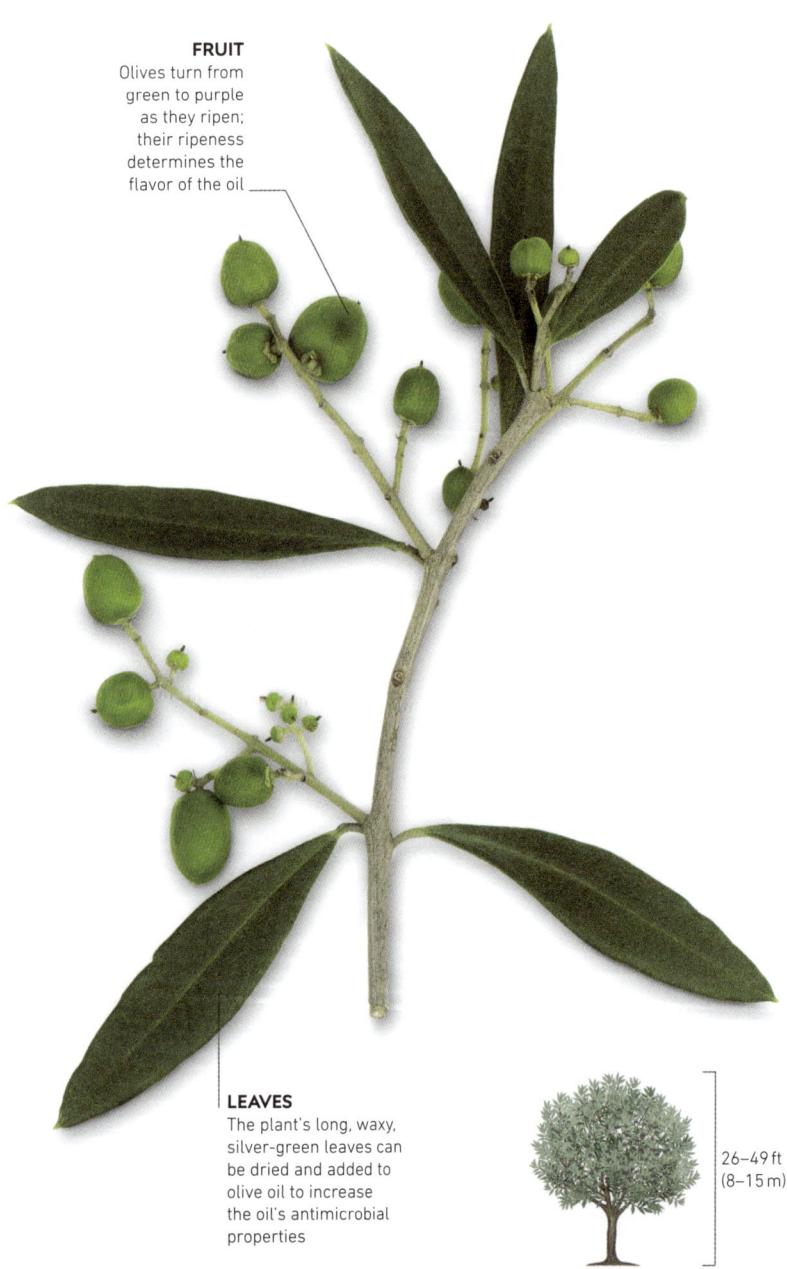

FRUIT
Olives turn from green to purple as they ripen; their ripeness determines the flavor of the oil

LEAVES
The plant's long, waxy, silver-green leaves can be dried and added to olive oil to increase the oil's antimicrobial properties

26–49 ft
(8–15 m)

GROWTH HABIT
Evergreen tree with a spread of around 30 ft (10 m).

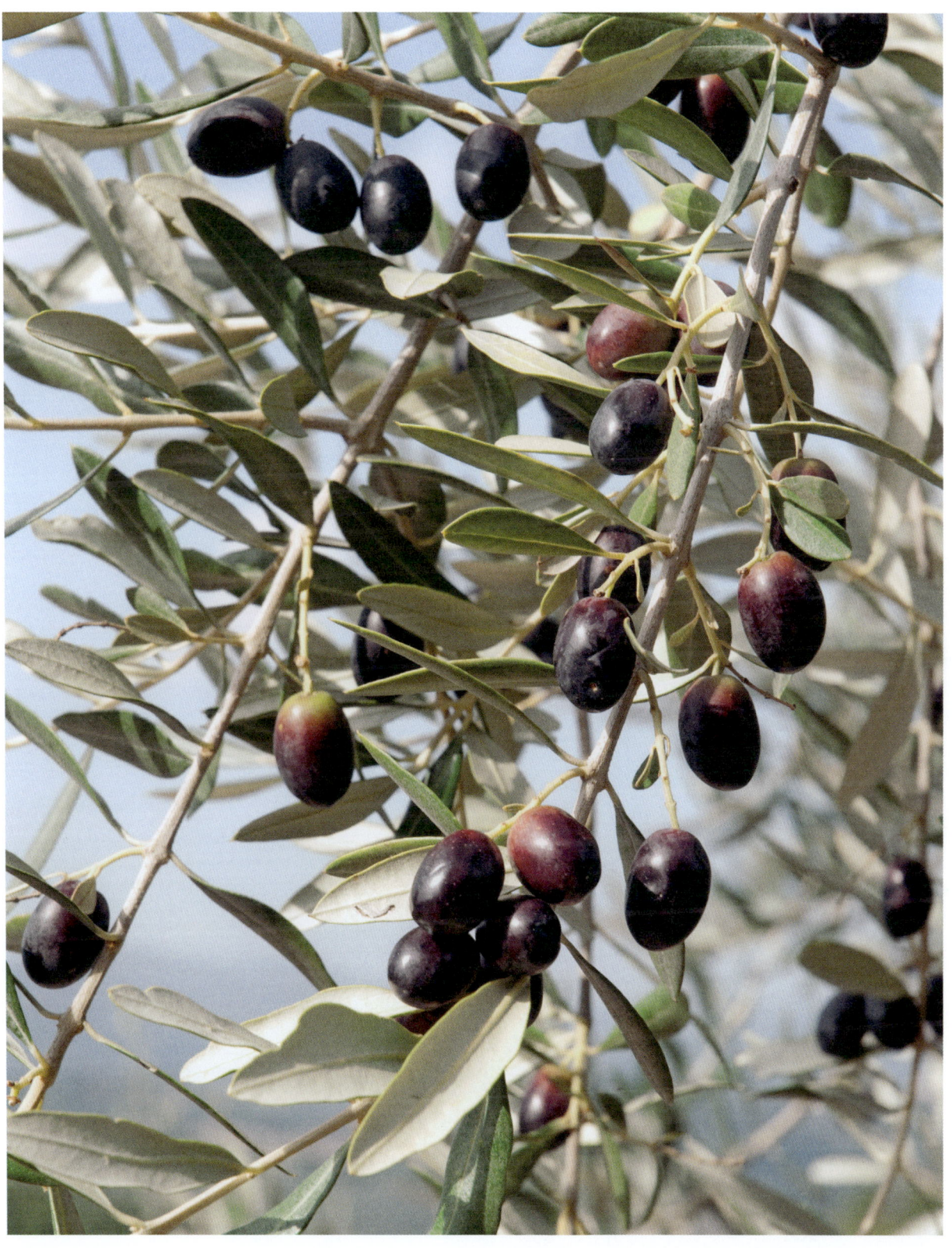

Panax japonicus
JAPANESE GINSENG

Found in mountainous woodland areas of Japan, Japanese ginseng is one of several related species used medicinally, and is largely used for coughs. The most popular is Korean ginseng (*Panax ginseng*) which, like American ginseng (*Panax quinquefolius*), is an important energy tonic. San qi ginseng (*Panax pseudo-ginseng*) is used to control bleeding.

PARTS USED Root
MAIN CONSTITUENTS Saponins, steroidal glycosides, sterols, volatile oil
ACTIONS Expectorant, tonic, febrifuge

HOW TO USE

TABLETS/CAPSULES Available in Japan. Can be used as a substitute for Korean ginseng, although the tonic effect is significantly reduced. Take 600 mg daily.
DECOCTION Recent research suggests that Japanese ginseng may have a mild stimulatory effect on the immune system. Take ½–1 cup of a decoction, made by heating ¼ oz (10 g) of root in 1 pint (600 ml) of water for 20 minutes, 2–3 times daily for recurrent infections or as a general immune tonic. The decoction is used in Japanese folk medicine for non-insulin dependent diabetes and to combat obesity.
SYRUP Add 1 lb (450 g) of sugar to 1 pint (600 ml) of above decoction, bring to a boil, and simmer for 5–10 minutes. Take in 1 tsp (5 ml) doses for productive coughs.

HOW TO SOURCE

GROW Sow seeds in a shaded area in a cold frame as soon as they are ripe. Germination can be slow and erratic. Transplant to 3 in (7.5 cm) pots as soon as the seedlings are large enough to handle, and continue growing in a shady position in the greenhouse for at least the first winter. Plant into a permanent position in moist but well-drained soil in shade in late summer. Alternatively, propagate by root division in spring.
FORAGE Unlikely to be found outside its native habitat.
HARVEST The roots of plants that are at least four years old are dug in fall.

CAUTION Avoid during pregnancy. Do not take with drinks containing caffeine. Japanese ginseng has been little researched and can be of poor quality.

FRUITS
Umbels of green-yellow flowers appear in spring and are followed by fruits, which are initially green and ripen to red

LEAVES
The whorls of five divided leaves grow on upright stems

2 ft (60 cm)

GROWTH HABIT
Perennial with aromatic rootstock and divided bright green leaves.

Passiflora incarnata
PASSIONFLOWER

Native to woodlands in the eastern United States, passionflower, a species of which is shown below, is known locally as "maypop" and was used by many Native American people for swellings, fungal infections, and as a blood tonic. Today it is generally regarded as a sedative and used for problems ranging from hyperactivity in children to the tremors of Parkinson's disease.

PARTS USED Leaves and stems
MAIN CONSTITUENTS Flavonoids (incl. rutin and apigenin), cyanogenic glycosides, alkaloids, sapanarin
ACTIONS Analgesic, antispasmodic, bitter, cooling, hypotensive, sedative, heart tonic, relaxes blood vessels

HOW TO USE

INFUSION Drink 1 cup made from equal amounts of passionflower and raspberry leaf (1 tsp each) twice daily for period pain. For insomnia, take ½–1 cup of an infusion made from ½ tsp of dried passionflower to 1 cup of boiling water infused for 15 minutes, at night. For period pain or tension headaches, take 3 times daily; reduced doses are suitable for hyperactivity in children.
TINCTURE Take 40–80 drops (2–4 ml) in water 3 times daily for nervous tension, high blood pressure associated with nervous stress, or to reduce the severity of attacks in Ménière's disease.
FLUID EXTRACT Take up to 40 drops (2 ml) in water twice a day to ease the pain associated with shingles and toothache.
TABLETS/CAPSULES Take 1–2 x 200 mg tablets or capsules night and morning for anxiety, tension, and nervous headaches.

HOW SOURCE

GROW Prefers poor, sandy soil that is slightly acidic. Sow the seeds at 64–70°F (18–21°C) in trays in spring and transplant to 3 in (7.5 cm) pots when large enough. Plant in final growing positions when well established in summer. Alternatively, take semi-ripe cuttings in summer. Shelter the plants from cold, wet winds in winter.
FORAGE Unlikely to be found growing wild outside its native habitat. The fruits are edible and can be collected in summer, but are only suitable for jams or jellies.
HARVEST Collect aerial parts when flowering or in fruit.

CAUTION May cause drowsiness.

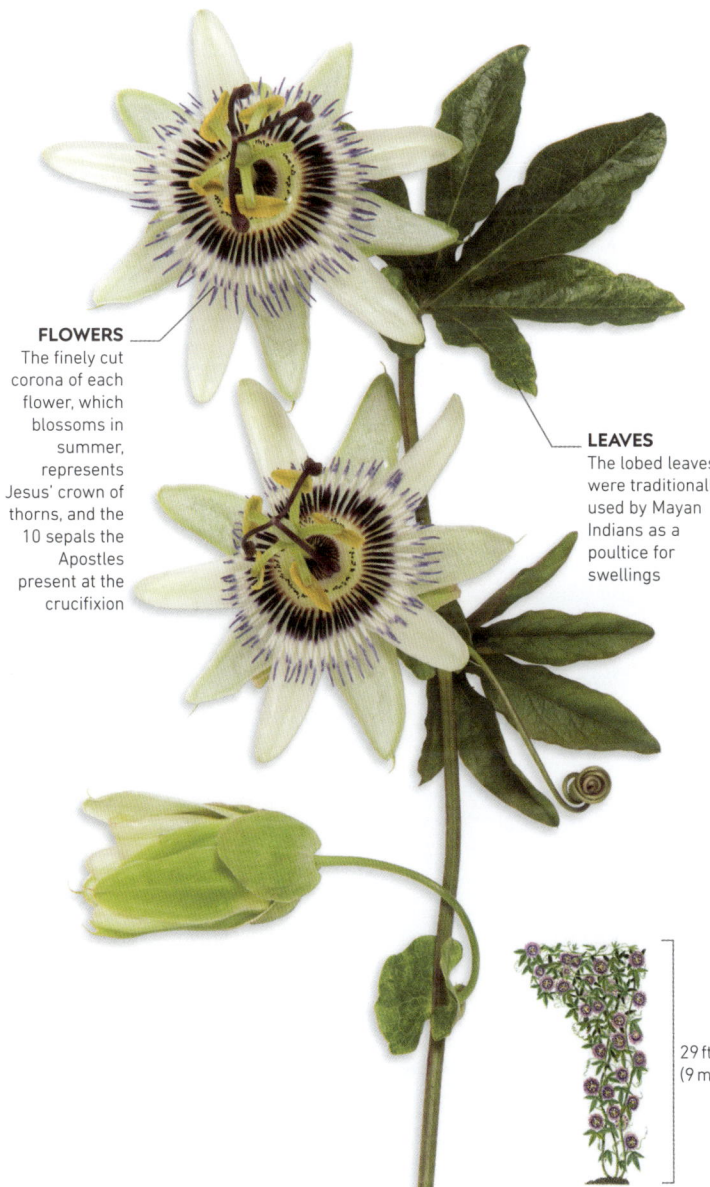

FLOWERS
The finely cut corona of each flower, which blossoms in summer, represents Jesus' crown of thorns, and the 10 sepals the Apostles present at the crucifixion

LEAVES
The lobed leaves were traditionally used by Mayan Indians as a poultice for swellings

29 ft (9 m)

GROWTH HABIT
Climbing perennial vine with ornate flowers and egg-shaped orange fruits.

Plantago lanceolata
RIBWORT PLANTAIN

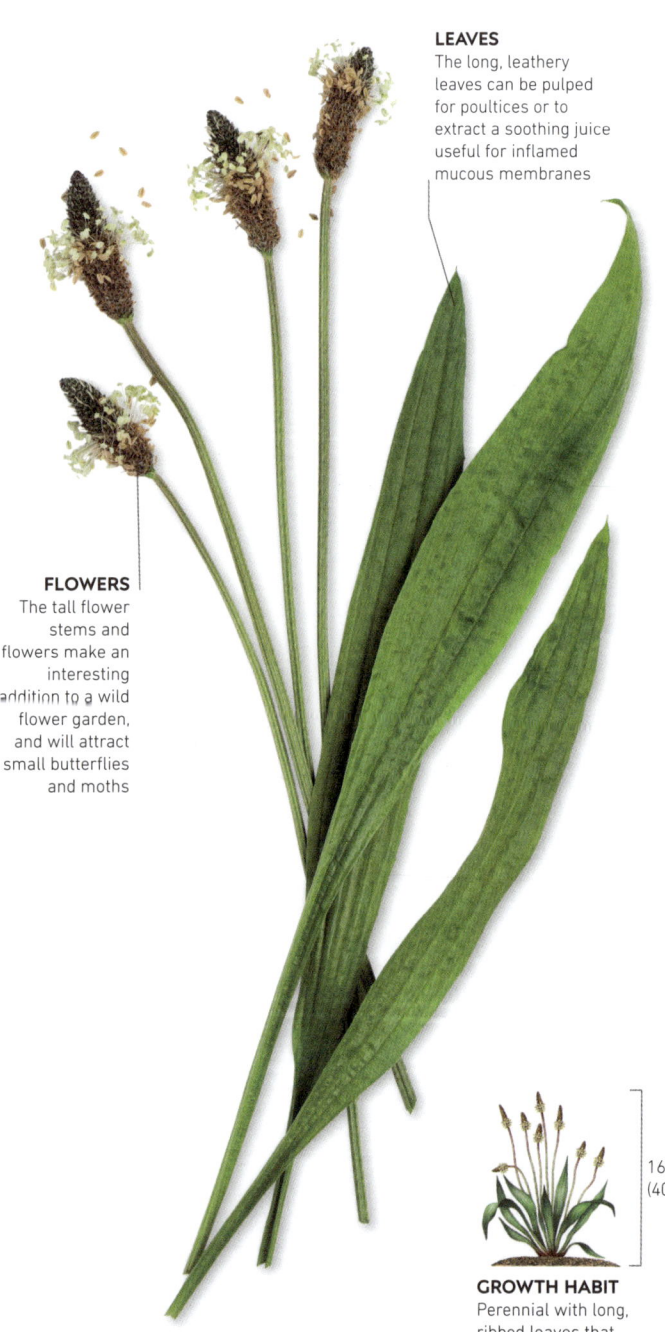

LEAVES
The long, leathery leaves can be pulped for poultices or to extract a soothing juice useful for inflamed mucous membranes

FLOWERS
The tall flower stems and flowers make an interesting addition to a wild flower garden, and will attract small butterflies and moths

GROWTH HABIT
Perennial with long, ribbed leaves that form a rosette shape.

16 in (40 cm)

Both ribwort plantain and its broad-leaved cousin common plantain (*Plantago major*) are among the most common European weeds likely to be found anywhere, from pavement cracks to hedges. The plants are also found in the temperate regions of Asia, and were introduced by settlers into North America and Australia. Plantain is a first-aid standby in folk tradition.

PARTS USED Leaves
MAIN CONSTITUENTS Flavonoids, iridoids, mucilage, tannins, minerals
ACTIONS Relaxing expectorant, toning to mucous membranes, anticatarrhal, antispasmodic, topically healing, hemostatic

HOW TO USE

TINCTURE Take 60 drops–1 tsp (3–5 ml) 3 times daily for catarrhal conditions or digestive problems, including gastritis and irritable bowel syndrome.
JUICE Use fresh leaves to make a juice and take in 2 tsp (10 ml) doses 3 times daily to soothe cystitis, diarrhea, and lung infections. The juice can also be applied to wounds and sores.
INFUSION Drink 1 cup (2 tsp herb per cup boiling water) 3 times daily for catarrhal conditions or use as a gargle for sore throats.
SYRUP Add 8 oz (225 g) of honey to 10 fl oz (300 ml) of above infusion and take in 1 tsp (5 ml) doses as required for sore throats or productive coughs.
POULTICE Use fresh leaves, mashed into a pulp, for slow-healing wounds and chronic ulcers, or apply the fresh leaves to insect bites and stings.

HOW TO SOURCE

GROW Prefers moist, poor to moderately fertile soil in sun, or partial shade. Usually found as a self-seeded garden weed, although seeds can be obtained from wild flower specialists. Sow seeds where you want them to grow in spring or in 3 in (7.5 cm) pots in a cold frame, and plant when established. Flowers, usually produced in the second year, appear from early spring until first frosts. It is generally included in wild meadow plantings, but self-seeds enthusiastically and can easily become invasive.
FORAGE Easily found growing on wasteland, hedges, roadsides, and grassy areas. It is best to choose plants growing in uncultivated areas well away from traffic to reduce the risk of collecting contaminated specimens.
HARVEST Gather leaves in summer.

Plantago psyllium
PSYLLIUM

Both black psyllium seeds, and the pale beige ispaghula seeds from its near relative, *Plantago ovata*, are commonly used over-the-counter remedies for constipation. Psyllium originates in the Mediterranean region, while ispaghula is native to India and Pakistan. The seeds swell in water to produce a mucilaginous mass, which is used as a bulking laxative.

PARTS USED Seeds
MAIN CONSTITUENTS Mucilage, fixed oil (incl. linoleic, oleic, and palmitic acids), starch, vitamins, minerals
ACTIONS Demulcent, bulking laxative, antidiarrheal, anti-inflammatory

HOW TO USE

MACERATION Soak two rounded teaspoons of the seeds in a mug of warm water overnight. Take as a single dose in the morning for constipation. The mixture can be flavored with fruit juice or mixed with oatmeal or yogurt, which some people find more palatable. Drink a glass of water or fruit juice after taking the seeds.
POULTICE Mix 1 tsp of psyllium husks with ½ tsp of slippery elm powder, add a little water to make a paste, and apply to boils or abscesses.
POWDER The husks are generally sold in powdered form: stir ½ tsp into a cup of water and take 3 times daily for diarrhea or to help reduce blood cholesterol levels.

HOW TO SOURCE

GROW Prefers well-drained soil in full sun. Sow seeds in spring in trays on the surface of compost; keep in a propagator at 59–70°F (15–21°C) and transplant to final growing positions in early summer when large enough to handle. The plant flowers about 60 days after planting and needs high temperatures to set seed.
FORAGE Likely to be found in southern Europe, North Africa, and western Asia in waste places and dry, shrubby ground. Both psyllium and ispaghula are widely cultivated commercially.
HARVEST Harvest the seeds when ripe in late summer or early fall.

CAUTION Always take with plenty of water and do not exceed the stated dose. Although sometimes recommended for irritable bowel syndrome, psyllium can exacerbate symptoms in some cases, so use with caution. Take at least 1 hour before any other medication.

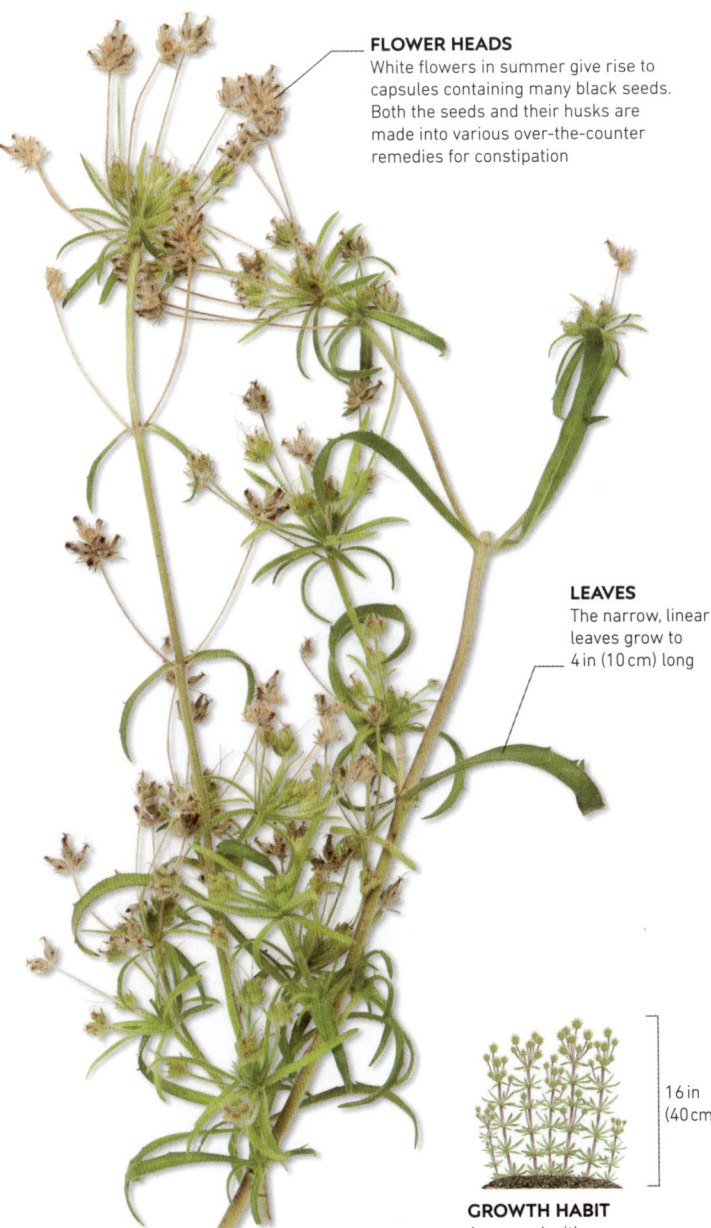

FLOWER HEADS
White flowers in summer give rise to capsules containing many black seeds. Both the seeds and their husks are made into various over-the-counter remedies for constipation

LEAVES
The narrow, linear leaves grow to 4 in (10 cm) long

16 in (40 cm)

GROWTH HABIT
An annual with lance-shaped leaves, small white flowers, and a spread of 12 in (30 cm).

Platycodon grandiflorus
CHINESE BALLOON FLOWER

Listed in the *Shennong Ben Cao Jing*—China's oldest herb book attributed to the legendary founder of herbal medicine, Shennong, who is said to have lived 5,000 years ago—the balloon flower, which is native to eastern Asia, is considered an important respiratory remedy in traditional Chinese medicine. In the West it is better known as a garden ornamental.

PARTS USED Root
MAIN CONSTITUENTS Saponins, stigmasterol, inulin, platycodin
ACTIONS Antifungal, antibacterial, expectorant, hypoglycemic, reduces cholesterol levels

HOW TO USE

DECOCTION Drink 1 cup (1–2 tsp root per cup of boiling water) 3 times daily for productive coughs and sore throats associated with common colds.
SYRUP Combine 1 lb (450 g) of sugar or honey with 1 pint (600 ml) of above decoction, bring to a boil, and simmer gently 10 minutes; take in 1–2 tsp (5–10 ml) doses as required for bronchitis and other coughs producing profuse phlegm. Seek medical help if a productive cough does not improve after 2–3 days.
PATENT REMEDY Included in a number of commercially available pills and powders used in traditional Chinese medicine, including *sang ju yin* (a decoction of mulberry leaf with chrysanthemum), which is used for coughs, bronchitis, and the early stages of some feverish diseases.
GARGLE Use 1 cup of above decoction 2–3 times daily as a gargle for laryngitis and sore throats.

HOW TO SOURCE

GROW Prefers a well-drained site in sun or partial shade and forms in broad clumps 18 in (45 cm) in diameter when well established. Sow seeds in a seed tray in spring or early summer and transplant to 3 in (7.5 cm) pots when large enough to handle. Transplant to a permanent position when large enough to handle.
FORAGE Unlikely to be found naturalized outside China and Japan, although cultivated plants that self-seed may occur.
HARVEST Dig the root of established plants in fall.

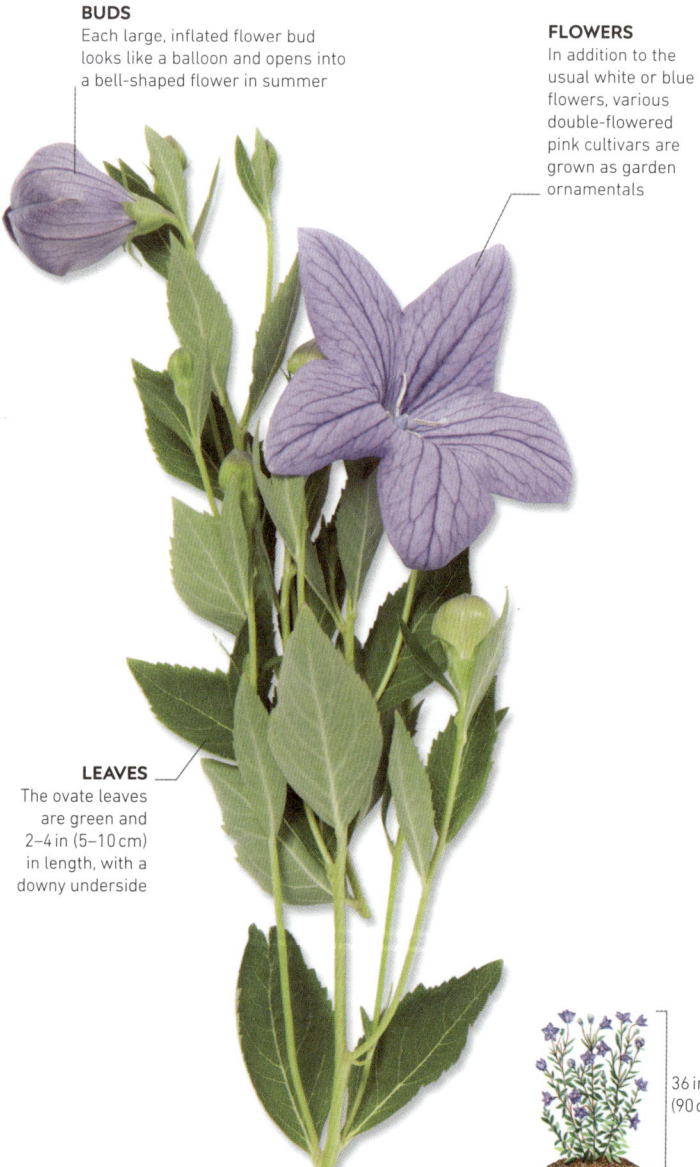

BUDS
Each large, inflated flower bud looks like a balloon and opens into a bell-shaped flower in summer

FLOWERS
In addition to the usual white or blue flowers, various double-flowered pink cultivars are grown as garden ornamentals

LEAVES
The ovate leaves are green and 2–4 in (5–10 cm) in length, with a downy underside

36 in (90 cm)

GROWTH HABIT
Erect, clump-forming perennial with a spread of 12 in (30 cm).

CAUTION Avoid this herb if there is blood in the phlegm.

Prunella vulgaris
SELF-HEAL

As with so many plants, the common name of this herb—self-heal—gives a good indication as to its use; it was once highly regarded as a wound remedy and cure-all. Native to Europe and Asia, self-heal is used as a wound healer and general tonic, and the flowers are a significant remedy in traditional Chinese medicine for soothing liver problems.

PARTS USED Aerial parts, flowers
MAIN CONSTITUENTS Flavonoids (incl. rutin); vitamins A, B1, C, K; fatty acids; volatile oil; bitter principle
ACTIONS Aerial parts: antibacterial, hypotensive, diuretic, astringent, hemostatic, wound herb. Flower spikes: liver stimulant, hypotensive, antibacterial, febrifuge

HOW TO USE

TINCTURE Best made from the freshly gathered leaves and stems. Take 1 tsp (5 ml) 3 times daily for all sorts of bleeding, including heavy periods, blood in the urine, or traumatic injuries.
MOUTHWASH/GARGLE Use ½ tsp of dried herb to 1 cup of boiling water and allow to cool; use for bleeding gums and mouth inflammations or as a gargle for sore throats.
INFUSION Drink 1 cup (1–2 tsp aerial parts per cup boiling water) 3 times daily for liver problems linked to anger, over-excitability, high blood pressure, headaches, or hyperactivity in children. (Consult an herbalist to treat children.) Often combined with Chinese chrysanthemum flowers, another herb used in Chinese medicine for liver problems.
POULTICE Use fresh leaves on wounds.
CREAM/OINTMENT Use for bleeding hemorrhoids.

HOW TO SOURCE

GROW Prefers moist, well-drained soil in full sun or partial shade, but will tolerate a wide range of conditions. Propagate from seeds sown in a cold frame in spring and transplant when established or by root division in spring or fall. A prolific self-seeder that can become invasive.
FORAGE A common weed throughout Europe and many parts of Asia, it is found in grassland, roadsides, and sunny meadows. Collect the leaves and stems in early summer or harvest the flowers while in full bloom in mid- to late summer.
HARVEST In the West the leaves and young shoots are traditionally gathered before flowering.

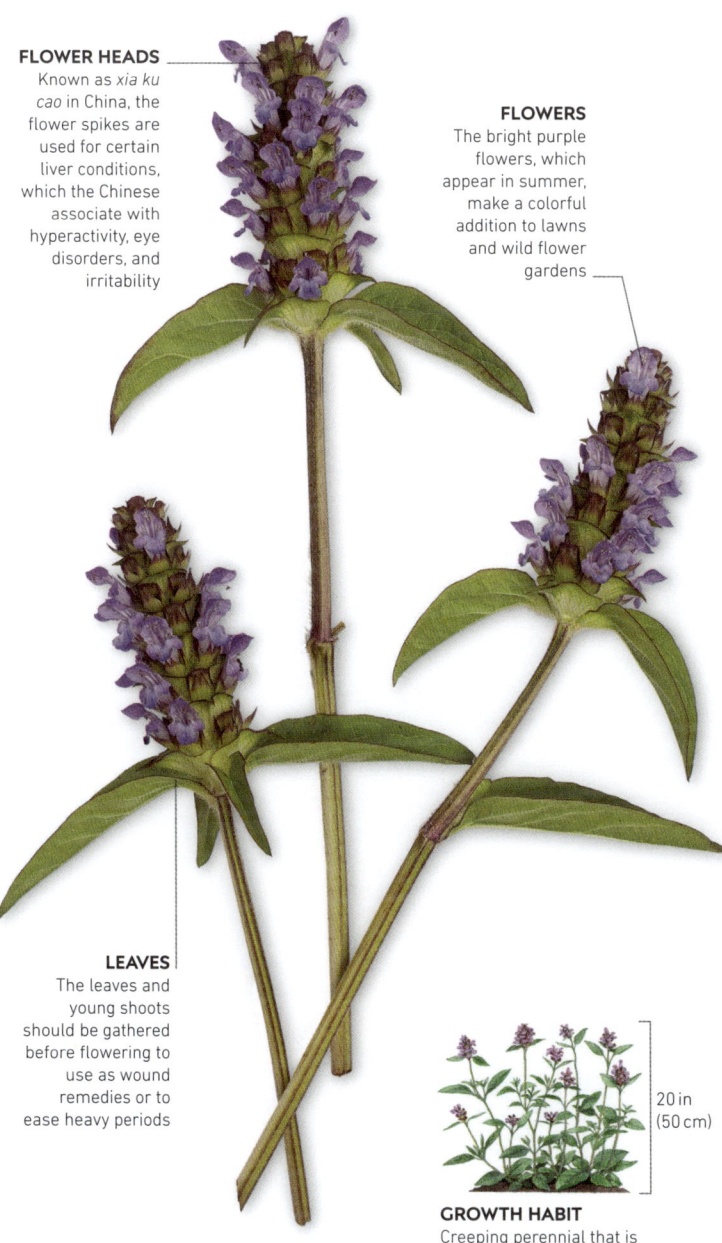

FLOWER HEADS
Known as *xia ku cao* in China, the flower spikes are used for certain liver conditions, which the Chinese associate with hyperactivity, eye disorders, and irritability

FLOWERS
The bright purple flowers, which appear in summer, make a colorful addition to lawns and wild flower gardens

LEAVES
The leaves and young shoots should be gathered before flowering to use as wound remedies or to ease heavy periods

20 in
(50 cm)

GROWTH HABIT
Creeping perennial that is usually low growing and has an indefinite spread.

Ribes nigrum
BLACK CURRANT

Native to temperate regions of Europe and Asia, black currants are extensively cultivated for their juice and as a flavoring. Demand for the juice is so high that the fruits are rarely available in stores and should be grown in gardens for home use. While the fruits are rich in vitamin C, the leaves are largely used as a diuretic.

PARTS USED Leaves, fruits, seed oil
MAIN CONSTITUENTS Leaves: volatile oil, tannins. Fruits: flavonoids, anthocyanosides, tannins, vitamin C, potassium.
Seeds: Essential fatty acids incl. gamma-linolenic acid
ACTIONS Astringent, mild febrifuge, diuretic, antirheumatic; the fruits are a rich source of vitamin C

HOW TO USE

INFUSION Drink ½–1 cup (1–2 tsp leaves per cup of boiling water) as desired during the early stages of colds and feverish infections.
SEED OIL Rich in gamma-linolenic acid, black currant seed oil capsules are available commercially as an alternative to evening primrose oil for treating eczema, menstrual irregularities, arthritis, etc. Follow dosage directions on the package.
JUICE Take 2 tsp (10 ml) 3 times daily (ideally as freshly made, unsweetened juice) for diarrhea and digestive upsets; also provides additional vitamin C for infections such as flu or pneumonia.
GARGLE/MOUTHWASH Use 1 cup of the above leaf infusion 2–3 times daily for sore throats and mouth ulcers
TINCTURE Take 1 tsp (5 ml) of leaf tincture in a little water 3 times daily to increase elimination of fluids in high blood pressure.

HOW TO SOURCE

GROW Prefers full sun and rich, well-drained soil, but tolerates other conditions. Usually propagated by hardwood cuttings in fall. Pot until well established and plant in final positions in early winter or up to mid-March. Plant bushes 2 in (5 cm) deeper than the top of their pot; they produce stems from just below the surface: Water regularly and keep well weeded.
FORAGE Rarely found growing wild in Europe, although bushes may grow in hedges. Unlikely to be found growing wild in the US (it is host to a rust fungi and is therefore banned in some states).
HARVEST Pick fruits in midsummer when ripe and leaves through the growing season.

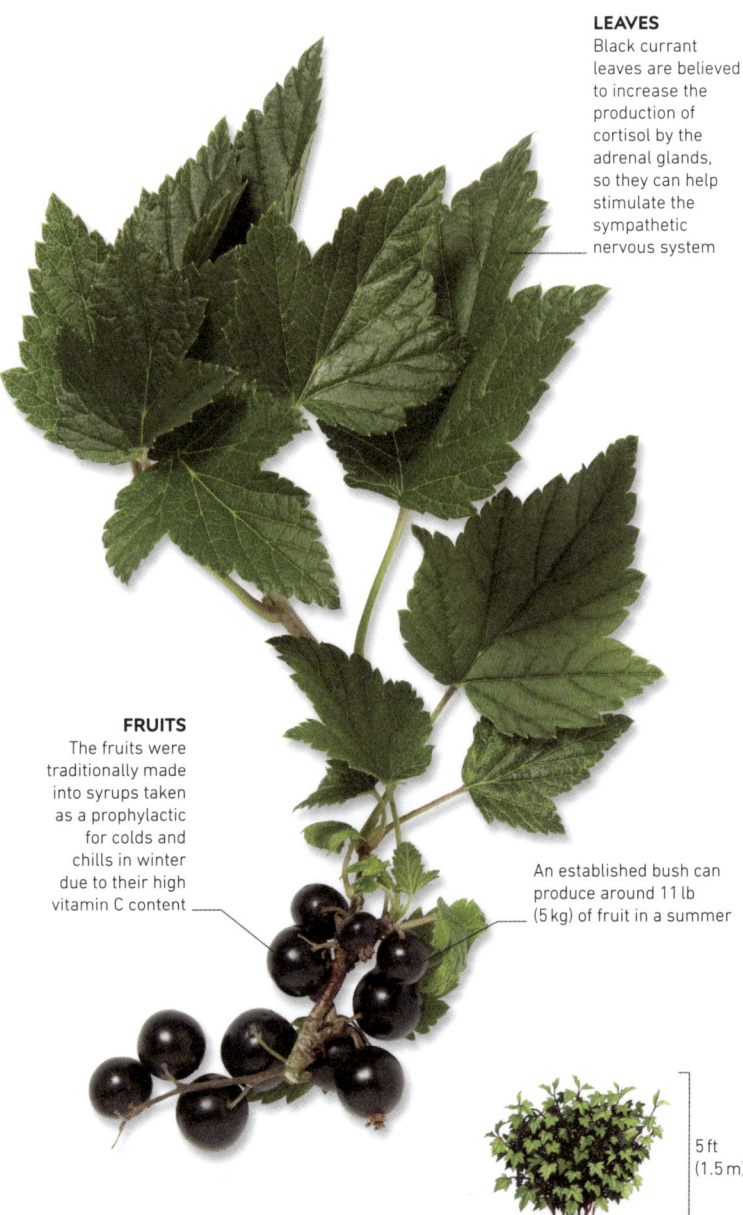

LEAVES
Black currant leaves are believed to increase the production of cortisol by the adrenal glands, so they can help stimulate the sympathetic nervous system

FRUITS
The fruits were traditionally made into syrups taken as a prophylactic for colds and chills in winter due to their high vitamin C content

An established bush can produce around 11 lb (5 kg) of fruit in a summer

5 ft (1.5 m)

GROWTH HABIT
Small deciduous perennial shrub with a spread of around 5–6 ft (1.5–2 m).

Rosa canina
DOG ROSE

Native to Europe, western Asia, and northwest Africa, dog roses are now found throughout North America and New Zealand, where they are regarded as an invasive weed. The name reputedly derives from a Roman tradition that the root was, erroneously, a cure for rabies caused by dog bites. The hips are rich in vitamins, especially vitamin C, and can be made into syrups and jellies.

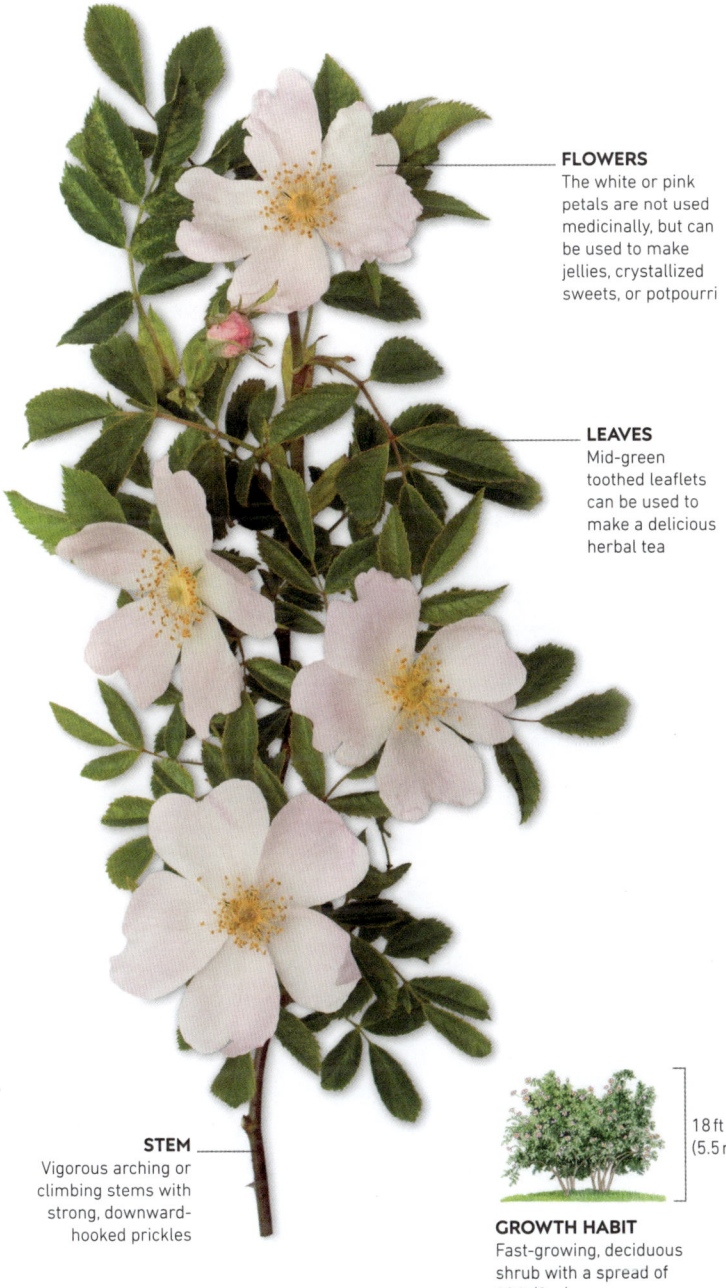

FLOWERS
The white or pink petals are not used medicinally, but can be used to make jellies, crystallized sweets, or potpourri

LEAVES
Mid-green toothed leaflets can be used to make a delicious herbal tea

STEM
Vigorous arching or climbing stems with strong, downward-hooked prickles

GROWTH HABIT
Fast-growing, deciduous shrub with a spread of 10 ft (3 m).

18 ft (5.5 m)

PARTS USED Fruits (hips), leaves
MAIN CONSTITUENTS Vitamins (A, B1, B2, B3, C, and K), flavonoids, tannins, polyphenols, carotenoids, volatile oil
ACTIONS Nutrient, astringent, diuretic, anti-inflammatory, mild laxative

HOW TO USE

SYRUP Popular form of nutritional supplement for young children. It is also used to flavor other medicines, and is added to cough mixtures. Put 5 tsp (25 ml) of hips in 2 cups of water, bring to a boil, and simmer gently until reduced in volume by half. Strain through a fine sieve to remove the hairs from the seeds, then add 8 oz (225 g) of honey to the decoction of hips and take 1 tsp (5 ml) doses as required.
TINCTURE Take up to 1 tsp (5 ml) of rose hip tincture 3 times daily for diarrhea, gastritis, to relieve colicky pains, or as a mild diuretic.
FRESH HIPS The ripe hips can be eaten as a food supplement (remove the seeds before eating). They were traditionally baked in tarts or made into fruit jellies, often combined with apples
INFUSION Once used as a substitute for tea, infused rose leaves can be made into a pleasant herbal tea for everyday drinking.

HOW TO SOURCE

GROW Usually grown from softwood cuttings in summer, it will self-seed freely once established. Often regarded as a weed by gardeners, dog rose is fast-growing and can be invasive. It will grow well in any well-drained moist soil in sun or partial shade, although it does not generally grow well in coastal areas. It is often grown as part of a mixed hedge.
FORAGE Found in hedges, roadside borders, and wasteland. The hips are best gathered in late fall when they start to fall from the plant. If picked any earlier, they can be hard and will need to be cooked before use.
HARVEST Gather the bright red hips in fall when ripe, and the leaves at any time for tea. Gather the rose petals in the summer to use in jam and jelly making.

Rosa x *damascena*
DAMASK ROSE

FLOWERS
The petals were once used in tinctures as an astringent remedy for sore throats and to flavor other medicines

THORNS
The thorns can be particularly vicious

7 ft (2.2 m)

GROWTH HABIT
A deciduous shrub with sprawling growth; spread 5 ft (1.5 m).

Damask roses originated in western Asia and were introduced into Europe in the 13th century. Today, they are regarded as a cross between *Rose gallica* and *Rosa moschata*. The flowers vary in color from pink to light red. Rose oil—known as rose otto—is extracted by steam distillation, mainly in Bulgaria and Turkey, and is said to be good for "the skin and the soul."

PARTS USED Flowers, essential oil, hydrosol
MAIN CONSTITUENTS Geraniol, nerol, citronellol, geranic acid (rose oil contains around 300 chemicals, of which about 100 have been identified)
ACTIONS Sedative, antidepressant, anti-inflammatory, reduces cholesterol levels, astringent

HOW TO USE

MASSAGE OIL Use 1 drop of rose oil in 1 tsp (5 ml) of almond oil to massage into the temples and neck for stress or exhaustion.
BATHS Add 2 drops of rose oil to bath water for depression, sorrows, or insomnia.
CREAM Made from the petals, or by adding a few drops of rose oil to a base cream. For dry or inflamed skin conditions.
LOTION Rosewater—the waste water from the steam distillation process (hydrosol)—can be used as the basis of various lotions: add 10% lady's mantle tincture for vaginal itching, or mix 50:50 with distilled witch hazel as a cooling lotion for skin prone to spots or acne.
TINCTURE Take 20–40 drops (1–2 ml) of a tincture made from the rose petals for nervous disorders, poor digestion, or to help reduce cholesterol levels.

HOW TO SOURCE

GROW Prefers fertile, moist, but well-drained soil and needs at least 5 hours of sunlight a day during the growing season. Will tolerate temperate to subtropical temperatures. Usually propagated by hardwood cuttings in fall.
FORAGE May be found growing wild, but more likely to be cultivated in hedges.
HARVEST Gather flowers in summer.

CAUTION Avoid during pregnancy. Do not take essential oils internally without professional advice. Rose oil is often adulterated or synthesized, so only buy from reputable sources.

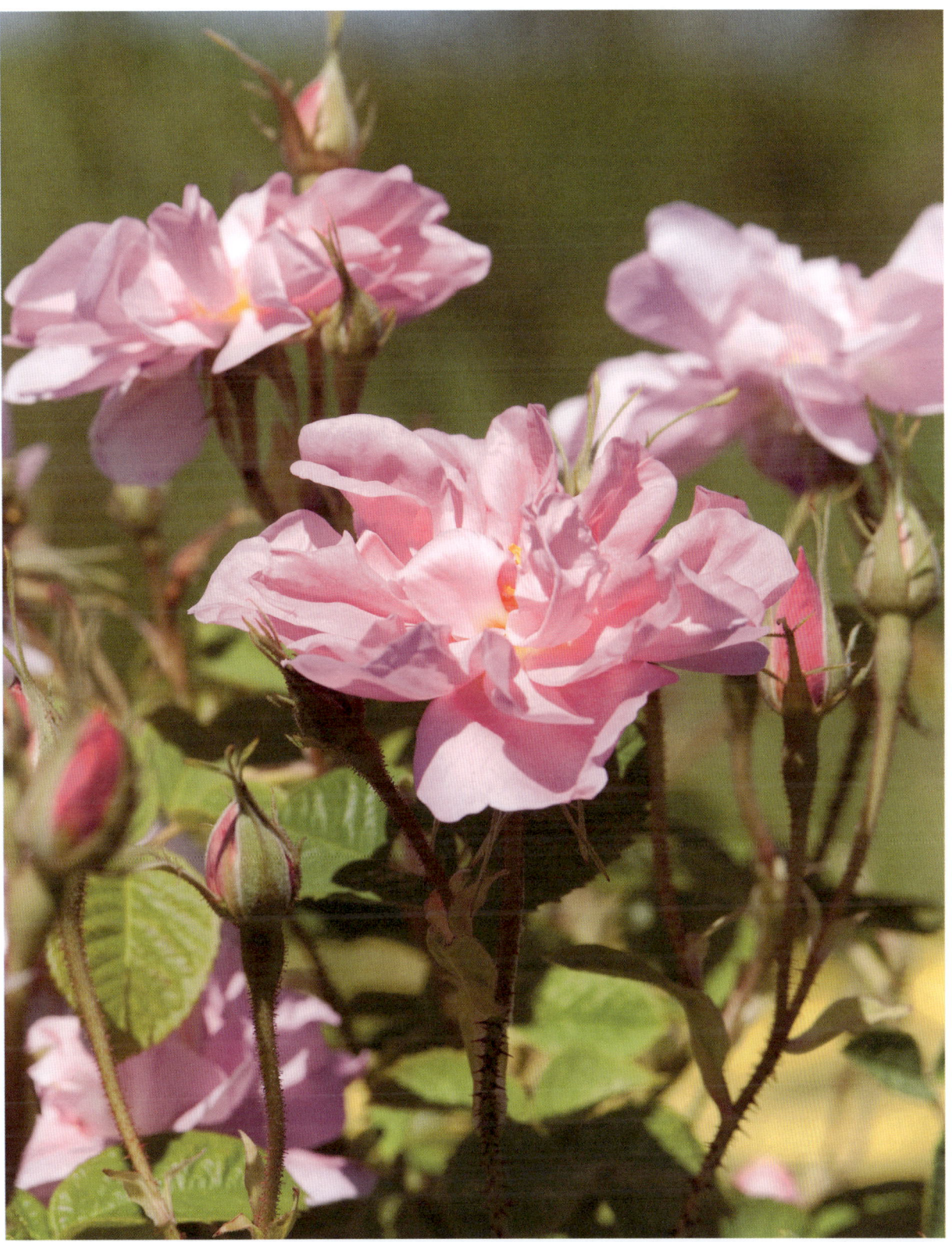

Rosmarinus officinalis
ROSEMARY

Originally found in dry coastal areas around the Mediterranean region, rosemary is now cultivated worldwide and is grown both as a culinary herb and for its essential oil. Medicinally, the herb is largely used as a stimulating tonic and digestive remedy, while the oil is used for arthritic pains. It is an important ingredient in the cosmetics and fragrance industry.

PARTS USED Leaves, flowers, essential oil
MAIN CONSTITUENTS Volatile oil (incl. borneol, camphene, cineole), flavonoids, rosmarinic acid, tannins
ACTIONS Astringent, nervine, carminative, antiseptic, diaphoretic, antidepressive, circulatory stimulant, antispasmodic, cholagogue, diuretic
ESSENTIAL OIL Topically rubefacient, analgesic

HOW TO USE

INFUSION A standard infusion (p.176) can taste unpleasant, so use a weaker mix; Pour 1 cup of boiling water over 1–2 tsp (5–10 ml). Take 1 cup for tiredness and headaches.
HAIR RINSE Use a standard infusion, strained, as a final rinse for dandruff.
INHALATION Inhaling a drop of essential oil from a tissue is an energizing brain stimulant and concentration aid.
TINCTURE Take up to 50 drops/½ tsp (2.5 ml) 3 times daily for tiredness and nervous exhaustion; combine with an equal amount of wild oat or vervain tincture for depression.
MASSAGE RUB Add 5 drops (¼ ml) of the essential oil to 1 tbsp (15 ml) of almond oil and massage aching joints and muscles. Massage also into the temples to ease tension headaches.
COMPRESS Use 1 cup of hot standard infusion in a compress to ease sprains. Alternating a very hot infusion with an ice pack every 2–3 minutes works best.

HOW TO SOURCE

GROW Can be grown from seed, although cultivars do not come true and must be propagated from semi-ripe cuttings. Prefers neutral to alkaline soil.
FORAGE Found in native areas—shrub and open woodland around the Mediterranean.
HARVEST Gather in spring and summer.

CAUTION Avoid therapeutic doses of the herb during pregnancy.

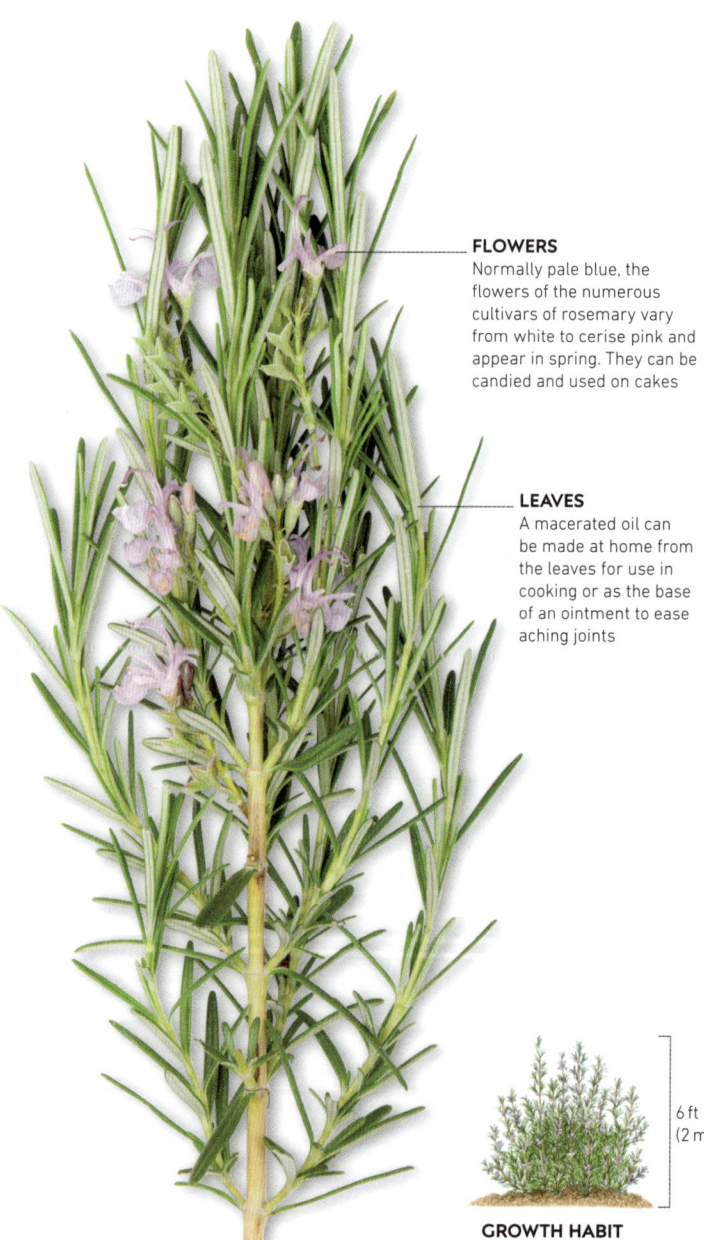

FLOWERS
Normally pale blue, the flowers of the numerous cultivars of rosemary vary from white to cerise pink and appear in spring. They can be candied and used on cakes

LEAVES
A macerated oil can be made at home from the leaves for use in cooking or as the base of an ointment to ease aching joints

6 ft
(2 m)

GROWTH HABIT
Bushy evergreen upright shrub with a spread of 5 ft (1.5 m).

Rubus idaeus
RASPBERRY

Familiar as a summer fruit, raspberry is native to Europe, Asia, and North America, and has been cultivated in kitchen gardens since at least the 16th century. The leaves are commonly taken in tea to strengthen the womb for childbirth, while the fruits can be made into vinegar to use in salad dressings or to add to cough mixtures.

PARTS USED Leaves, fruit
MAIN CONSTITUENTS Leaves: fragarine (uterine tonic), tannins, polypeptides.
Fruit: vitamins A, B, C, and E, sugars, fruit acids, pectin
ACTIONS Astringent, prepares the womb for childbirth, stimulant, digestive remedy, increases urination, laxative

HOW TO USE

INFUSION 1 cup (2–3 tsp leaves per cup boiling water) can be taken daily in the last two months of pregnancy to help strengthen and prepare the womb for childbirth; drink the infusion as often as needed during labor. Take 1 cup 3 times daily to ease painful or heavy menstruation.
TINCTURE Take 60 drops–1 tsp (3–5 ml) of the tincture 3 times daily for mild diarrhea, or add to 3½ fl oz (100 ml) of warm water and use to bathe wounds, varicose veins, or skin inflammations. Put 2–5 drops into an eye bath of boiled, cooled water for conjunctivitis and eye inflammations.
MOUTHWASH/GARGLE Use 1 cup of an infusion for mouth ulcers or sore throats.
JUICE Take 2 tsp (10 ml) 3–4 times daily of the juice (made from pulped berries) as a cooling remedy in mild fevers.

HOW TO SOURCE

GROW Prefers moist, slightly acidic soil. Propagate from rooted suckers, root division, or softwood cuttings, and plant in winter/early spring; prune canes to 10 in (25 cm) above ground after planting. Cut fruited canes back to ground level after harvesting, and select and support young canes for the following year's crop.
FORAGE Found on shrubland and waste areas. Collect the leaves in early- to midsummer, and the berries when ripe.
HARVEST Gather the fruits in summer or fall and the leaves in early summer.

CAUTION Therapeutic doses of raspberry leaf should only be taken in the last trimester of pregnancy; consult your doctor about use in the early stages.

FRUITS
Both summer and fall varieties of raspberry are available, and the fruits, which can be red or yellow, are astringent and nutritious

LEAVES
The leaves can be used for both menstrual cramps and to strengthen the womb for childbirth. The leaves are gathered in early summer

GROWTH HABIT
Deciduous shrub with prickly, woody stems and a spread of 3–6 ft (1–2 m).

6 ft
(2 m)

Rumex crispus
YELLOW DOCK

Native throughout Europe and Africa, yellow dock is a common wayside plant and garden weed that thrives on shrubby waste ground and grass verges. Its main use today is as a detoxifying herb and as a mild laxative. It is often combined with other herbs, such as burdock root, in the treatment of chronic skin conditions.

PARTS USED Root
MAIN CONSTITUENTS Anthraquinones (incl. emodin and chrysophanol), tannins, oxalates, volatile oil
ACTIONS Blood and lymphatic cleanser, bitter tonic, stimulates bile flow, laxative

HOW TO USE

DECOCTION Take ½–1 cup 3 times daily of a decoction made from ½ oz (15 g) of root to 17 fl oz (550 ml) of water simmered gently for 20 minutes for mild constipation, or to stimulate bile flow to improve the digestion and help clear toxins from the system.
TINCTURE Take 20–40 drops (1–2 ml) of tincture 3 times daily as part of a cleansing regimen for conditions such as irritant skin rashes and eczema, boils, acne, shingles, rheumatism, and osteoarthritis.
MOUTHWASH Use ½ cup of the decoction (made as above) diluted with an equal amount of warm water 2–3 times daily for mouth ulcers.
HOMEOPATHIC EXTRACTS In homeopathy, yellow dock root is used for coughs, sore throats, and hoarseness made worse by cold air and damp weather. Take 1–2 tablets up to 3 times daily.

HOW TO SOURCE

GROW A perennial weed that self-seeds enthusiastically, and which few people would want to cultivate in their gardens. Seeds can be gathered from hedges in fall if required and scattered where you want them to grow. Once established, the plant can be difficult to eradicate thanks to its tough root. It will tolerate any soil and grows in both sun and shade.
FORAGE The roots are long and can be difficult to dig up unless the ground has been well wetted first. Gather in fall.
HARVEST Dig up the roots in fall, wash thoroughly, chop, and dry.

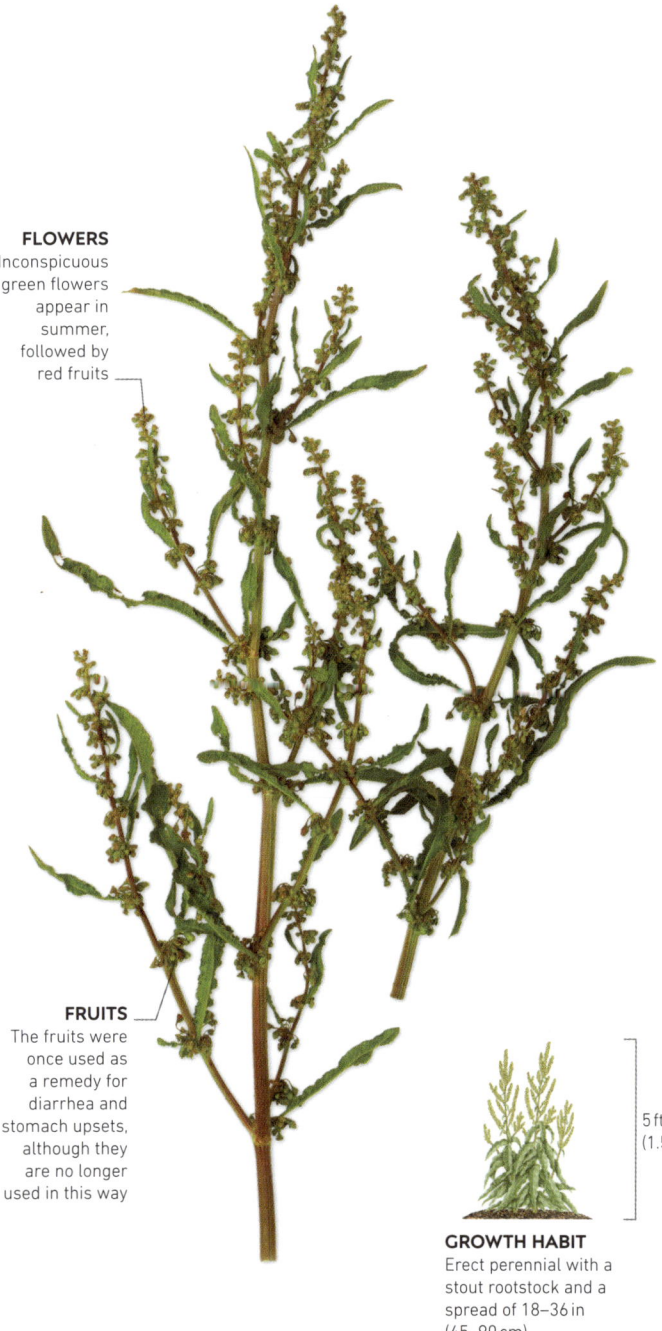

FLOWERS
Inconspicuous green flowers appear in summer, followed by red fruits

FRUITS
The fruits were once used as a remedy for diarrhea and stomach upsets, although they are no longer used in this way

GROWTH HABIT
Erect perennial with a stout rootstock and a spread of 18–36 in (45–90 cm).

5 ft (1.5 m)

CAUTION Do not take during pregnancy or when breastfeeding. Use for occasional constipation; for chronic constipation, consult an herbalist.

Salix alba
WHITE WILLOW

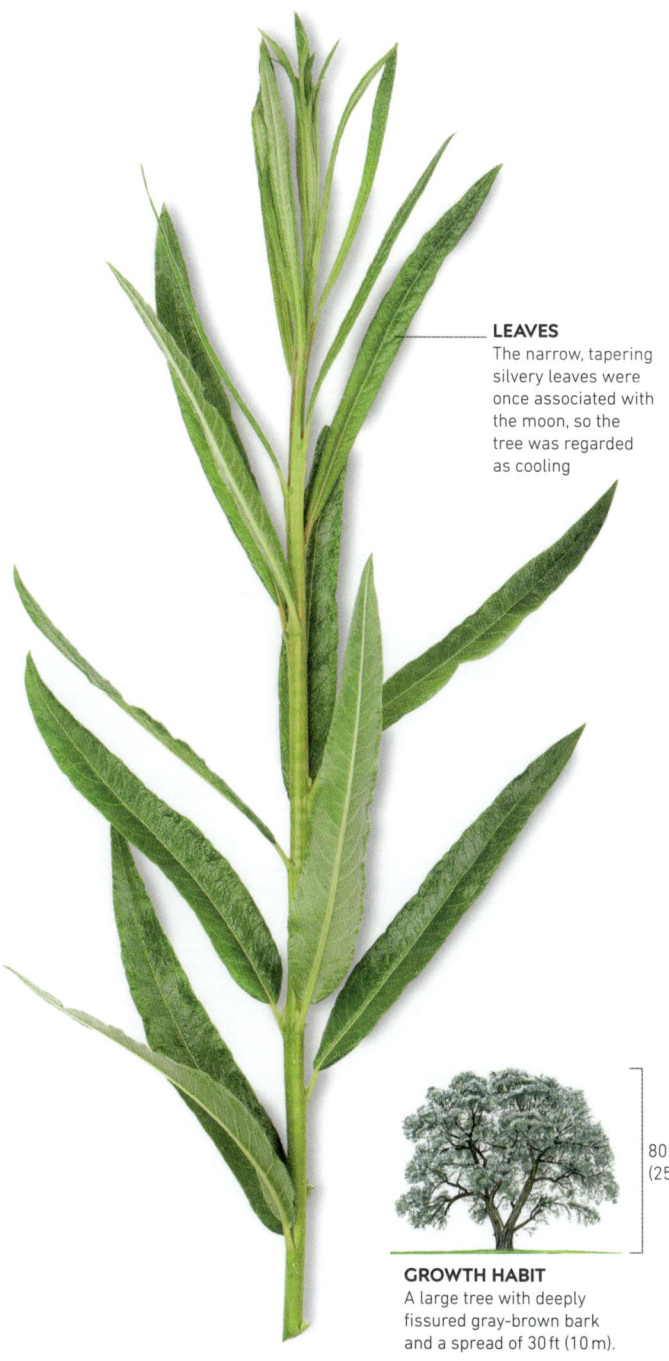

LEAVES
The narrow, tapering silvery leaves were once associated with the moon, so the tree was regarded as cooling

GROWTH HABIT
A large tree with deeply fissured gray-brown bark and a spread of 30 ft (10 m).

80 ft
(25 m)

Originally found in temperate or cold regions in the northern hemisphere, white willow was classified as a cool and moist remedy due to its preference for growing near water. In 1828, the Bavarian pharmacist, Johann Buchner (1783–1852), extracted bitter-tasting crystals—which he named salicin—from the bark; these were synthesized as aspirin by Bayer in 1899.

PARTS USED Bark, leaves
MAIN CONSTITUENTS Salicin, salicylic acid, tannins, flavonoids
ACTIONS Antirheumatic, anti-inflammatory, febrifuge, antihidrotic (reduces sweating), analgesic, antiseptic, astringent, bitter digestive tonic

HOW TO USE

FLUID EXTRACT Take 20–40 drops (1–2 ml) of the bark extract in water 3 times daily for rheumatic conditions, lumbago, sciatica, and neuralgia. Combine with an equal amount of rosemary tincture for headaches.
TINCTURE Use 1–2 tsp (5–10 ml) doses of the bark tincture (p.177) 3 times daily for fevers: generally combined with other herbs such as boneset (*Eupatorium perfoliatum*) or elderflower. Add 20–40 drops to menopausal remedies to help reduce night sweats and hot flashes.
DECOCTION Drink 1 cup (1–2 tsp bark per cup of boiling water) 3 times daily for feverish chills, headaches, or as part of arthritic treatments with herbs such as St. John's wort and cramp bark.
INFUSION Drink 1 cup (1–2 tsp leaves per cup of boiling water) after meals for indigestion.

HOW TO SOURCE

GROW Prefers moist but well-drained soil. Propagate from semi-ripe cuttings in summer or hardwood cuttings in winter, although it can be grown from seed.
FORAGE Often found growing near water such as rivers or canals. The leaves were once collected in summer and used in infusions as a fever remedy, for colicky pains, or for digestive problems, although they are no longer commercially harvested. The bark should not be stripped from wild trees.
HARVEST The bark is stripped in spring from branches of two- to five-year-old trees that have been pollarded.

CAUTION Avoid if allergic to aspirin or salicylates. Avoid during pregnancy.

Salvia officinalis
SAGE

Saliva officinalis originates in Mediterranean regions, and is well known as a culinary and medicinal herb. It is largely used for digestive and menopausal problems, particularly hot flashes, and is traditionally associated with longevity: modern research has shown that it can slow the progress of Alzheimer's disease.

PARTS USED Leaves, essential oil
MAIN CONSTITUENTS Volatile oil (incl. thujone, linalool, and borneol), diterpene bitter, tannins, flavonoids, estrogenic substances
ACTIONS Carminative; antispasmodic; astringent; antiseptic; reduces sweating, salivation, and lactation; uterine stimulant; stimulates bile flow

HOW TO USE

INFUSION Drink 1 cup (1–2 tsp leaves per cup of boiling water) 3 times daily for diarrhea; to help improve digestive function in debility; or to ease menopausal symptoms, including night sweats. It can also help dry off milk at the weaning stage.
GARGLE/MOUTHWASH Use 1 cup of above infusion as a gargle for sore throats, tonsillitis, quinsy, or as a mouthwash for mouth ulcers, gingivitis, etc.
TINCTURE Take 20–40 drops (1–2 ml) of tincture 3 times daily for menopause or as a tonic for digestive function.
HAIR RINSE Use 16 fl oz (500ml) of above infusion as a final rinse to control dandruff or restore color to graying hair.
CREAM/OINTMENT/LOTION Used as a household standby in many parts of Europe for treating minor cuts and scrapes.

HOW TO SOURCE

GROW Prefers neutral to alkaline soil and full sun. Sow seeds in 3 in (7.5 cm) of compost in spring or summer and plant out the following year when sturdy, or propagate from softwood cuttings in summer. Prune after flowering and in early spring to stop the plant becoming too straggly.
FORAGE Found growing wild on dry, sunny hillsides in temperate regions.
HARVEST Cropped just before flowering in summer, or collect the leaves to use in cooking throughout the year.

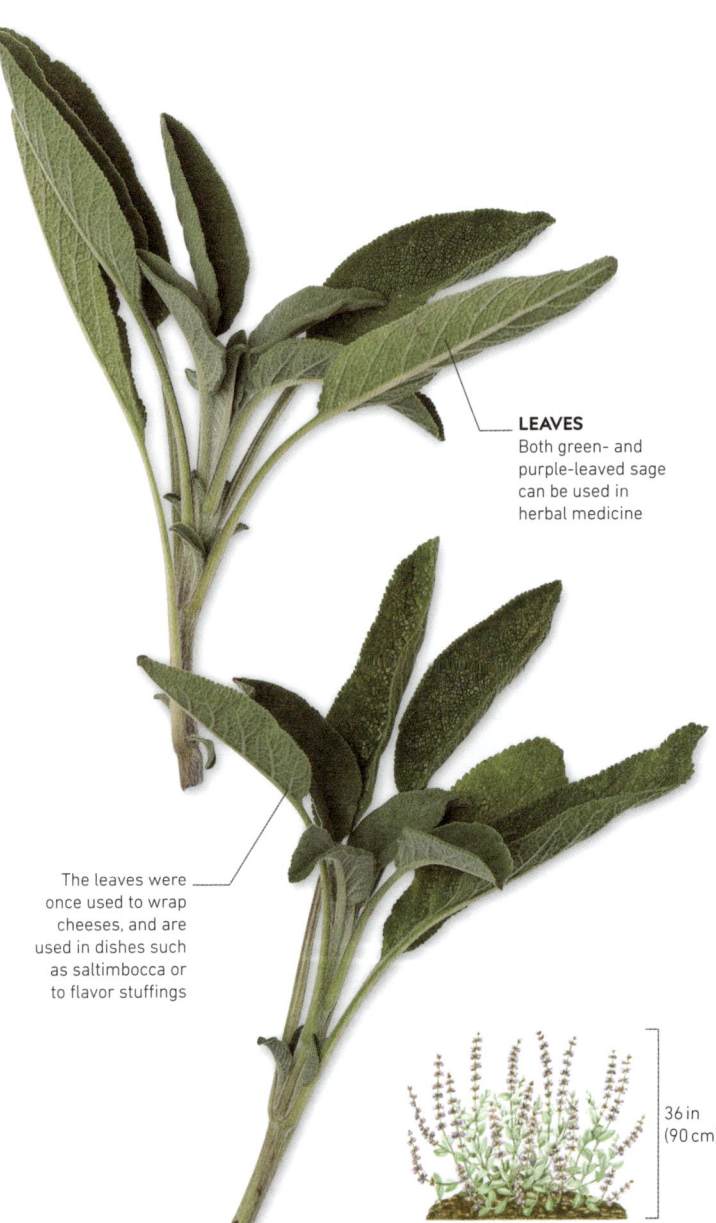

LEAVES
Both green- and purple-leaved sage can be used in herbal medicine

The leaves were once used to wrap cheeses, and are used in dishes such as saltimbocca or to flavor stuffings

36 in (90 cm)

GROWTH HABIT
Shrubby evergreen perennial with usually blue flowers in early summer; spread 3 ft (1 m).

CAUTION Due to its high thujone content, sage should not be taken in therapeutic doses by epileptics. Avoid therapeutic doses during pregnancy.

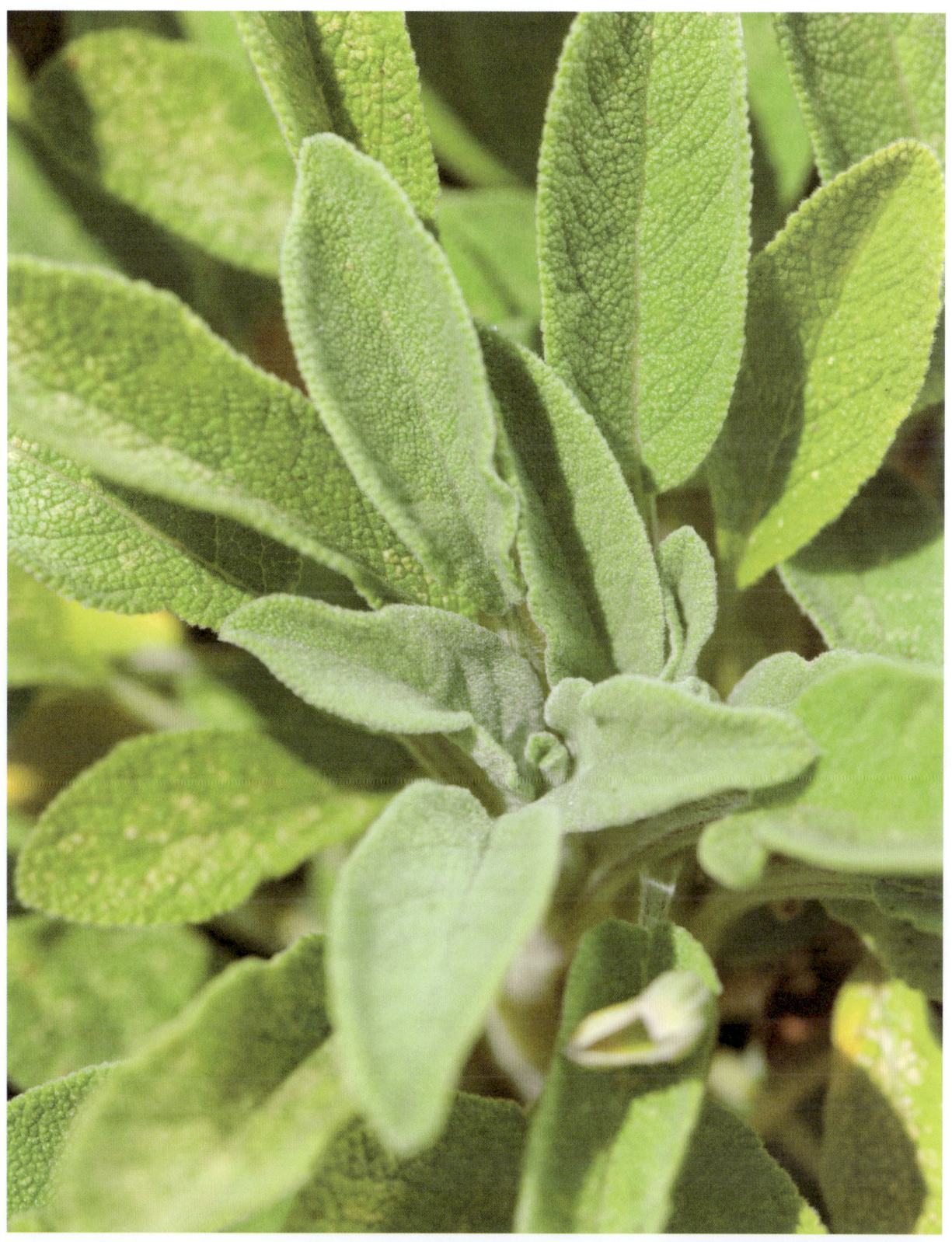

Sambucus nigra
ELDER

A common woodland tree throughout Europe, North Africa, and southwest Asia, elder was once regarded as a complete medicine chest: the root and bark made strong purgatives, while the leaves were made into a green ointment for use on bruises and sprains. Today, the flowers are most commonly used in refreshing elderflower cordials and medicinal brews.

PARTS USED Leaves, flowers, fruits
MAIN CONSTITUENTS Volatile oil, flavonoids, mucilage, tannins, cyanogenic glycosides, viburnic acid, phenolic acid, sterols; berries contain vitamins A and C
ACTIONS Flowers: expectorant, anticatarrhal, circulatory stimulant, diaphoretic, antiviral, topically anti-inflammatory.
Berries: diaphoretic, diuretic, laxative.
Leaves: topically wound-healing

HOW TO USE

INFUSION Make an infusion (p.176) of 1 cup of boiling water over 2 tsp flowers. Drink 1 cup 3 times daily for feverish conditions and coughs; combine with yarrow, boneset, and peppermint in equal proportions for seasonal colds.
MOUTHWASH/GARGLE Use 1 cup of a standard infusion of the flowers as a mouthwash and gargle for mouth ulcers, sore throats, or tonsillitis.
CREAM/OINTMENT Made from the flowers to soothe inflamed or chapped hands, or from the leaves for bruises, sprains, chilblains, or hemorrhoids.
SYRUP Add 1 pint (600 ml) of a standard decoction of berries to 1 lb (450 g) honey and take in 2 tsp (10 ml) doses for colds.
TINCTURE Take 40–80 drops (2–4 ml) elderberry tincture three times a day for coughs, colds, and flu symptoms. Combines well with echinacea.

HOW TO SOURCE

GROW Tolerates almost any soil, but prefers a moist, well-drained site. Propagate from hardwood cuttings in winter or ripe seeds sown in a cold frame; it will also self-seed easily. Can be invasive.
FORAGE Collect from hedges away from busy roads to avoid pollutants.
HARVEST Gather flowers in early summer and berries in early fall, removing them from the stem before use.

CAUTION Excessive consumption of fresh berries can have a laxative effect.

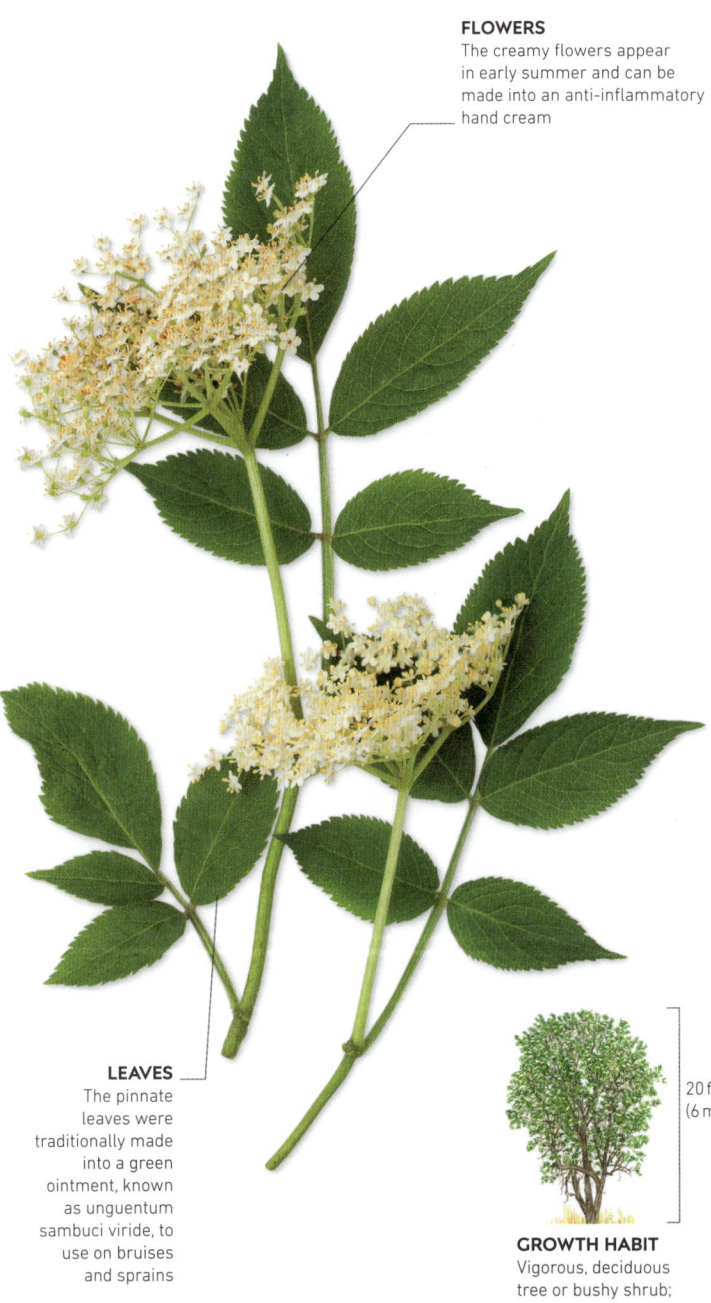

FLOWERS
The creamy flowers appear in early summer and can be made into an anti-inflammatory hand cream

LEAVES
The pinnate leaves were traditionally made into a green ointment, known as unguentum sambuci viride, to use on bruises and sprains

GROWTH HABIT
Vigorous, deciduous tree or bushy shrub; spread 20 ft (6 m).

20 ft (6 m)

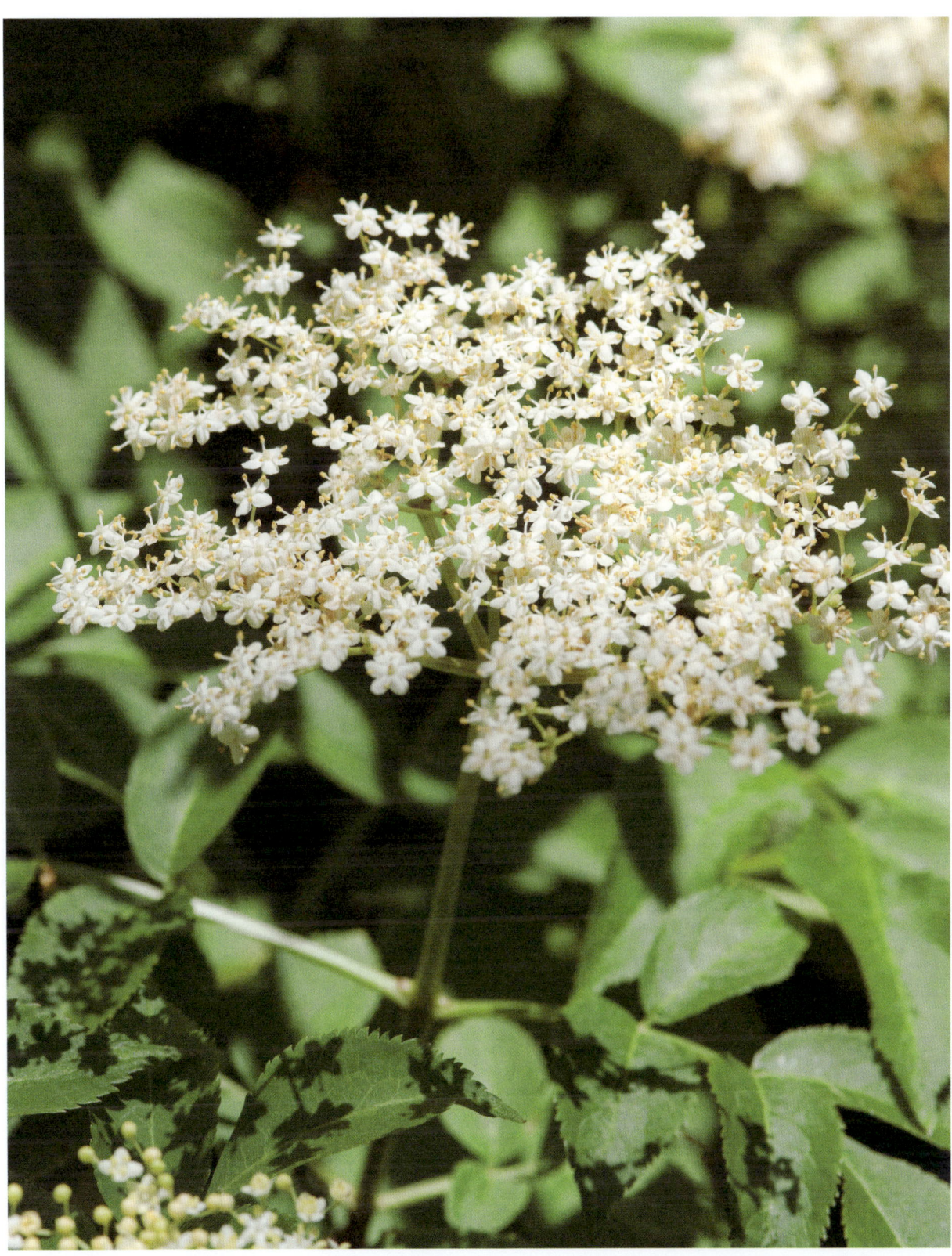

Saussurea costus
COSTUS

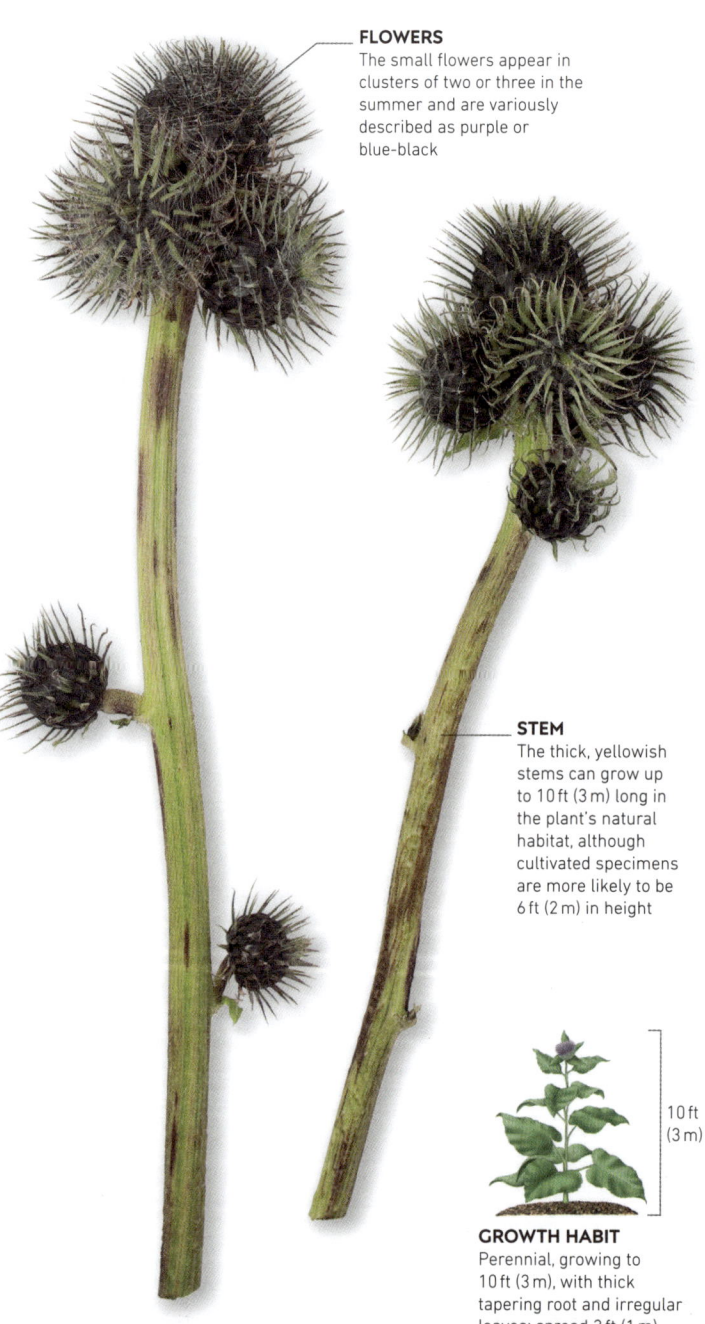

FLOWERS
The small flowers appear in clusters of two or three in the summer and are variously described as purple or blue-black

STEM
The thick, yellowish stems can grow up to 10 ft (3 m) long in the plant's natural habitat, although cultivated specimens are more likely to be 6 ft (2 m) in height

10 ft (3 m)

GROWTH HABIT
Perennial, growing to 10 ft (3 m), with thick tapering root and irregular leaves; spread 3 ft (1 m).

Native to the eastern Himalayas, costus has been used in the Ayurvedic tradition (in which it is known as *kuth*) for digestive and respiratory problems for at least 2,500 years. It was exported to China (where the root is called *mu xiang*) and also to the Middle East, where it is still used in Unani Tibb medicine.

PARTS USED Root, essential oil
MAIN CONSTITUENTS Alkaloid (sausserine), volatile oil (incl. linalool, terpenes and sesquiterpenes), stigmasterol, inulin, tannins
ACTIONS Antispasmodic, anodyne, aphrodisiac, astringent, bronchodilator, carminative, stimulant, stomachic, tonic

HOW TO USE

DECOCTION Generally used in Chinese medicine in combination with other herbs, such as cardamom (*Elettaria cardamomum*) or tangerine peel (*Citrus reticulata*), to relieve abdominal distention and pain, or for poor appetite, nausea, and vomiting. Typical dosage is ½–1 tsp (1–5 g) of root, usually added in the last 5 minutes of heating.
PATENT REMEDIES Included in patent pills and powders marketed by Chinese pharmaceutical companies. These include *mu xiang shun qi wan* and *mu xiang bing lang wan* for digestive problems. Usual dosage is 8 tiny pills 3 times daily.
OINTMENT Kuth oil is traditionally used in ointments in Ayurvedic medicine for wounds, ulceration, and skin disease.
HAIR RINSE Use 1 cup of a decoction made from ½–1 tsp of dried root to 1 pint (600 ml) of water.

HOW TO SOURCE

GROW Prefers moist soil in sun or partial shade. Sow seeds in a cold frame when ripe and transplant when large enough to handle or by root division in spring.
FORAGE Unlikely to be found growing wild outside its native region. As it is listed as "most endangered" (Appendix I) by CITES, it should not be gathered in the wild.
HARVEST The roots of mature plants are gathered in spring or fall.

CAUTION Avoid during pregnancy. Seek professional advice before taking patent Chinese remedies. As costus is so endangered, substitutes are often used. Only use costus plants from sustainable sources.

Schisandra chinensis
SCHISANDRA

Native to northeastern China and Japan, schisandra is valued as an aphrodisiac, although it is also used for coughs, diarrhea, insomnia, and skin rashes. The berries are called *wu wei zi* in Mandarin, which translates as "five taste seeds," as the pulp, skin, and seeds combine the five classic tastes identified in traditional Chinese medicine.

PARTS USED Fruit
MAIN CONSTITUENTS Phytosterols (incl. stigmasterol and beta-sitosterol), lignans, volatile oil, vitamins C and E
ACTIONS Antibacterial, astringent, tonic, aphrodisiac, circulatory stimulant, digestive stimulant, expectorant, hypotensive, sedative, uterine stimulant

HOW TO USE

LOTION Dilute 1 fl oz (30 ml) of tincture with 10 fl oz (300 ml) of water to make a lotion to bathe irritant skin rashes.
BERRIES Traditionally, a few berries are chewed as a tonic every day for 100 days.
DECOCTION Drink 1 cup (1–4 tsp dried berries per cup boiling water), with a tiny pinch of powdered ginger added, 3 times daily for coughs and wheezing For insomnia, drink ½–1 cup without ginger before bedtime.
TINCTURE Take 1 tsp (5 ml) in water 3 times daily for poor liver function.
TONIC WINE Put 4 oz (115 g) of berries in a jar and cover with 1 pint (600 ml) of rice wine. Seal and leave in a cool place for 1 month, shaking the bottle occasionally. Strain and take a sherry-glass dose daily as a tonic or to improve sexual energy.

HOW TO SOURCE

GROW Prefers rich, well-drained, moist soil against a sheltered, shady wall. Sow ripe seeds in fall in a cold frame; soak seeds sown in spring overnight first. Grow until well established before planting in final positions. Must be trained against a wall or fence; remove unwanted shoots in late winter. Both male and female plants are required to produce berries.
FORAGE Unlikely to be found growing wild outside its native habitat, although it is cultivated as a garden ornamental.
HARVEST Collect the fruits after the first frosts and sun-dry them.

CAUTION Avoid during pregnancy or in feverish chills and conditions involving heat. Large doses may cause heartburn.

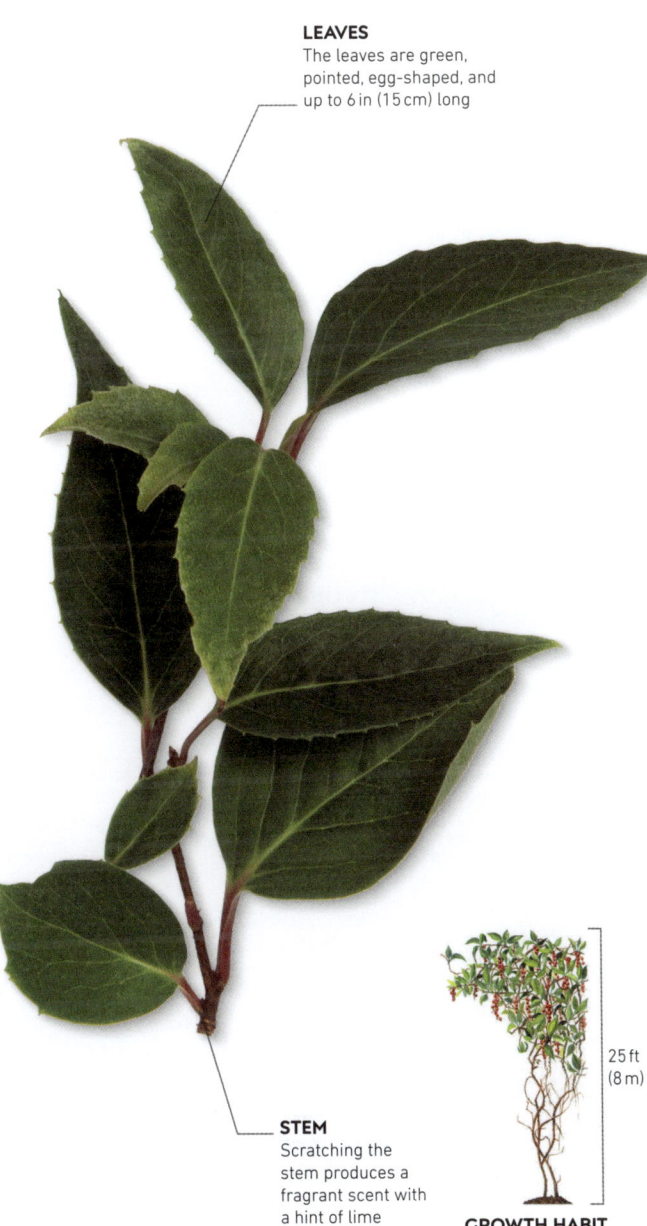

LEAVES
The leaves are green, pointed, egg-shaped, and up to 6 in (15 cm) long

STEM
Scratching the stem produces a fragrant scent with a hint of lime

25 ft (8 m)

GROWTH HABIT
Deciduous, dioecious, climbing shrub with solitary flowers that appear in late spring.

Scutellaria lateriflora
VIRGINIAN SKULLCAP

Native to North America, Virginian skullcap was once known as "mad dog herb" due to an erroneous belief that it could cure rabies. Today it is mainly used as a sedative. Its European relative, marsh, or hooded, skullcap (*Scutellaria galericulata*) has similar properties, while the root of the Chinese species (*Scutellaria baicalensis*), known as *huang qin*, is used in hot, feverish conditions.

PARTS USED Aerial parts
MAIN CONSTITUENTS Flavonoids, tannins, bitter iridoids, volatile oil, minerals
ACTIONS Relaxing and restorative nervine, sedative, antispasmodic, mild bitter

HOW TO USE

INFUSION Drink 1 cup (1–2 tsp dry herb per cup of boiling water) 3 times daily for nervous exhaustion, excitability, anxiety, or stress. In cases of insomnia, drink 1 cup (1–2 tsp herb per cup of boiling water) before bedtime for a soothing tea to ease tensions at the end of the working day or to ease emotional upsets associated with premenstrual syndrome.
TINCTURE Take 20–40 drops (1–2 ml) in a little water 3 times daily for nervous tension, stress, anxiety, or associated headaches.
TABLETS/CAPSULES Commercially available, and often combining skullcap with passionflower. Follow dosage directions on the package and use for anxiety and stress.

HOW TO SOURCE

GROW Prefers moist but well-drained soil in sun or partial shade. Sow seeds in fall or spring in seed trays and transplant to 3 in (7.5 cm) pots when large enough to handle. Grow until well established before planting in their final positions. Alternatively, divide plants in spring. Self-seeds enthusiastically and can become invasive.
FORAGE Found in hedges or riverbanks in the US and Canada; likely elsewhere only in isolated groups that may have self-seeded in grass verges or hedges from neighboring herb gardens. Common skullcap (*Scutellaria galericulata*) can be used in similar ways and is likely to be found along riverbanks or in fens.
HARVEST Cut while flowering and dry immediately; the aerial parts will contain both flowers and seed pods.

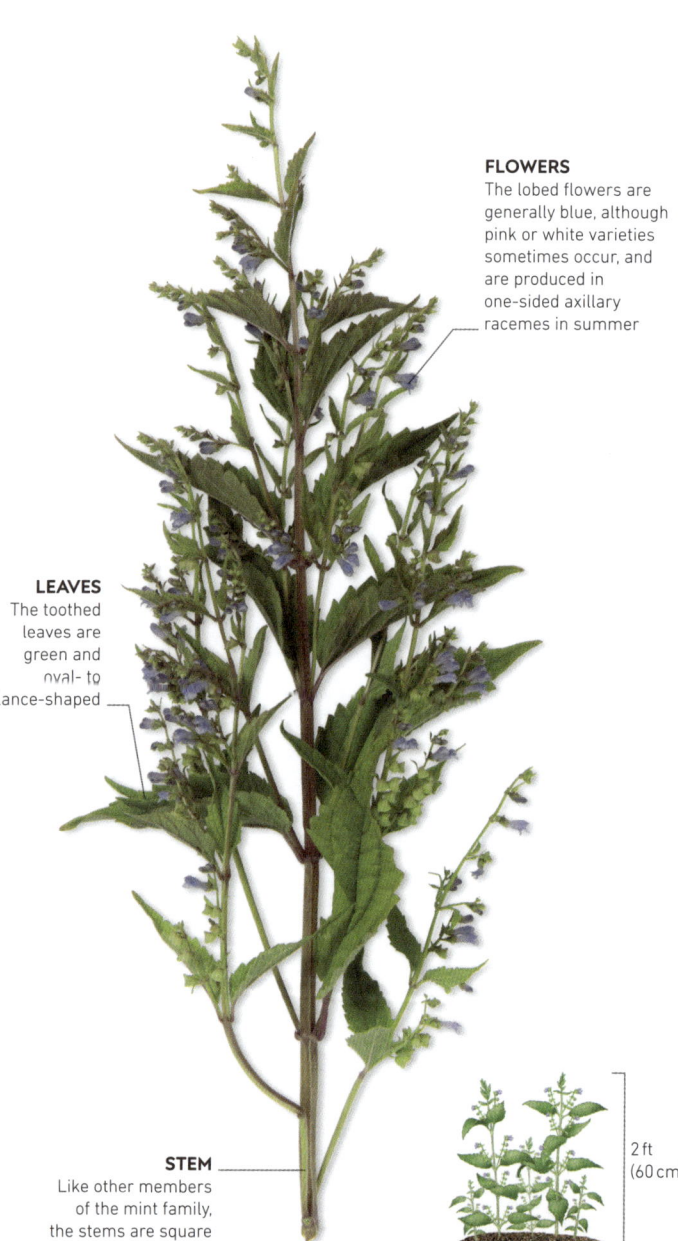

FLOWERS
The lobed flowers are generally blue, although pink or white varieties sometimes occur, and are produced in one-sided axillary racemes in summer

LEAVES
The toothed leaves are green and oval- to lance-shaped

STEM
Like other members of the mint family, the stems are square

2 ft (60 cm)

GROWTH HABIT
Herbaceous perennial spreading to 8 in (45 cm), often with blue flowers.

Senna alexandrina
SENNA

Native to Egypt, Sudan, Somalia, and Arabia, senna was used in the 9th century by Arabian physicians as a cathartic, or strong laxative. Its use soon spread, and both pods and leaves are still used as laxatives. The leaves are known as *fan xie ye* in traditional Chinese medicine, while their Indian name, *rajavriksha*, translates as "king of trees."

PARTS USED Leaves, pods
MAIN CONSTITUENTS Anthraquinone glycosides (incl. sennosides, dianthrone diglycosides) polysaccharides, mucilage, flavonoids (incl. kaempferol), salicylic acid
ACTIONS Stimulating laxative, antibacterial, anthelmintic, cooling

HOW TO USE

INFUSION For constipation, soak 3–6 pods (15–30 mg) in 1 cup of warm water and drink last thing at night. Add a slice of fresh ginger root or 1 tsp of fennel seeds to combat griping pains caused by an increase in bowel movement. Use half the adult dose for children over 10 years.
FLUID EXTRACT Take 5–10 drops (¼–½ml) of senna leaf extract in a little water at night for constipation.
TINCTURE Take 10–30 drops (½–1½ml) in a little water at night for constipation.
TABLETS/POWDERS Take 1–2 tsp of granules or 2–4 tablets at night for occasional constipation.

HOW TO SOURCE

GROW Prefers rich, moist, sandy soil in full sun. Requires a minimum of 41°F (5°C) to grow, but can be grown in containers in cooler regions. Sow seeds in spring and transplant to containers or final growing positions when well established, or take semi-ripe cuttings in spring.
FORAGE Unlikely to be found growing wild outside its native habitat.
HARVEST Pick leaves before and during flowering; gather pods in fall when ripe.

LEAVES
Hand-collected senna leaves are known as Tinnevelly senna, while leaves that have been harvested and graded mechanically are called Alexandria senna

The hairy, divided leaves are used in Ayurveda for constipation following fevers. They have a stronger action than the pods, so are less commonly used

STEM
The stem is branched, erect, and pale green

36 in
(90 cm)

GROWTH HABIT
Low-branching, shrubby perennial with small yellow flowers in spring; spread 20–24 in (50–60 cm).

CAUTION Can cause abdominal cramps. Do not take in cases of inflammatory bowel disease (such as Crohn's disease or ulcerative colitis), or if pregnant or breastfeeding. Avoid in intestinal obstruction. Excessive use can cause diarrhea and can damage the colon. Do not take leaf extracts or infusions for more than seven days at a time and take a break of at least two weeks before repeating the treatment.

Serenoa repens
SAW PALMETTO

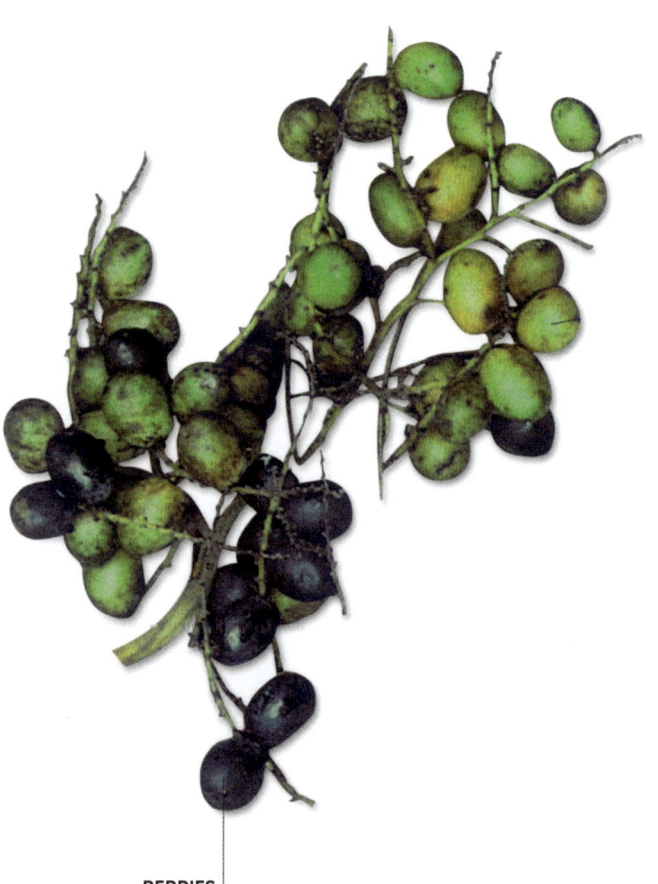

BERRIES
Used to treat urinary
disorders, the fresh
berries are said to taste
a little like blue cheese

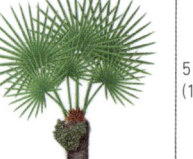

5 ft
(1.5 m)

GROWTH HABIT
Waxy, evergreen, sharp-
toothed spines with a flat
edge, palm-shape leaves;
spread 5 ft (1.5 m). It
has a horizontal
creeping stem.

Native Americans have used saw palmetto for centuries to treat a wide range of conditions, including poor digestion, colds, male baldness, benign prostatic hyperplasia (BPH), and low libido. Historically, it has been used to treat urinary infections, and recent studies show success in treating polycystic ovaries and hirsutism in women by inhibiting the elevation of androgen levels that contribute to these conditions.

PARTS USED Fruit
MAIN CONSTITUENTS Volatile oil, steroids and fixed oils (found in the seed resin), dextrose, enzymes
ACTIONS Anti-inflammatory, antiprostatic, diuretic, male tonic, urinary antiseptic, spasmolytic

HOW TO USE

FRESH BERRIES Eat 4–5 fresh berries raw like olives (take care, as they do contain pips).
DECOCTION Simmer ½–1 tsp (1–3 g) of dried fruit in 1 pint (600 ml) of water for 15 minutes (p.176) and take ½–1 cup 2–3 times daily as a urinary antiseptic.
TINCTURE Take 40 drops–1 tsp (2–5 ml) twice daily to improve symptoms of BPH and urinary infections such as cystitis.
CAPSULES Take 325–480 mg of a 10:1 liposterolic saw palmetto extract twice daily for 4–6 weeks for to treat frequent urination and prostate enlargement.

HOW TO SOURCE

GROW Seeds prefer sandy soil but sometimes take years to germinate. They can be activated by fire and usually flourish in fire-prone environments. Root cuttings planted in well-drained soil in full sun or partial shade can be easier to grow. The plant is a low, slow-growing palm, growing only 1 in (2.5 cm) a year.
FORAGE Plants can be found in southeast America, particularly from South Carolina to Florida, in a wide variety of habitats, including swamps, prairies, and sand dunes. It is important to note that it is illegal to harvest without a written permit from the landowner or local authority.
HARVEST Fruits are collected when partly dried, like a prune, from August to January. Wear gloves, as the leaves are razor-sharp, and shake berries from the stem into a container.

CAUTION May interfere with blood-thinning medication; seek professional advice before using.

Silybum marianum
MILK THISTLE

Native to stony areas in the Mediterranean region and southwest Asia, milk thistle is also known as Mary thistle, as the white veins on its leaves are reputedly due to splashes of the Virgin Mary's milk falling on them while she fed the Christ child. Although it encourages milk flow, it is probably now better known for its liver-protective qualities.

PARTS USED Seeds, leaves, flower heads
MAIN CONSTITUENTS Flavolignans (incl. silymarin), bitters, polyacetylenes
ACTIONS Bitter tonic, cholagogue, antiviral, choleretic, antidepressant, antioxidant, galactagogue, liver protector

HOW TO USE

TINCTURE Take 20–50 drops of the seed tincture with a little water 3 times daily for piles, liver and gall bladder problems, or to stimulate the digestion. Take up to 1 tsp (5 ml) daily in water as a preventative if you have a history of gallstones or liver disease. Treatment of gallstones requires professional advice.
CAPSULES Regular use of milk thistle capsules may help in the treatment of liver diseases.
INFUSION Drink 1–2 cups of a standard leaf infusion (p.176) daily to stimulate milk production when breastfeeding. The infusion can be used to stimulate a sluggish digestion.
DECOCTION Take ½ cup of a standard decoction (p.176) of the cracked seeds daily for liver disorders, including infections.

HOW TO SOURCE

GROW Prefers full sun in poor to moderately fertile soil that is well drained and neutral to alkaline. Sow seeds where you want to grow them in spring for annual growth or in late summer or early fall for flowers the following year. Thin to at least 18 in (45 cm) between plants.
FORAGE May be found in hedgerows and waste areas in many parts of Europe, North and East Africa, and western Asia. The flower heads can be cooked and eaten as a vegetable (rather like globe artichoke), the young leaves are used as a spinach substitute, and the root tastes rather like salsify.
HARVEST Collect the seeds in late summer; other parts of the plant can be gathered for culinary use during the summer.

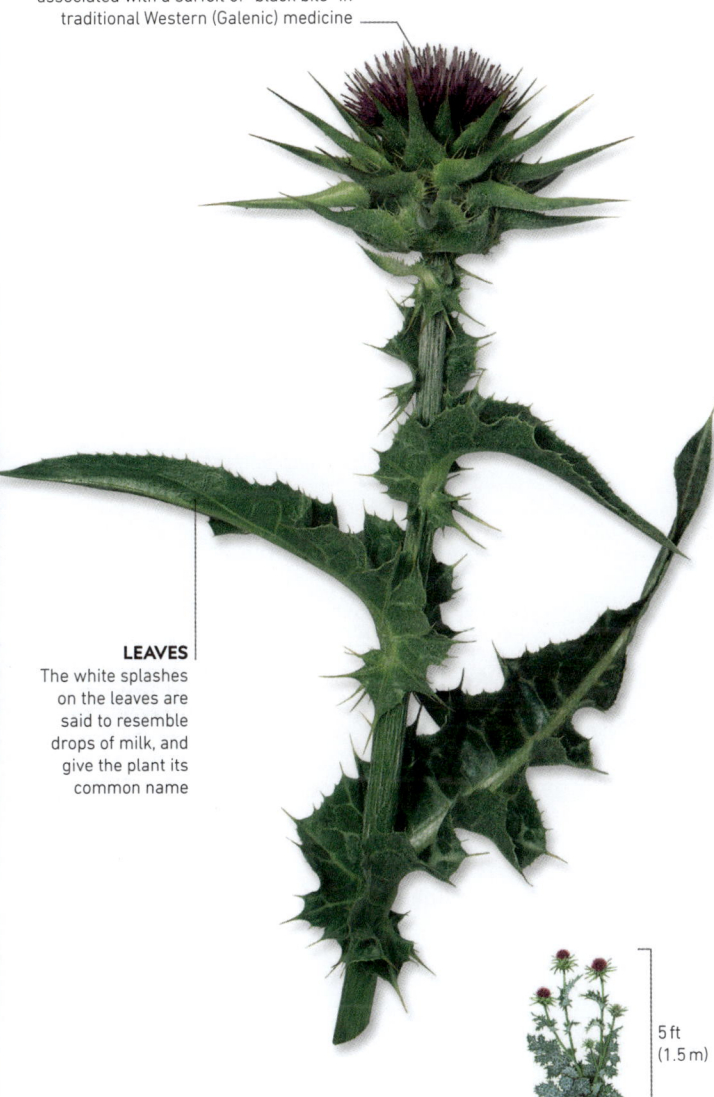

FLOWER HEADS
The flower heads, which can be boiled and eaten as a vegetable, were once taken for "melancholia" a condition associated with a surfeit of "black bile" in traditional Western (Galenic) medicine

LEAVES
The white splashes on the leaves are said to resemble drops of milk, and give the plant its common name

5 ft
(1.5 m)

GROWTH HABIT
Biennial with spiny green leaves marbled with white; spread 24–36 in (60–90 cm).

Stellaria media
CHICKWEED

Found throughout Europe and Asia, chickweed has long been used as a soothing and healing remedy for skin problems and wounds. Regarded by many as a weed, it is a favorite food for chickens—as the name implies—and other small birds: in the 16th century it was regularly fed to caged linnets.

PARTS USED Aerial parts
MAIN CONSTITUENTS Mucilage, saponins, coumarins, minerals, vitamins A, B, and C
ACTIONS Astringent, antirheumatic, wound herb, demulcent, emollient, mild laxative

HOW TO USE

INFUSED OIL Fill a jar with fresh chickweed and cover completely with sunflower oil; steep for 2 weeks, then strain and use on eczema and irritant skin rashes—or add 5 tsp (25 ml) to bath water for eczema sufferers.
CREAM/OINTMENT Use regularly on itching skin rashes and eczema. Can also soothe minor burns and be used to draw out thorns and splinters—put a little on the embedded splinter, cover with an adhesive bandage, and leave overnight; the next morning the splinter can usually be found on the bandage pad.
INFUSION Take 1 cup of a standard infusion (p.176) 3 times daily for muscular rheumatism, urinary tract inflammations, or whenever a cooling and cleansing remedy is required.
POULTICE Apply the crushed, fresh plant on gauze or in a muslin bag for boils, abscesses, skin sores, or gout.

HOW TO SOURCE

GROW Prefers moist soil and full sun, but will tolerate many conditions. Sow seeds directly at any time. Usually regarded as a weed, but worth growing as a useful source of food for domestic chickens.
FORAGE Generally found in hedgerows, ditches, waste areas, or grassy areas. Cut the aerial parts as required through the growing period. Chickweed can be sweated like spinach as a vegetable and served with butter.
HARVEST Can be cut throughout the growing period and used fresh or dried.

FLOWER BUDS
The buds open into the star-shaped flowers that give the plant its botanical name, *Stellaria*, from the Latin, *stella*, meaning "star"

LEAVES
The plant and its leaves are a useful source of vitamin C, and can be eaten in salads or cooked as a vegetable

16 in
(40 cm)

GROWTH HABIT
Spreading annual weed with small, white, star-shaped flowers; spread 2–16 in (5–40 cm).

CAUTION If taken in excess, it may cause nausea and vomiting.

Symphytum officinale
COMFREY

Growing throughout Europe, comfrey has been used to heal broken bones since ancient times. In the 1970s, it became popular as a remedy for arthritis when taken internally, which led to extensive animal studies using the plant and a realization that the alkaloids it contains may cause liver cancer. Since then it has been banned in a number of countries.

PARTS USED Aerial parts, root
MAIN CONSTITUENTS Mucilage, steroidal saponins (root), allantoin, vitamin B12, tannin, pyrrolizidine alkaloids, rosmarinic acid
ACTIONS Cell proliferator, astringent, demulcent, anti-inflammatory, expectorant, wound herb

HOW TO USE

MACERATED OIL Use night and morning to massage arthritic joints, sprains, bruises, and other traumatic injuries.
OINTMENT Use on clean cuts and grazes, or on skin sores such as diaper rash. Also useful for boils, acne, and psoriasis.
POULTICE Use pureed leaves as a poultice for minor breaks (broken toes, etc) not normally set in plaster. Make a paste with powdered root and a little water, and use on varicose ulcers, stubborn wounds, or bleeding piles.
COMPRESS Apply a pad soaked in a standard decoction of the root to bruises and sprains.

HOW TO SOURCE

GROW Prefers moist soil in a sunny or partially shaded site. Can be propagated from seed sown in fall or spring, by root division in spring, or root cuttings in winter. Does not tolerate dry winters. Once established, it can be difficult to eradicate.
FORAGE Usually found in damp field borders or hedgerows. When not in flower, the plant can be confused with foxglove.
HARVEST Gather leaves and flowering tops in summer and roots in fall.

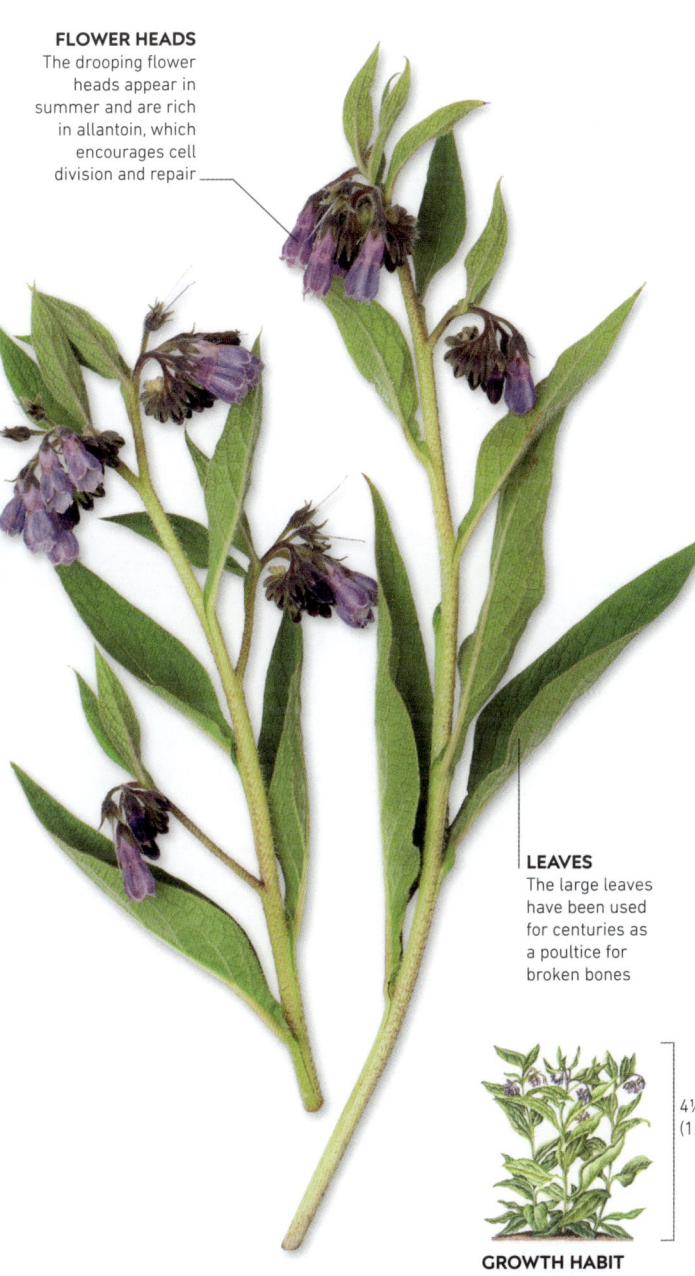

FLOWER HEADS
The drooping flower heads appear in summer and are rich in allantoin, which encourages cell division and repair

LEAVES
The large leaves have been used for centuries as a poultice for broken bones

4½ ft (1.3 m)

GROWTH HABIT
Vigorous rhizomatous perennial spreading to 6 ft (2 m) or more.

CAUTION Avoid during pregnancy. Do not take comfrey internally; it contains compounds that may be carcinogenic when taken internally. Do not use on dirty wounds, as rapid healing may trap pus or dirt.

Tabebuia impetiginosa
PAU D'ARCO

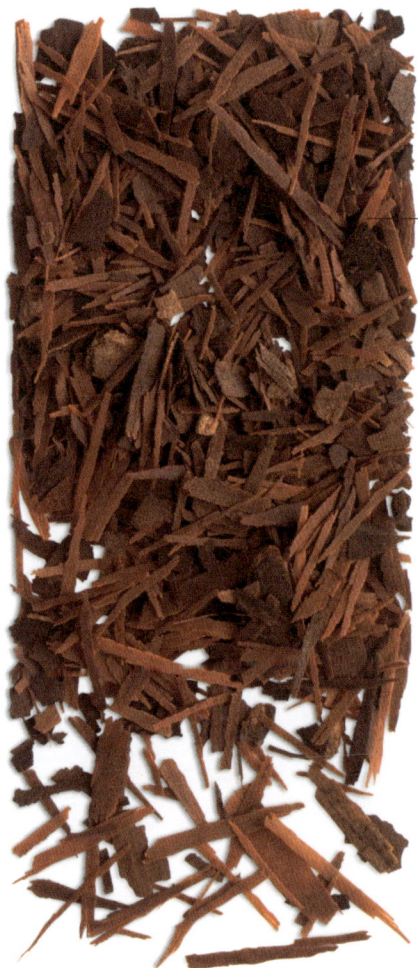

BARK
The pink-brown inner bark of the tree is peeled from the trunk in strips, and has a cocoa-like aroma

Used in traditional South American herbal medicine for more than a thousand years, and now widely planted throughout the tropics of South America, pau d'arco has renowned antibiotic and antifungal properties. It is used to treat the fungal infection candidiasis (the cause of thrush and athlete's foot, among other ailments), as well as weakened immunity, arthritis, and rheumatism.

PARTS USED Inner bark and leaves
MAIN CONSTITUENTS Quinones, flavonoids (incl. quercetin), steroidal saponins, alkaloids
ACTIONS Antiparasitic, anti-inflammatory, antifungal, immunostimulant, antimicrobial, antitumorous, antiviral

HOW TO USE

DECOCTION Take ½–1 cup of a decoction (p.176), made by heating ½ oz (15 g) of bark in 1 pint (600 ml) of water, 3 times daily to treat fever and a weakened immune system.
TINCTURE Take 40 drops–1 tsp (2–5 ml) in a little hot water 3 times daily to help reduce inflammation of skin infections or fungal disease.
POULTICE Soak a piece of gauze or cloth in a decoction to treat skin diseases such as eczema, psoriasis, or inflammatory conditions.
GARGLE/MOUTHWASH Use 1 cup of a standard decoction 2–3 times a day as a gargle for mouth, throat, or gum infections.
TABLETS/CAPSULES Take 2–4 x 500 mg tablets or capsules 1–2 times per day to reduce symptoms of arthritis and candidiasis.

HOW TO SOURCE

GROW Seeds prefer to grow in well-drained soil in tropical areas at 77–82°F (25–28°C). Keep seeds moist and plant in a permanent position in full sun or partial shade.
FORAGE Often grown in commercial plantations in tropical areas. However, take care to forage responsibly as the exploitation of this plant has led to significant decline in the wild.
HARVEST Inner bark is harvested all year round.

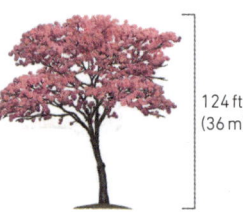

124 ft
(36 m)

GROWTH HABIT
A hardwood tree with purple flowers; spread 9 ft (3 m).

CAUTION Large doses may cause gastrointestinal upset or nausea.

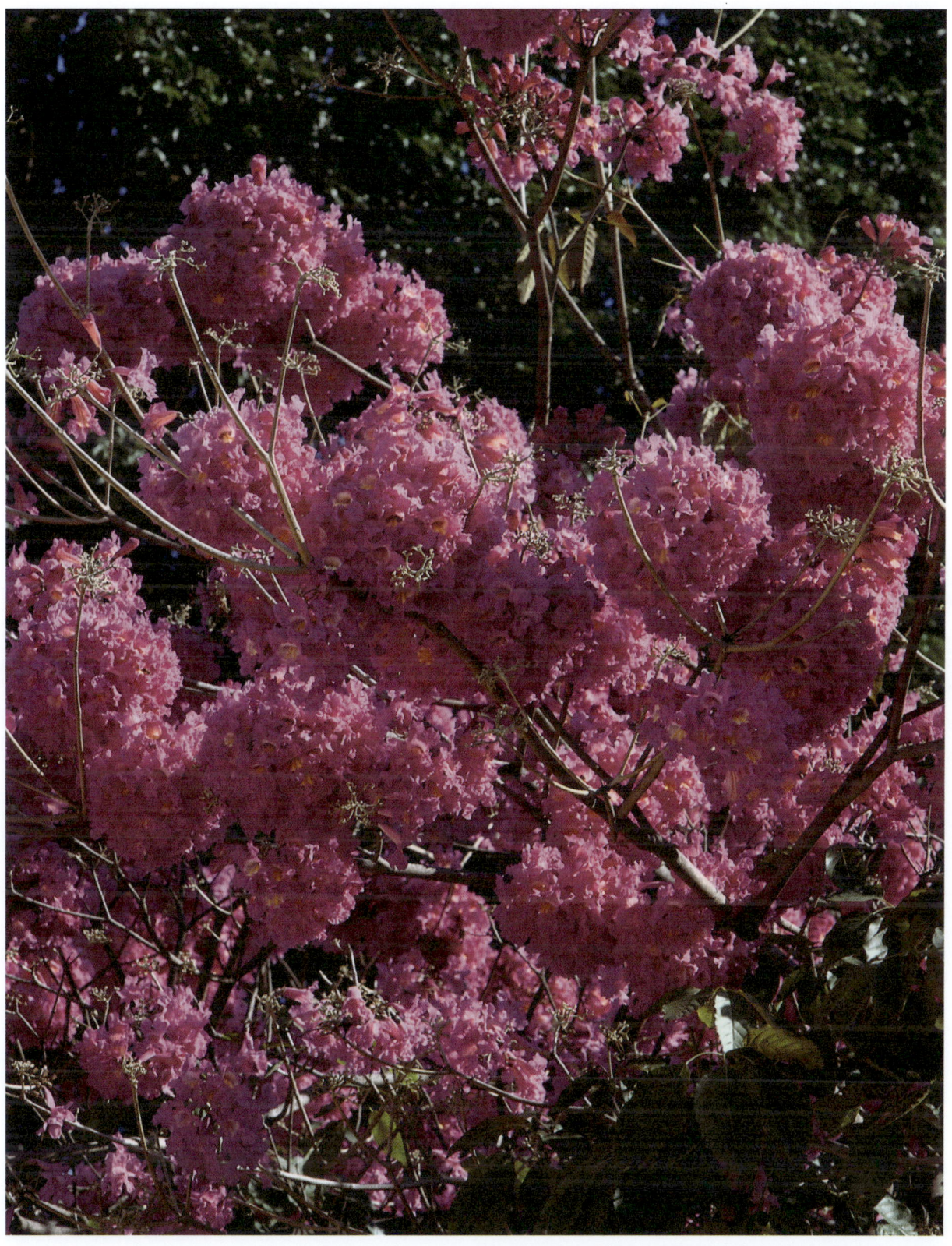

Tanacetum parthenium
FEVERFEW

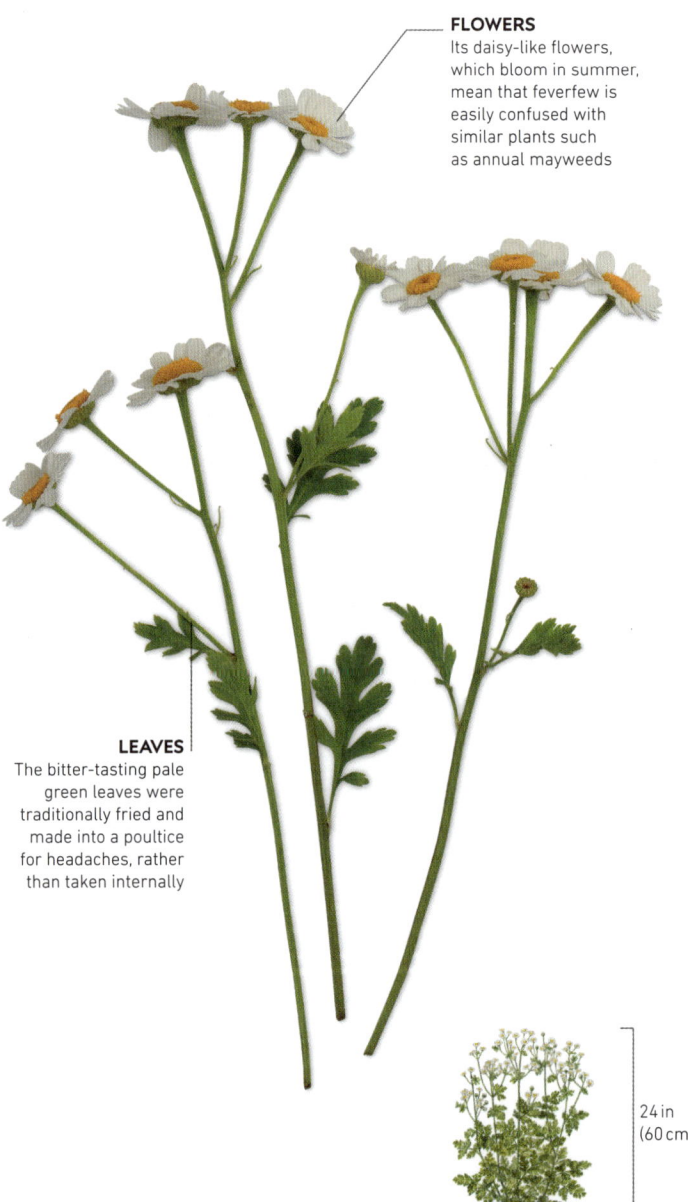

FLOWERS
Its daisy-like flowers, which bloom in summer, mean that feverfew is easily confused with similar plants such as annual mayweeds

LEAVES
The bitter-tasting pale green leaves were traditionally fried and made into a poultice for headaches, rather than taken internally

GROWTH HABIT
Short-lived, bushy perennial with deeply scalloped leaves and a spread of 24 in (60 cm).

24 in
(60 cm)

Found throughout northern temperate regions, feverfew is widely used today as a migraine remedy. Earlier herbalists thought of it as "a general strengthener of the womb" (Nicholas Culpeper, 1653). It has also traditionally been used to treat arthritis and rheumatism. Numerous cultivars have been developed as garden ornamentals.

PARTS USED Aerial parts
MAIN CONSTITUENTS Sesquiterpene lactones (parthenolide), volatile oil, pyrethrin, tannins, camphor
ACTIONS Anti-inflammatory, vasodilator, relaxant, digestive stimulant, emmenagogue, anthelmintic, bitter

HOW TO USE

TINCTURE Use 5–10 drops at 30-minute intervals at the onset of a migraine. It is most effective for preventing and treating "cold" type migraines involving vasoconstriction, which are eased by applying a hot towel to the head. For the acute stages of rheumatoid arthritis, add up to 40 drops (2 ml) 3 times a day to herbal remedies such as celery seed, white willow, or devil's claw (*Harpagophytum procumbens*).
POULTICE Fry a handful of leaves in a little oil and apply to the abdomen as a poultice for colicky pains.
INFUSION Drink 1–2 cups of a weak infusion made from ½ oz (15 g) of the aerial parts to 1 pint (600 ml) of water after childbirth to encourage cleansing and toning of the womb; take 1 cup 3 times daily for period pain associated with sluggish flow and congestion.

HOW TO SOURCE

GROW Prefers full sun and well-drained soil, but tolerates a range of conditions. Sow seeds in a propagator at 50–64.4°F (10–18°C) in late winter or early spring, or take softwood cuttings in early summer. A prolific self-seeder that can be invasive.
FORAGE Often found in hedgerows and waste places. Easily confused with other daisy-like plants; look for its characteristic leaves, which have a very bitter taste.
HARVEST Collect the leaves as required throughout the growing period and the whole plant in summer while flowering.

CAUTION Mouth ulcers can occur after eating the fresh leaves. Avoid if taking anticoagulant drugs such as warfarin. Avoid during pregnancy.

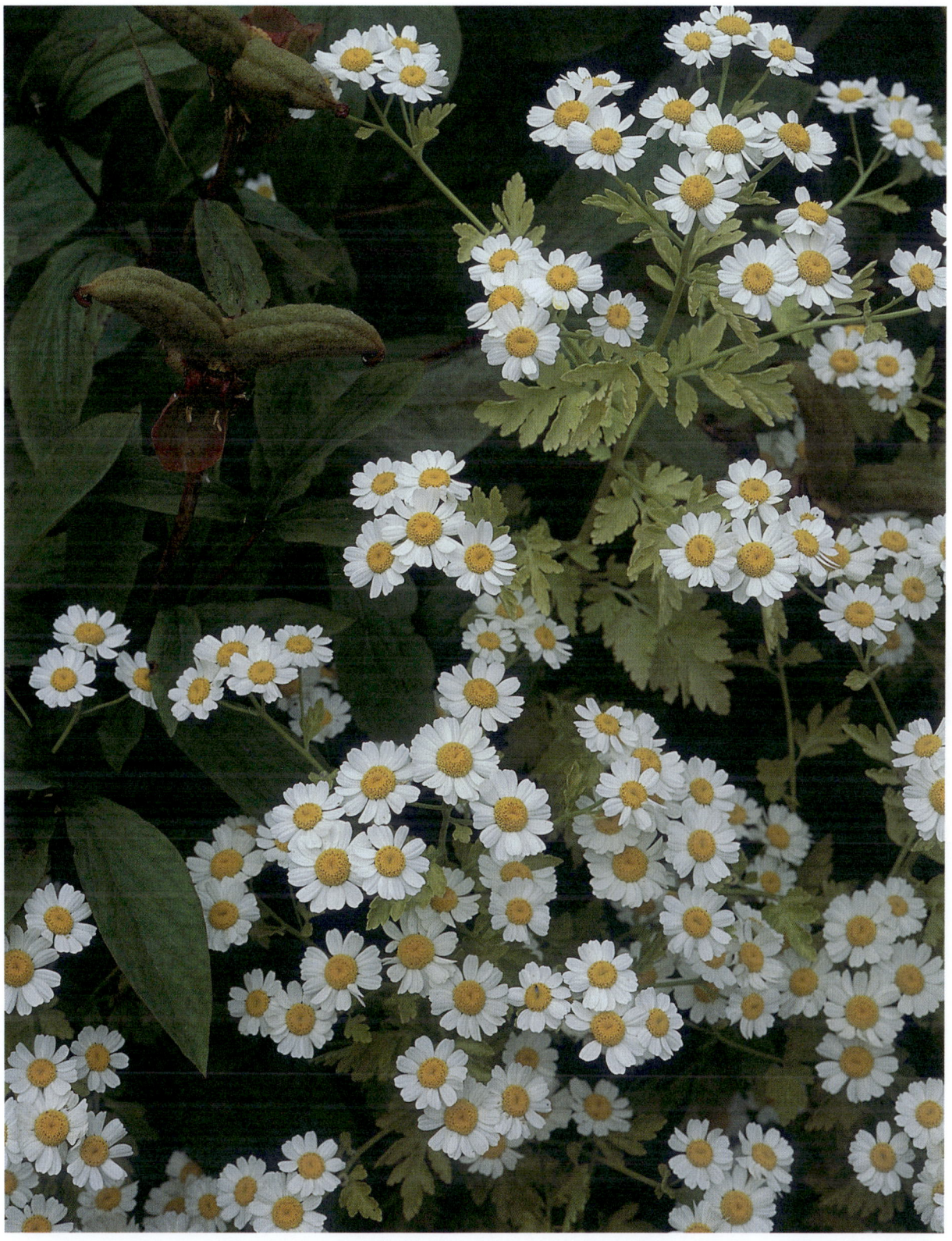

Taraxacum officinale
DANDELION

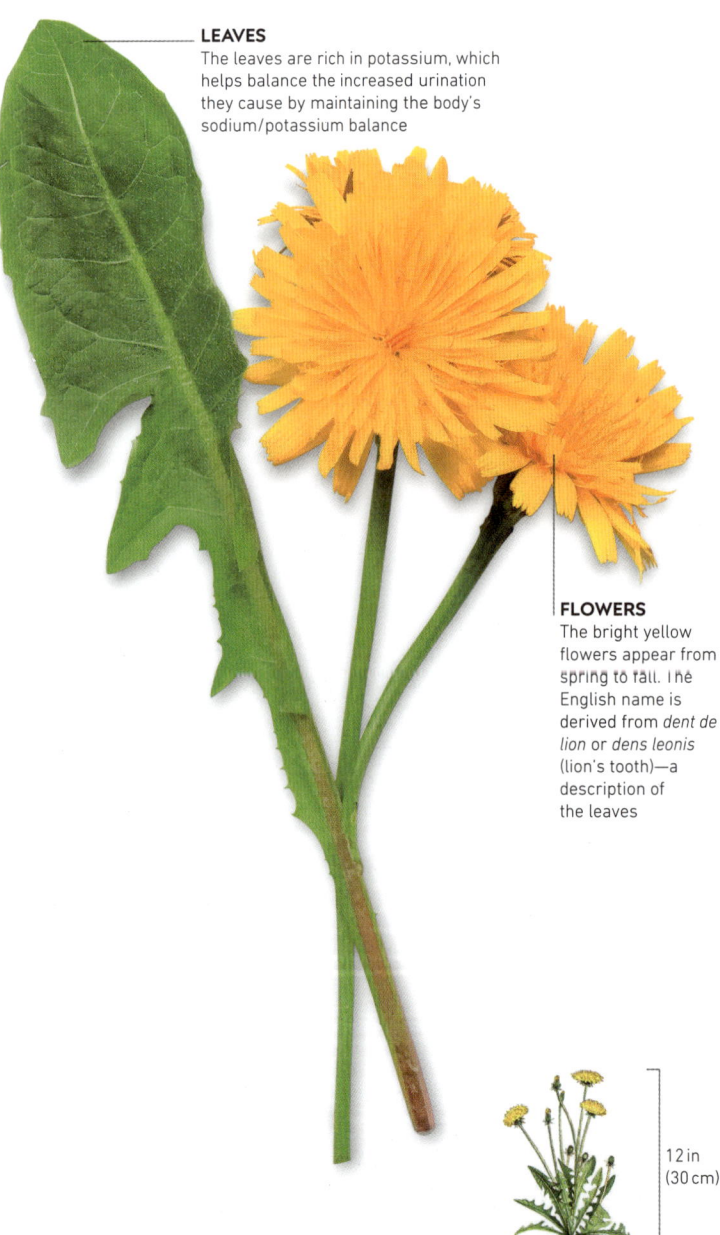

LEAVES
The leaves are rich in potassium, which helps balance the increased urination they cause by maintaining the body's sodium/potassium balance

FLOWERS
The bright yellow flowers appear from spring to fall. The English name is derived from *dent de lion* or *dens leonis* (lion's tooth)—a description of the leaves

GROWTH HABIT
Tap-rooted perennial; spread 18 in (45 cm).

12 in (30 cm)

Several species of dandelion are found throughout the temperate regions of Europe, Asia, and South America. The plant is a comparative newcomer to the medicinal repertoire, and was first mentioned in Arabic herbals in the 11th century, as a remedy to increase urination. The root, an effective liver tonic, was not used until much later.

PARTS USED Leaf, root
MAIN CONSTITUENTS Sesquiterpene lactones; vitamins A, B, C, D; choline; minerals (incl. potassium). Leaf only: coumarins, carotenoids, potassium Root only: taraxacoside, phenolic acids, iron
ACTIONS Diuretic, liver and digestive tonic, cholagogue, stimulates pancreas and bile duct, mild laxative (root only)

HOW TO USE

DECOCTION Put 2–3 tsp (5–10 ml) root into 1 cup of water and bring to a boil. Simmer for 10-15 minutes. Drink 1 cup 3 times daily for any condition—such as osteoarthritis, rheumatism, acne, and psoriasis—where liver stimulation and detoxification may help.
INFUSION Make an infusion (p.176) of 1 cup boiling water over 2 tsp dry leaves. Drink 1 cup 3 times daily to encourage urination in conditions such as cystitis, fluid retention, or high blood pressure.
JUICE Process the leaves in a juicer and take up to 4 tsp (20 ml) 3 times daily as a stronger alternative to the infusion.
TINCTURE Take 40 drops–1 tsp (2–5 ml) of combined root and leaf tincture 3 times daily to stimulate bile flow, act as a mild laxative, or help dissolve small gallstones.

HOW TO SOURCE

GROW Tolerates a wide range of soils and will grow in full sun or partial shade. Sow the seeds in spring. It self-seeds enthusiastically. The plant is also cultivated for salad leaves in parts of Europe.
FORAGE Found in many parts of the world growing in hedges, field borders, waste areas, and even in city pavement cracks. Avoid collecting plants where traffic pollution may be a problem.
HARVEST Gather young leaves for salads in the spring, and the larger leaves in summer for medicinal use. The two-year-old roots are collected in fall.

CAUTION If suffering from gallstones, only use dandelion root under professional supervision.

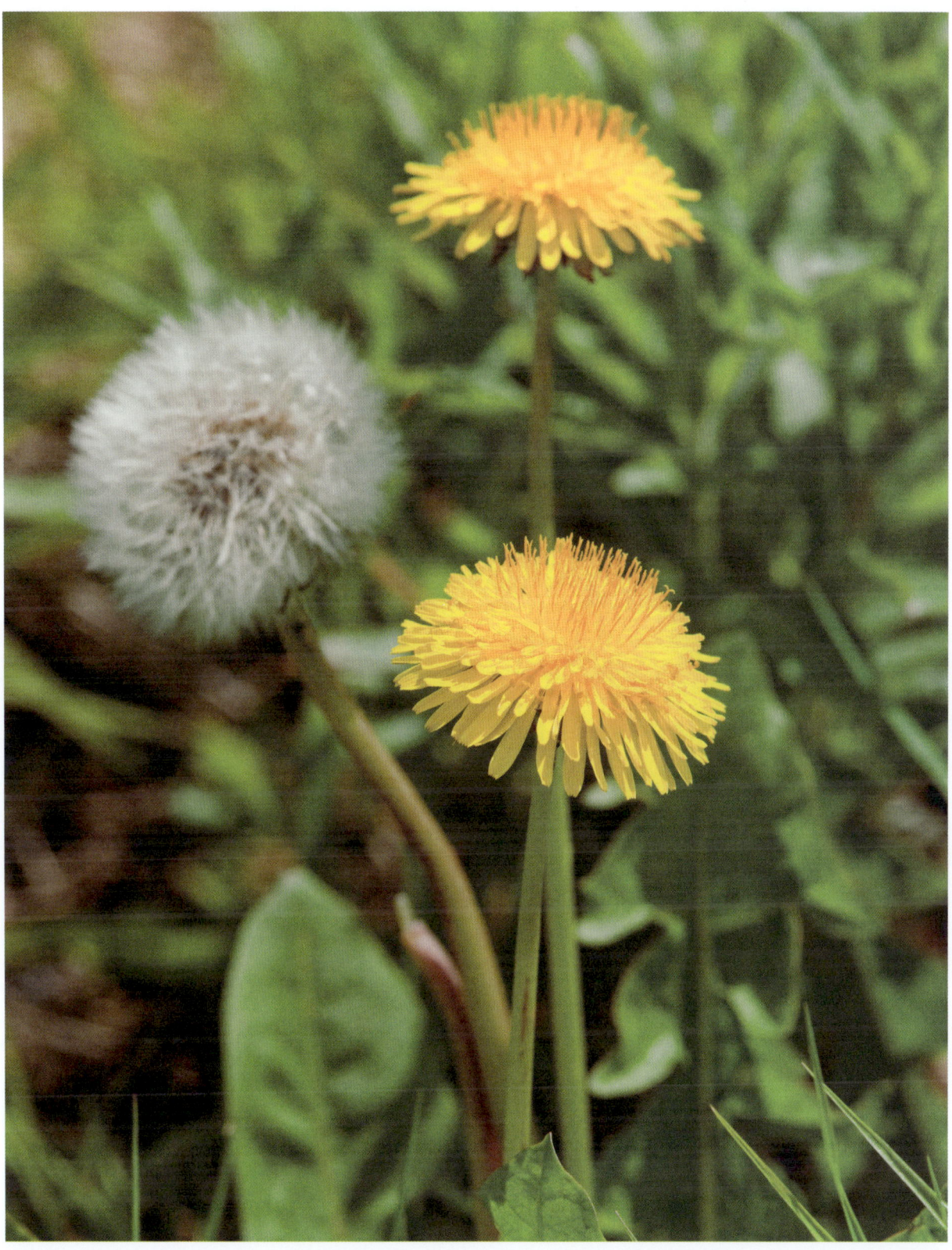

Thymus vulgaris
COMMON THYME

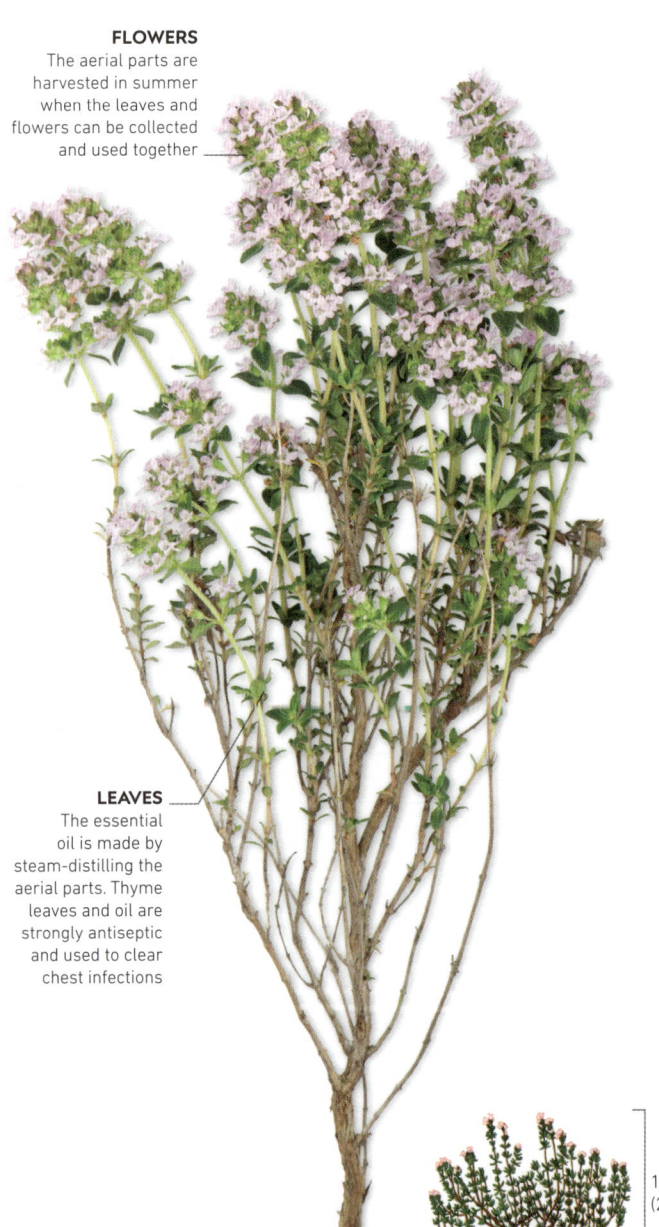

FLOWERS
The aerial parts are harvested in summer when the leaves and flowers can be collected and used together

LEAVES
The essential oil is made by steam-distilling the aerial parts. Thyme leaves and oil are strongly antiseptic and used to clear chest infections

10 in (25 cm)

GROWTH HABIT
Low-growing, evergreen, woody-based perennial; spread 16 in (40 cm).

Originating from the dry, grassy areas of southern Europe, thyme is now widely grown worldwide as a culinary herb. It is mainly used as an expectorant and antiseptic for the lungs to clear productive coughs and infections, while the essential oil is used in aromatherapy. Research in the 1990s also suggested antioxidant and anti-aging properties.

PARTS USED Aerial parts, essential oil
MAIN CONSTITUENTS Volatile oil (incl. thymol, cineole and borneol), flavonoids, bitter, tannins, saponins
ACTIONS Antiseptic expectorant, antispasmodic, antiseptic, astringent, antimicrobial, diuretic, antitussive, tonic, antibiotic, wound herb, topically rubefacient

HOW TO USE

INFUSION Drink 1 cup (2 tsp herb per cup boiling water) 3 times daily for colds, chest infections, mild asthma, hay fever, stomach chills, or irritable bowel syndrome.
SYRUP Add 1 lb (450 g) of honey to 1 pint (600 ml) of strained infusion (above) to make a syrup for coughs and chest infections. Take in 1 tsp (5 ml) doses as needed.
MOUTHWASH/GARGLE Use 1 cup of above infusion morning and night for gum disease and sore throats.
CHEST RUB/MASSAGE OIL Use 10 drops of thyme oil in 5 tsp (25 ml) of almond oil as a chest rub for bronchitis and infections. Use with an equal amount of lavender oil for rheumatic pains and strained muscles.
LOTION Dilute 20 drops (1 ml) of thyme oil in 2 fl oz (60 ml) of water and use for insect bites and infected wounds.

HOW TO SOURCE

GROW Prefers dry alkaline soil in full sun. Sow seeds in trays in a greenhouse or cold frame in spring, potted into 3 in (7.5 cm) pots when large enough to handle, and planted out when well established. Alternatively, take softwood cuttings in summer as flowering starts.
FORAGE Found in shrubby, rocky wasteland or dry grassland throughout Europe and Asia.
HARVEST Gather aerial parts in mid- to late summer, and sprigs for cooking throughout the growing period.

CAUTION Avoid therapeutic doses during pregnancy. Do not take the essential oil internally, and always use well diluted.

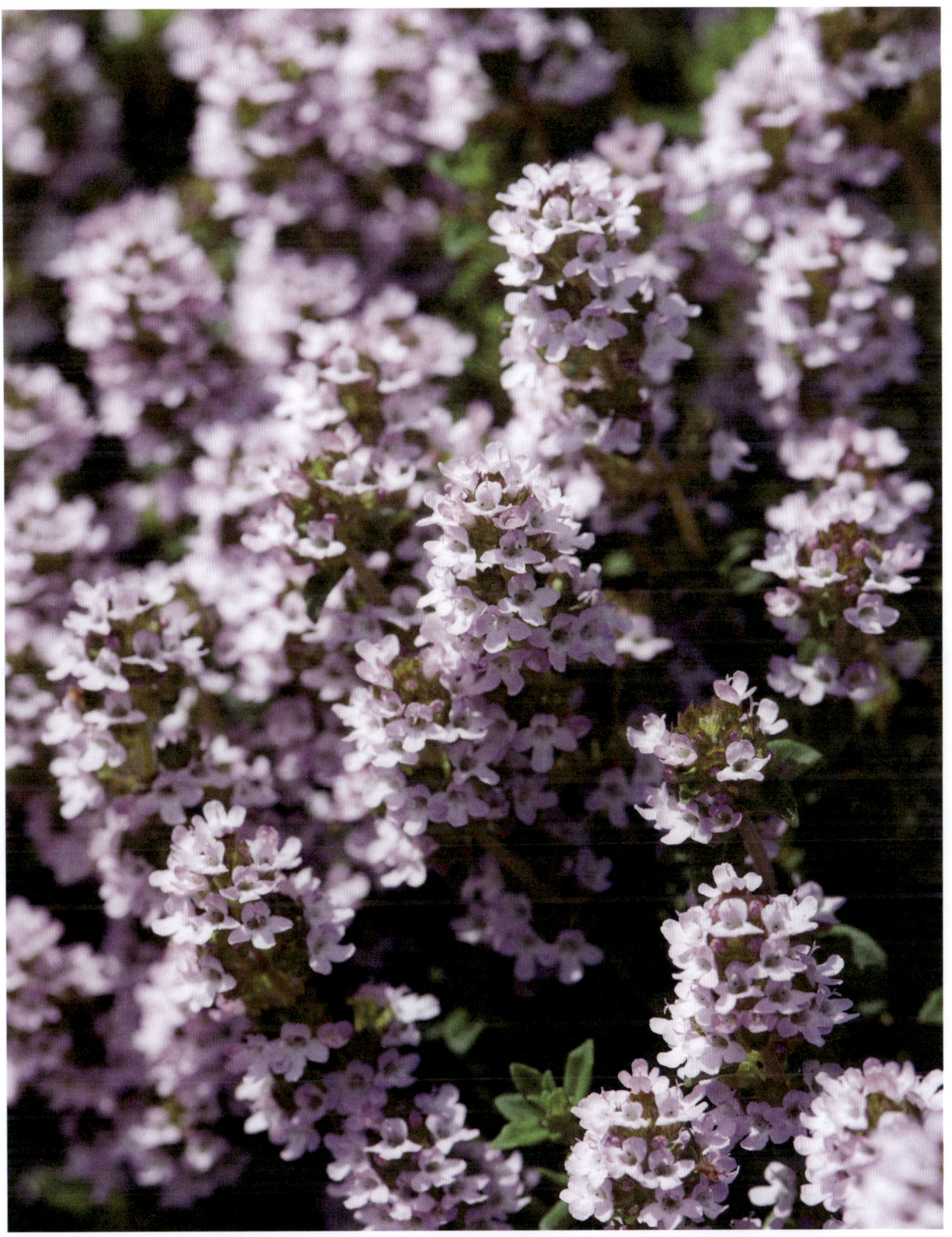

Tilia cordata
LINDEN

Native to central and eastern Europe, the linden, or lime tree, is popular in urban street plantings in many countries—perhaps most notably in the iconic avenue, the *Unter den Linden*, leading to the Brandenburg Gate in Berlin. The flowers are mainly used in sedative mixtures, although they can also be used in soothing lotions.

PARTS USED Flowers
MAIN CONSTITUENTS Flavonoids (incl. quercetin and kaempferol), caffeic acid, mucilage, tannins, volatile oil
ACTIONS Antispasmodic, diaphoretic, tonic, diuretic, sedative, hypotensive, anticoagulant

HOW TO USE

INFUSION Drink 1 cup (1 tsp herb per cup boiling water) up to 3 times daily to soothe tension or stress headaches, or to relieve colds, flu, and nasal catarrh. Commercial tea bags often combine linden with chamomile, or mix the dried flowers with equal amounts of lemon balm and chamomile and use 1–2 tsp of the dried mix in a cup of boiling water for a relaxing and calming tea.
TINCTURE Take 1 tsp (5 ml) of the tincture in water 3 times daily for high blood pressure associated with stress and anxiety or arteriosclerosis. Usually used n combination with other herbs such as valerian or hawthorn.
OINTMENT/LOTION Use as required for itching skin caused by rashes or insect bites.
CHILDREN'S TEA Can be used as a soothing remedy in the early stages of childhood infections such as flu, seasonal colds, or chicken pox. Consult an herbalist for advice on dosage.

HOW TO SOURCE

GROW Prefers fertile, moist, but well-drained soil that is neutral to alkaline. The seeds need to be stratified over winter and planted in a seed bed outside in the spring, but it can be slow to germinate. It is a large tree, so is not suitable for small or congested gardens.
FORAGE Lindens are found throughout Europe and in many other temperate zones, often as part of a street-planting scheme. The flowers can be collected in early to mid-summer, but it is best to avoid trees in high traffic areas to minimize pollution.
HARVEST Gather the flowers in midsummer. They can be collected with the sepals and crushed when dry.

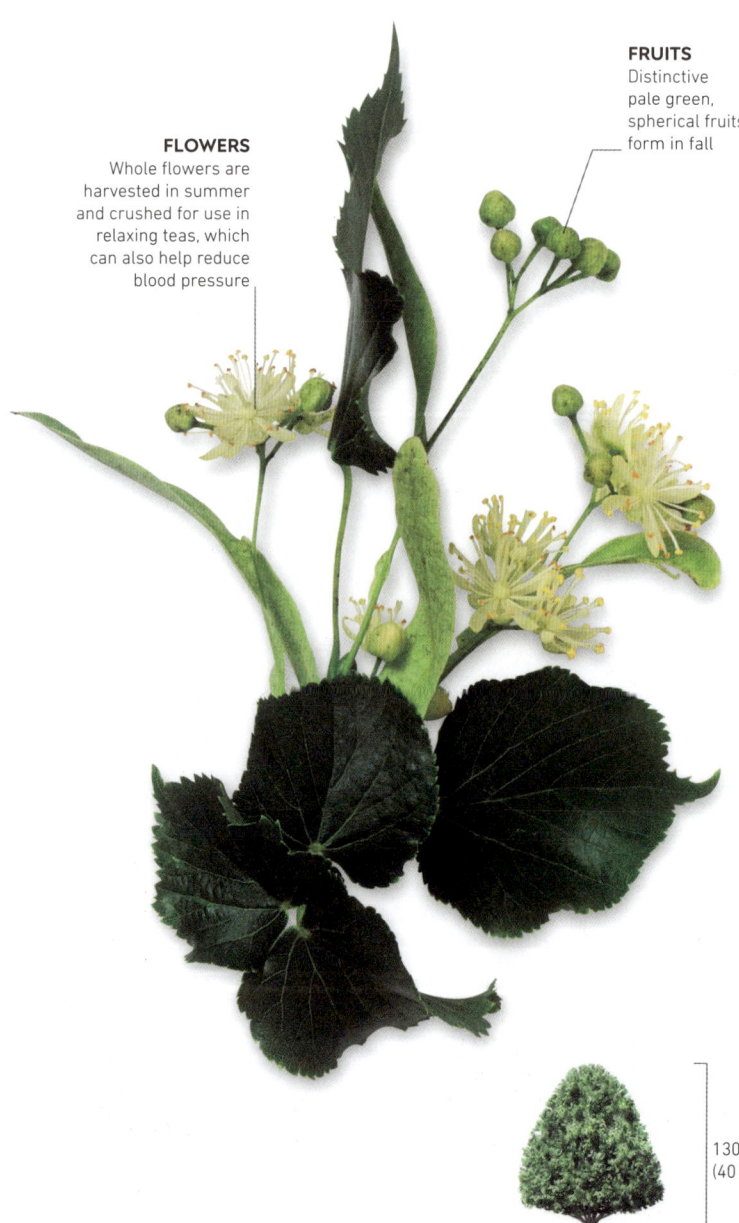

FLOWERS
Whole flowers are harvested in summer and crushed for use in relaxing teas, which can also help reduce blood pressure

FRUITS
Distinctive pale green, spherical fruits form in fall

130 ft
(40 m)

GROWTH HABIT
Medium–large columnar tree; spread 30–100 ft (10–30 m).

CAUTION Seek professional advice before taking for high blood pressure.

Trifolium pratense
RED CLOVER

Native to temperate regions of Europe and Asia, red clover is now naturalized in many parts of North America and Australia. The plant was known as "honey stalk," as children sucked the sweet sap from its stems. In the 1930s, it became popular for treating breast cancer. Today it is mainly used for coughs, skin problems, and menopausal symptoms.

PARTS USED Flower heads
MAIN CONSTITUENTS Flavonoids, salicylates, coumarins, phenolic glycosides, cyanogenic glycosides, volatile oil (incl. methyl salicylate and benzyl alcohol), sitosterol
ACTIONS Antispasmodic, diuretic, lymphatic cleanser, possible estrogenic activity, expectorant, sedative

HOW TO USE

INFUSION Make an infusion (p.176) of 1 cup boiling water over 1–3 tsp (5–15 ml). Drink 1 cup 3 times daily for coughs, menopausal problems, or for skin problems.
SYRUP Make a standard infusion (see above) and use 1 pint (600 ml) to make a syrup with 1 lb (450 g) of honey. Take in 1 tsp (5 ml) doses as required for stubborn coughs, especially whooping cough or bronchitis.
MOUTHWASH/GARGLE Use 1 cup of a standard infusion (see above) for mouth ulcers and sore throats.
TINCTURE Take 1–2 tsp (5–10 ml) 3 times daily for eczema, psoriasis, and old sores that are slow to heal. Combines well with heartsease for childhood eczema.
CREAM/OINTMENT Use frequently for lymphatic swellings.
FRESH HERB Use the crushed flowers directly on insect bites and stings.

HOW TO SOURCE

GROW Prefers moderate summer temperatures and adequate moisture throughout the growing period. Scatter seeds where you want them to grow in late winter or early spring, and then cover with a light dusting of good compost.
FORAGE Widely cultivated as a fodder crop and as part of a crop-rotation program, red clover can be found growing in many parts of the world. Look for it growing in hedges and meadows and collect the flower heads when they are newly opened.
HARVEST Gather throughout the summer, choosing newly opened flower heads.

CAUTION Avoid during pregnancy.

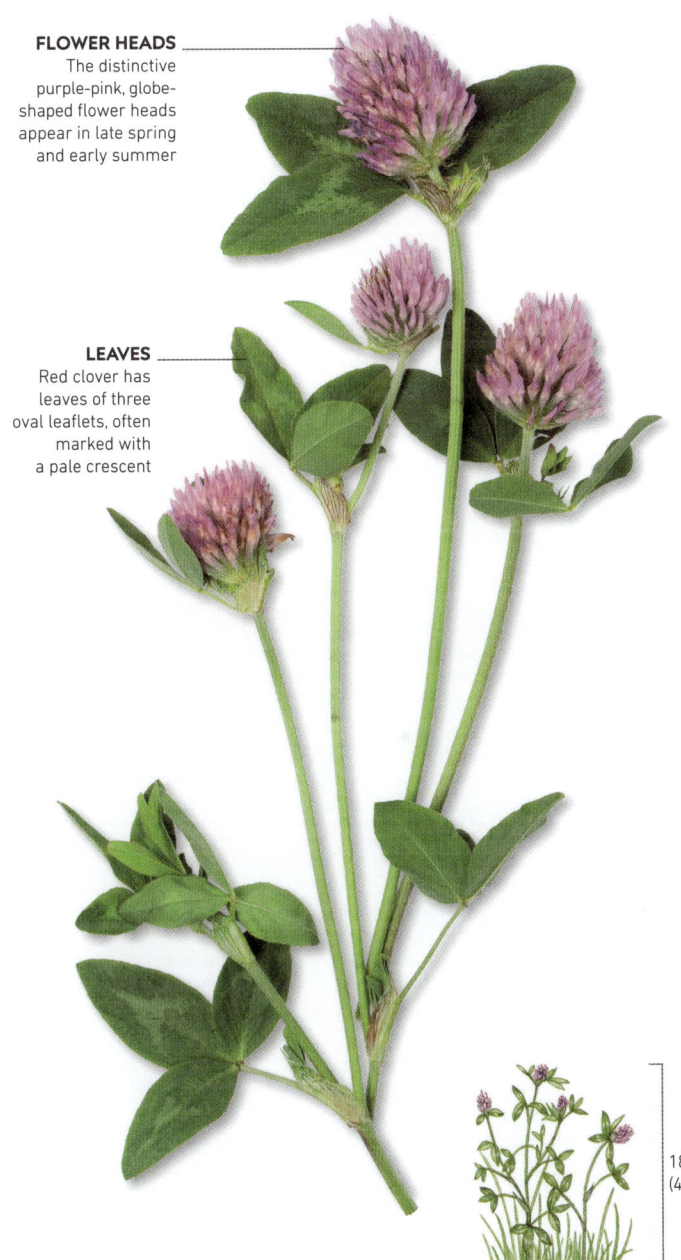

FLOWER HEADS
The distinctive purple-pink, globe-shaped flower heads appear in late spring and early summer

LEAVES
Red clover has leaves of three oval leaflets, often marked with a pale crescent

18 in (45 cm)

GROWTH HABIT
Biennial or perennial; spread 18 in (45 cm).

Tropaeolum majus
NASTURTIUM

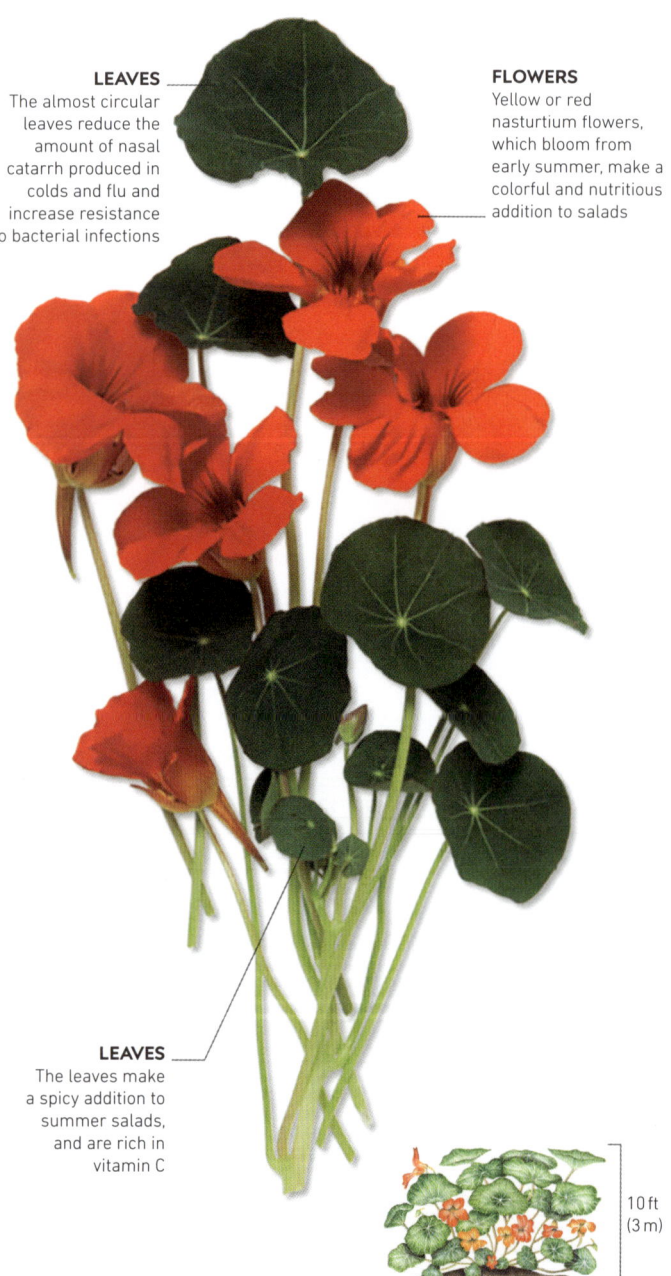

LEAVES
The almost circular leaves reduce the amount of nasal catarrh produced in colds and flu and increase resistance to bacterial infections

FLOWERS
Yellow or red nasturtium flowers, which bloom from early summer, make a colorful and nutritious addition to salads

LEAVES
The leaves make a spicy addition to summer salads, and are rich in vitamin C

GROWTH HABIT
Fast-growing trailing annual with a spread of 5–6 ft (1.5–2 m).

10 ft (3 m)

Originally found in the Andes from Bolivia to Colombia, nasturtiums have now spread worldwide as a popular and easy-to-grow garden ornamental. They naturalize readily and are classified as an invasive weed in New Zealand and other areas. Valued both as an antiseptic and respiratory remedy, the flowers and seeds also have many culinary uses.

PARTS USED Flowers, leaves, seeds
MAIN CONSTITUENTS Glucocyanates, spilanthol, myrosin, mineral salts (incl. iodine, iron, and phosphates), oxalic acid, vitamin C
ACTIONS Antibiotic, antitussive, diuretic, expectorant

HOW TO USE

INFUSION Drink 1 cup (1–2 tsp leaves per cup of boiling water) 3 times daily to increase resistance to bacterial infection; also effective for clearing catarrh due to colds and flu.
TINCTURE Take 1–2 tsp (5–10 ml) of a leaf tincture 3 times daily for colds, influenza, and dry coughs.
JUICE Pulp the whole plant in a food processor or juicer and take 4 tsp (20 ml) 3 times daily in a little milk for chronic lung conditions such as emphysema; the juice rubbed into the scalp is said to stimulate hair growth in alopecia.
LOTION Use 1 cup of above infusion of the leaves as an antiseptic wash for cuts and scrapes.
FRESH LEAVES AND FLOWERS Add both to salads—the leaves have a spicy flavor and are rich in vitamin C.

HOW TO SOURCE

GROW Nasturtiums will grow almost anywhere, but prefer well-drained soil and a sunny site. A rich soil encourages leaf growth rather than flowers. Sow the seeds where you want to grow them in early summer, or plant in trays in mid-spring at 55–61°F (13–16°C) and transplant when all danger of frost has passed.
FORAGE An invasive weed in some parts of the world, in temperate zones they may be found in urban areas outside gardens as self-seeded plants. Gather the flowers as required and the whole plant in late summer for use in tinctures.
HARVEST Gather leaves and flowers as required for salads, or the whole plant in summer for drying.

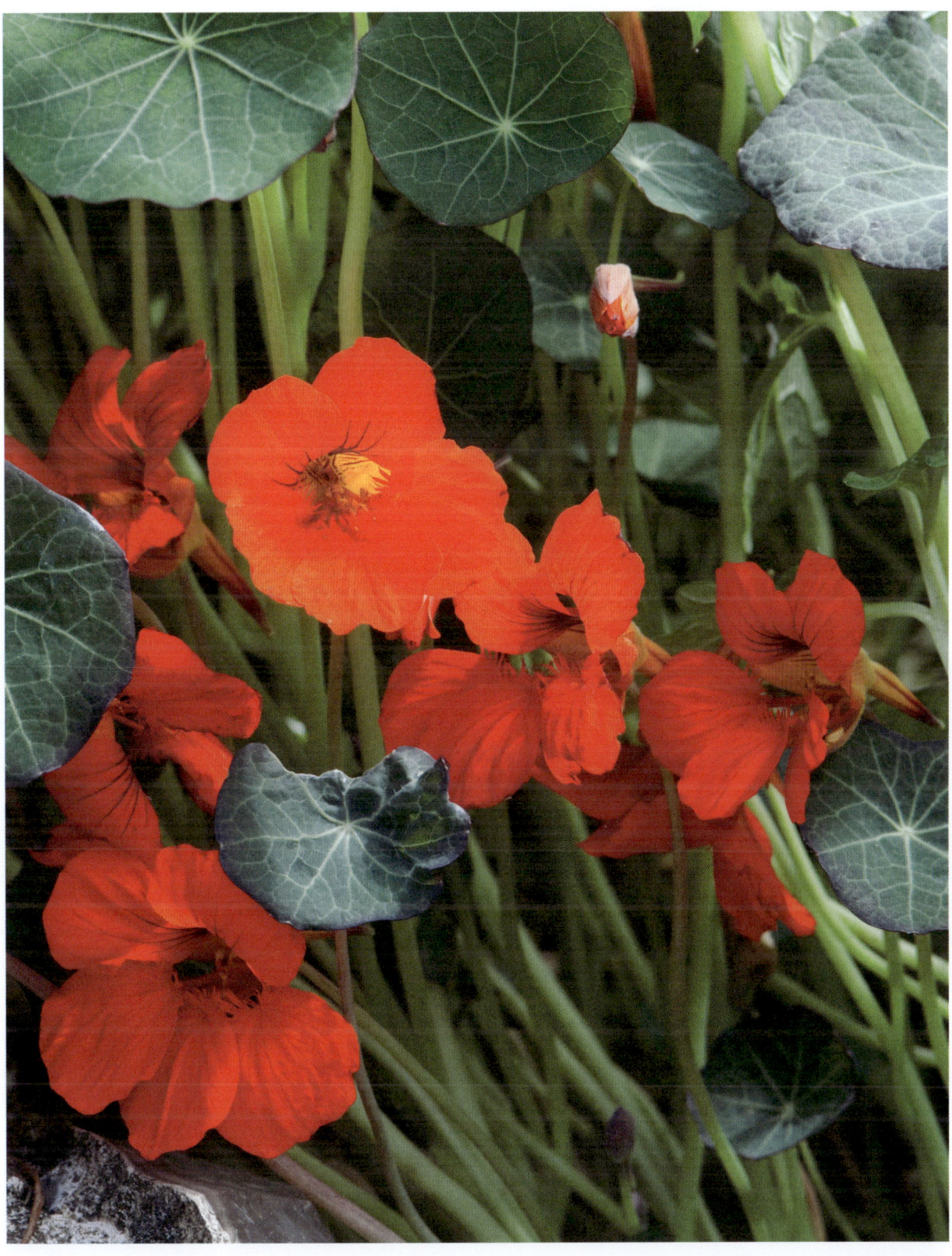

Turnera diffusa
DAMIANA

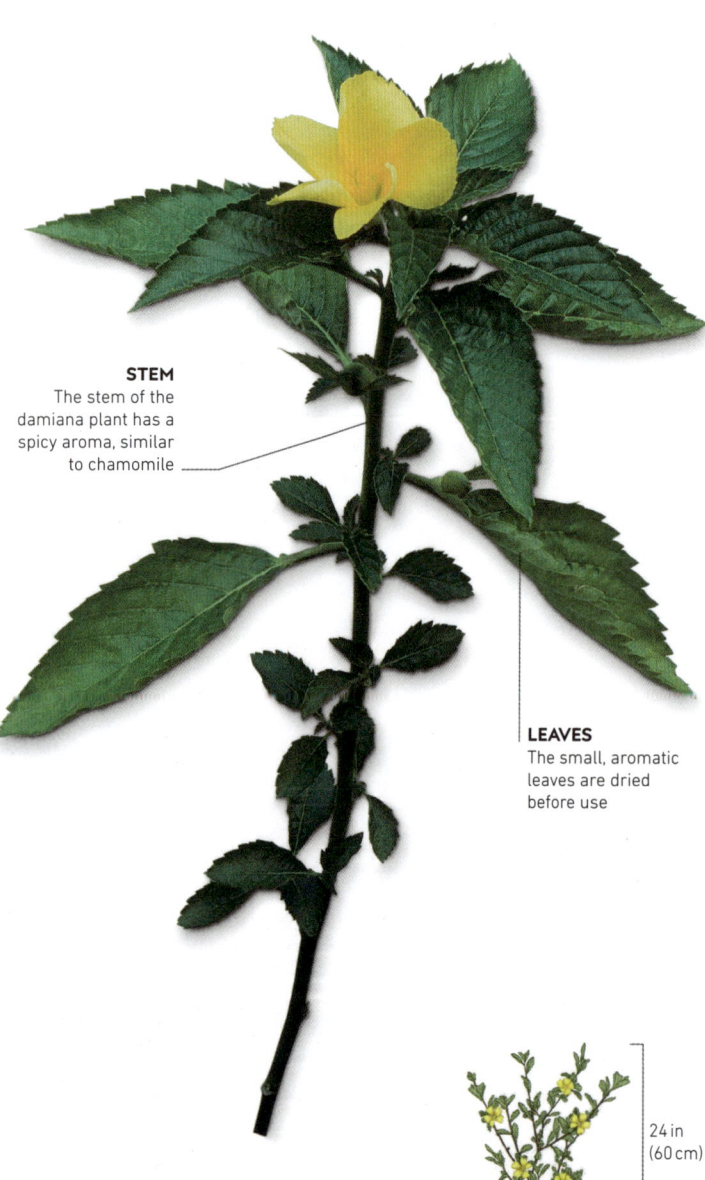

STEM
The stem of the damiana plant has a spicy aroma, similar to chamomile

LEAVES
The small, aromatic leaves are dried before use

GROWTH HABIT
Aromatic perennial growing up to 24 in (60 cm) tall; flowers in late summer.

24 in (60 cm)

Traditionally used by the Maya people of Central America for thousands of years, damiana is best known for its aphrodisiac and tonic properties. Highly aromatic, damiana is also used to flavor drinks, food, teas, and liqueurs; and men and women can both use it to enhance fertility, sexual desire, and well-being. It is native to South and Central America, Mexico, and the West Indies.

PARTS USED Dried leaves and stem
MAIN CONSTITUENTS Volatile oils, arbutin, cyanogenic glycosides, resins, starch, flavonoids, vitamins, minerals, tannins
ACTIONS Antidepressant, aphrodisiac, mild diuretic, mild laxative

HOW TO USE

INFUSION Add 1–1½ tsp (2–4 g) to a cup with some hot water. Take it as a tonic for the urinary and nervous system.
TINCTURE Take 20–60 drops (1–3 ml) in a little hot water 3 times daily (p.176) to help reduce anxiety and depression, improve libido, and relieve constipation.

HOW TO SOURCE

GROW Sow in the spring or summer in pots. The plant does not require fertilizer and can grow in acidic or alkaline soil.
FORAGE Damiana grows wild on rocky hillsides in Mexico and south Texas.
HARVEST Collect and dry the leaves in summer.

CAUTION May reduce iron absorption.

Ulmus rubra
SLIPPERY ELM

One of the most widely used herbal remedies, slippery elm is native to eastern areas of North America from Quebec to Mexico. It is used to heal and soothe damaged tissues—both external wounds and internal mucous membranes—and is also extremely nutritious, so is used as a food in debility and convalescence.

PARTS USED Inner bark
MAIN CONSTITUENTS Mucilage, starch, tannins
ACTIONS Soothing demulcent, emollient, laxative, expectorant, antitussive, nutritive

HOW TO USE

FOOD SUPPLEMENT Use as a food for infants or those recovering from recent illness. Mix ¼–1 level tsp of the powder with a little water to make a paste and add boiling water or hot milk, stirring constantly, to make up to 1 cup of thin gruel. Alternatively, sprinkle the powder on porridge or muesli.
OINTMENT Use to draw pus, thorns, or splinters to the surface; often combined with marshmallow powder.
POULTICE Mix 1 tsp of powder with a little water or calendula infusion to form a paste, spread on gauze, and apply to boils, abscesses, varicose ulcers, or suppurating wounds.
CAPSULES/TABLETS Take 200 mg 3 times daily for gastric or oesophageal inflammation or ulceration or chronic indigestion. Take 1 tablet or capsule before a journey to allay travel sickness.

HOW TO SOURCE

GROW Prefers moist, deep soil in full sun. Usually propagated by seed sown in fall, from suckers, or from semi-ripe cuttings in summer. Not generally grown in gardens. Susceptible to pests, fungal infections, and Dutch elm disease.
FORAGE Planted as a street tree in parts of the US, but rarely cultivated elsewhere, and unlikely to be found in the wild outside its native habitat. Stocks have been depleted by elm leaf beetle and Dutch elm disease, so great care needs to be taken when gathering the bark to avoid damaging trees further.
HARVEST Strip the inner bark from the trunks and branches of mature trees in spring. Always harvest from sustainable sources.

NOTE Availability of the whole bark is restricted in some countries.

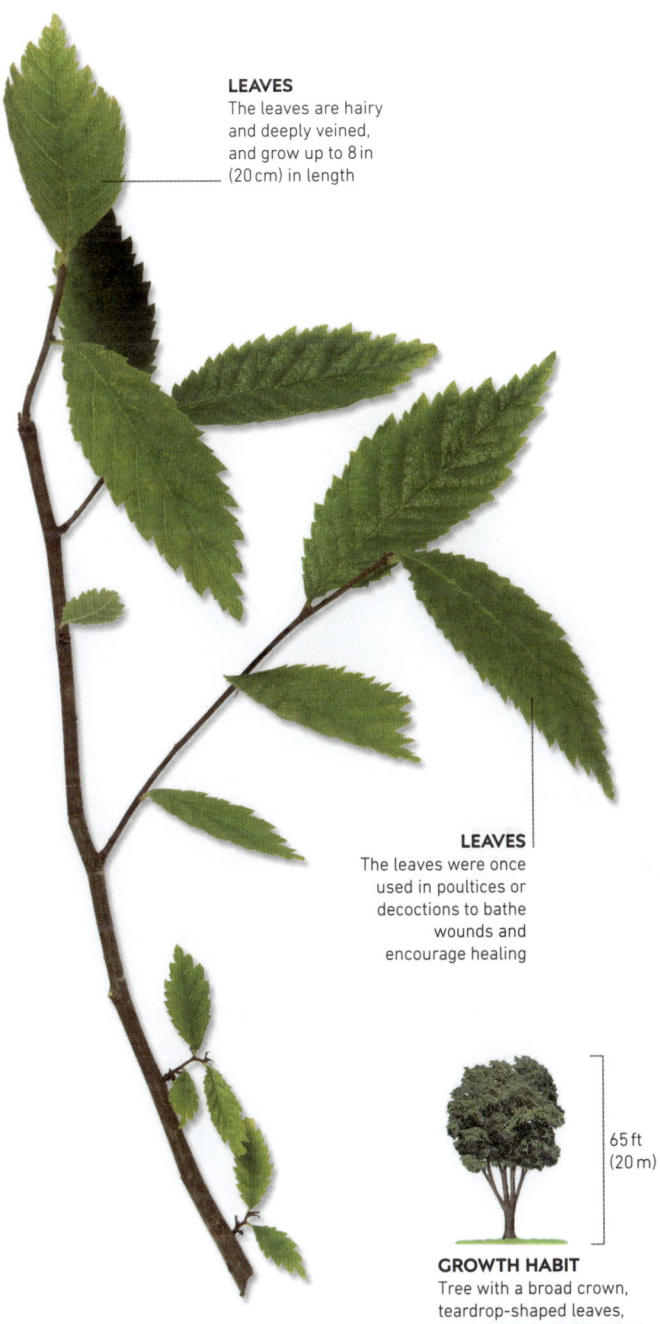

LEAVES
The leaves are hairy and deeply veined, and grow up to 8 in (20 cm) in length

LEAVES
The leaves were once used in poultices or decoctions to bathe wounds and encourage healing

65 ft
(20 m)

GROWTH HABIT
Tree with a broad crown, teardrop-shaped leaves, and a spread of 60 ft (18 m).

Urtica dioica
NETTLE

Found throughout the temperate regions of Europe and Asia, the stinging nettle is an all-too-familiar weed that thrives in the rich soil of cultivated land. The "sting" is caused by hairs on the plant that contain histamine and formic acid. Nettles are said to rob the soil of its minerals and vitamins by absorbing them and concentrating them in its leaves, making them highly nutritious.

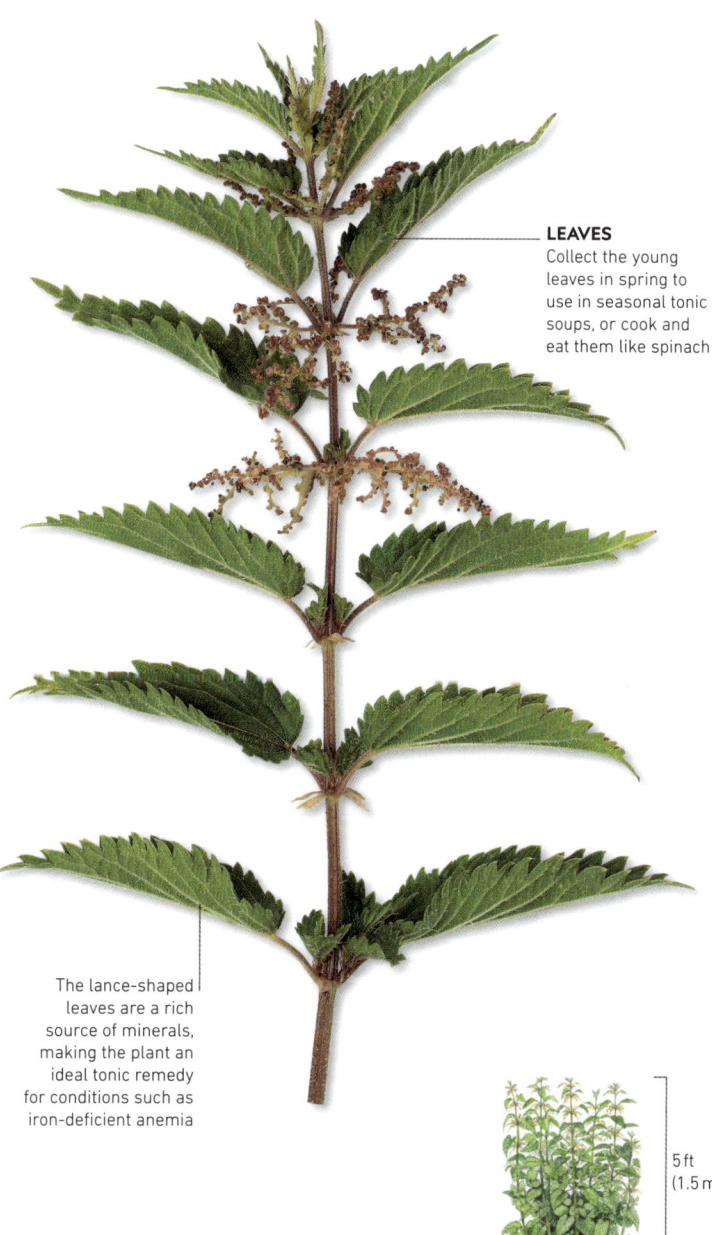

LEAVES
Collect the young leaves in spring to use in seasonal tonic soups, or cook and eat them like spinach

The lance-shaped leaves are a rich source of minerals, making the plant an ideal tonic remedy for conditions such as iron-deficient anemia

GROWTH HABIT
Creeping rhizomatous perennial.

5 ft
(1.5 m)

PARTS USED Aerial parts, root
MAIN CONSTITUENTS Amines (histamine, acetylcholine, choline, serotonin); flavonoids; formic acid; glucoquinones; minerals (incl. silica and iron); vitamins A, B, and C; tannins
ACTIONS Astringent, diuretic, tonic, nutritive, hemostatic, circulatory stimulant, galactogogue, hypotensive, antiscorbutic, anti-allergenic, alterative, rubefacient

HOW TO USE

JUICE Pulverize or process the whole fresh plant to obtain juice. Take in 2 tsp (10 ml) doses 3 times daily as a tonic for debilitated conditions and anemia.
INFUSION Make an infusion (p.176) of 1 cup boiled water over 1-3 tsp. Drink 1 cup 3 times daily as part of a cleansing regime in arthritis, rheumatism, gout, and eczema, or use as a final hair rinse for dandruff.
CREAM/OINTMENT Use for minor cuts and scrapes, skin rashes including eczema, or hemorrhoids.
FRESH LEAVES AND STEMS Lashing arthritic joints (urtication) is an uncomfortable but traditional remedy with some recent studies showing its efficacy. Compress: Use a pad soaked in a strong infusion or diluted tincture of leaves to relieve pain in arthritis, gout, neuralgia, sprains, tendonitis, and sciatica.
TINCTURE Take 40–80 drops (2–4 ml) of the root tincture 3 times daily for allergic skin conditions and hay fever. Take 40–80 drops (2–4 ml) of the root tincture 3 times daily for benign prostatic hypertrophy.

HOW TO SOURCE

GROW It is not usually necessary to cultivate nettles, as they grow freely in the wild.
FORAGE Found growing in hedges, waste areas, and shrubs.
HARVEST Gather aerial parts when in flower. Dig up roots in fall, and young leaves in spring.

CAUTION Wear rubber gloves when harvesting the plant.

Vaccinium myrtillus
BILBERRY

Native to temperate regions of Europe and Asia, bilberry is closely related to the North American blueberry. It has become renowned as a "superfood" thanks to the potent antioxidant proanthocyanidins contained in the fruit. Bilberry jam was eaten by fighter pilots during World War II as it was believed to improve night vision.

PARTS USED Fruit, leaves
MAIN CONSTITUENTS Tannins, sugars, fruit acids, anthocyanosides, glucoquinone, glycosides, vitamin A
ACTIONS Astringent, hypoglycemic, tonic, antiseptic, anti-emetic, anti-inflammatory, diuretic, venous tonic

HOW TO USE

MOUTHWASH Use 1 cup of the infusion below as a gargle or mouthwash for mouth ulcers and throat inflammation; 2 tsp (10 ml) of the fresh berry juice diluted in 4 fl oz (120 ml) of water can be used in the same way.
LOTION Mix 1 fl oz (30 ml) of unsweetened berry juice with 1 fl oz (30 ml) of distilled witch hazel and use as a cooling lotion for sunburn and other skin inflammations.
FRESH RAW BERRIES Eat a large bowl of fresh berries with sugar and milk or cream for constipation.
INFUSION Drink 1 cup (2 tsp dry berries per cup boiling water) 3 times daily for chronic diarrhea. To support dietary control in late-onset, non–insulin dependent diabetes mellitus, drink 1 cup (1 tsp leaves per cup boiling water) 3 times per day.

HOW TO SOURCE

GROW Prefers moist, very acid soil (pH 5.5 or less) in sun or partial shade and water, as it is shallow-rooted. Sow seeds in a cold frame in fall and transplant to final growing positions when large enough. Or propagate by semi-ripe cuttings in summer. Prune in spring to encourage bushy growth. Grow in a sheltered position. Best grown in large containers in alkaline soil areas.
FORAGE Grows wild in acidic, poor soil such as peat bogs, moors, and similar areas in temperate and sub-arctic regions.
HARVEST Gather the leaves in spring and the fruits when ripe in late summer.

CAUTION Insulin-dependent diabetics should not use bilberry leaf teas without professional guidance. Do not use the leaves for more than four weeks.

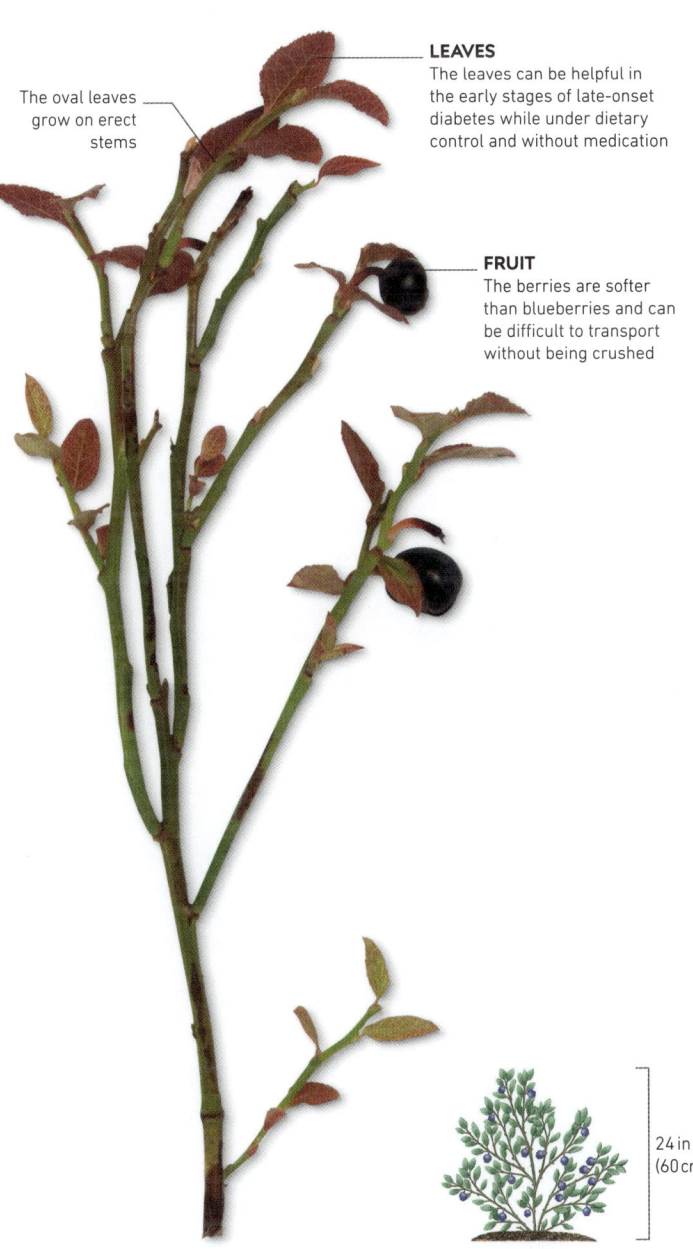

LEAVES
The leaves can be helpful in the early stages of late-onset diabetes while under dietary control and without medication

The oval leaves grow on erect stems

FRUIT
The berries are softer than blueberries and can be difficult to transport without being crushed

24 in (60 cm)

GROWTH HABIT
A deciduous shrub with creeping rhizomes and a spread of 24 in (60 cm) or more.

Valeriana officinalis
VALERIAN

Sometimes described as "nature's tranquilizer," valerian originates in temperate areas from Europe to Japan. It has been extensively researched in recent years. Chemicals called valepotriates, which seem to have a depressant effect on the nervous system, are now known to develop in extracts and the dried plant. The fresh plant is more sedating.

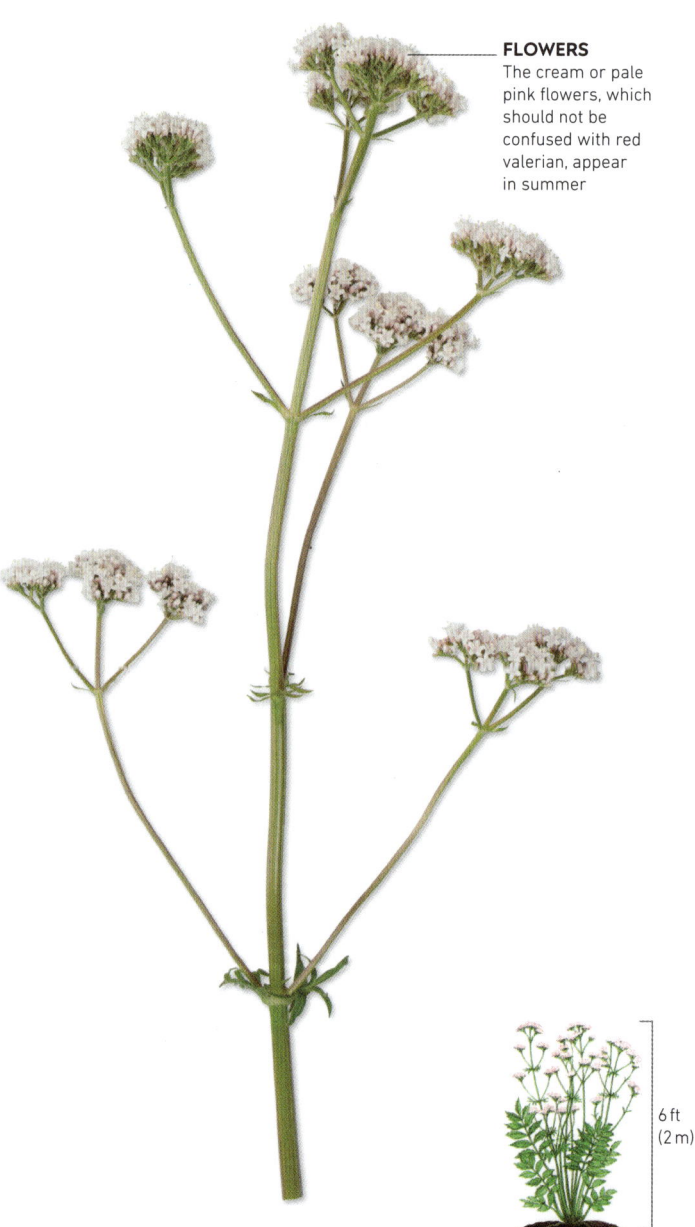

FLOWERS
The cream or pale pink flowers, which should not be confused with red valerian, appear in summer

GROWTH HABIT
Clump-forming rhizomatous perennial.

6 ft (2 m)

PARTS USED Root and rhizome
MAIN CONSTITUENTS Volatile oil (incl. isovaleric acid, borneol), valepotriates, alkaloids
ACTIONS Sedative, hypnotic, nervine, antispasmodic, expectorant, diuretic, hypotensive, carminative, mildly analgesic

HOW TO USE

MACERATION Valerian root is best made into a maceration rather than a decoction. Soak scant 1 oz (25 g) of the chopped, preferably fresh, root for 8–10 hours in 1 pint (600 ml) of cold water. Take 1 cup up to 3 times daily for anxiety, nervous tension, or high blood pressure linked to stress. Take a cup before bed for insomnia.
CAPSULES The ground root may be added to capsules (also commercially available).
TINCTURE Take 20 drops–1 tsp (1–5 ml) up to 3 times daily for nervous problems. Dosage can vary considerably between individuals, with higher doses causing headaches in some, so start with low doses.
COMPRESS Soak a pad in a cup of maceration or the diluted tincture and apply to muscle cramps or the abdomen for period pain and colic.

HOW TO SOURCE

GROW Prefers moist soil in a sunny or partially shaded area; suitable for a woodland garden. Sow seeds in a cold frame in spring, transplant to pots, and plant out when established, or propagate by root division in spring or fall.
FORAGE Usually found in woodland edges or damp grass. Easily confused with the popular garden plant red, or American, valerian (*Centranthus ruber*).
HARVEST Dig roots and rhizomes of plants that are at least 2 years old in fall.

CAUTION Enhances the action of sleep-inducing drugs, so avoid if taking such medication.

Verbascum thapsus
MULLEIN

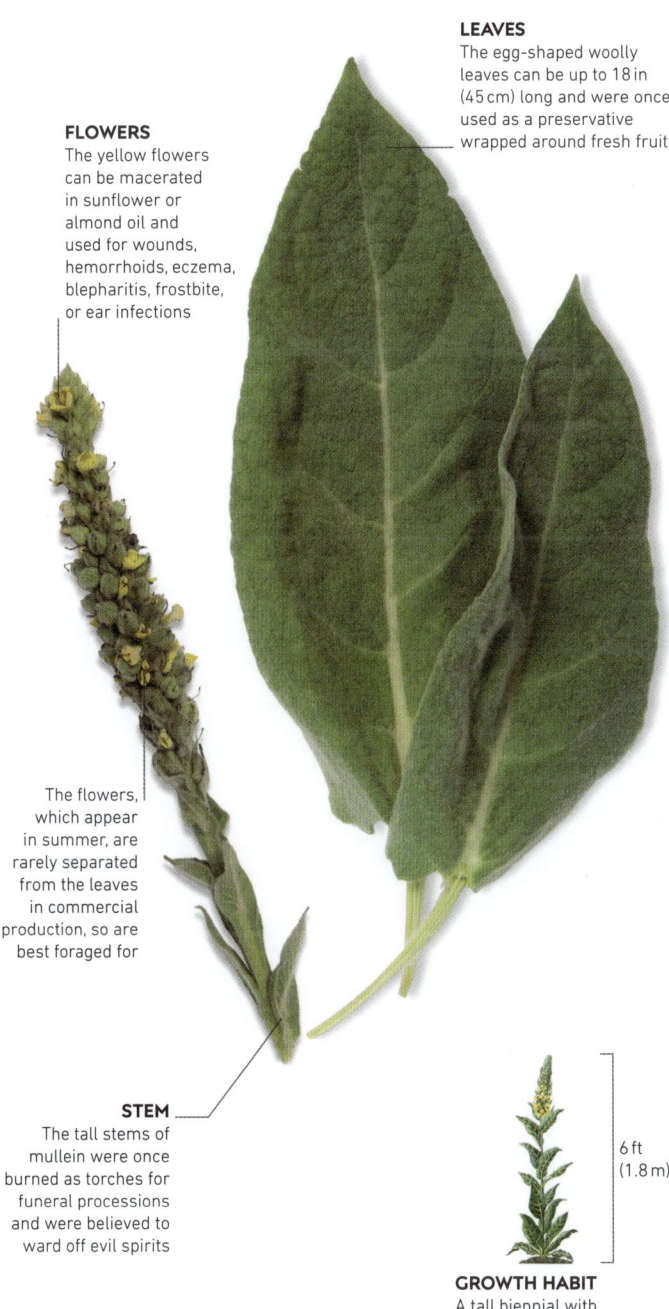

FLOWERS
The yellow flowers can be macerated in sunflower or almond oil and used for wounds, hemorrhoids, eczema, blepharitis, frostbite, or ear infections

LEAVES
The egg-shaped woolly leaves can be up to 18 in (45 cm) long and were once used as a preservative wrapped around fresh fruits

The flowers, which appear in summer, are rarely separated from the leaves in commercial production, so are best foraged for

STEM
The tall stems of mullein were once burned as torches for funeral processions and were believed to ward off evil spirits

GROWTH HABIT
A tall biennial with soft, gray-green downy leaves; spread 3 ft (1 m).

6 ft (1.8 m)

Found from Europe to western China, mullein was traditionally used to ward off evil spirits and cure wasting diseases, such as tuberculosis, which it was once believed such spirits caused. Simply carrying the plant or using it in an amulet was thought to be sufficient. Today it is mainly used in cough remedies and for respiratory disorders.

PARTS USED Flowers, leaves, aerial parts
MAIN CONSTITUENTS Mucilage, saponins, volatile oil, bitter, flavonoids (incl. rutin), glycosides (incl. aucubin)
ACTIONS Expectorant, demulcent, mild diuretic, sedative, wound herb, astringent, anti-inflammatory

HOW TO USE

SYRUP Make a syrup by combining 1 pint (600 ml) of below infusion of fresh flowers with 1 lb (450 g) of honey or golden syrup: combine the ingredients, bring to a boil, and simmer gently for 10–15 minutes. Take 1 tsp (5 ml) doses as required.
INFUSED OIL Macerate the fresh flowers in sunflower oil for 2 weeks, shaking daily. Strain and use to relieve the pain of ear infections (add 2 drops to a cotton ball and place in the outer ear) or as a salve on wounds, skin ulcers, hemorrhoids, eczema, frostbite, blepharitis, or as a chest rub for respiratory complaints.
INFUSION Drink 1 cup (1–2 tsp dry leaves or flowers per cup of boiling water) 3 times daily for chronic coughs, feverish chills with hard coughs, throat inflammation, and to tone the respiratory system.
TINCTURE Take 1–2 tsp (5–10 ml) 3 times daily of a tincture of the leaf or aerial parts for chronic respiratory disorders.

HOW TO SOURCE

GROW Prefers well-drained to dry soil in full sun, and will spread to 3 ft (90 cm). Sow seeds in a cold frame in fall or spring and transplant to 3 in (7.5 cm) pots when the seedlings are large enough to handle. Plant in their final positions when well-established. Self-seeds enthusiastically if growing conditions are ideal.
FORAGE Found in hedges; roadsides; and open, uncultivated land and can be easily spotted in summer by its statuesque flower spikes. Collect and dry the different parts separately for maximum use.
HARVEST Collect individual yellow blossoms when in full bloom. Cut the aerial parts while flowering and gather the leaves separately.

Verbena officinalis
VERVAIN

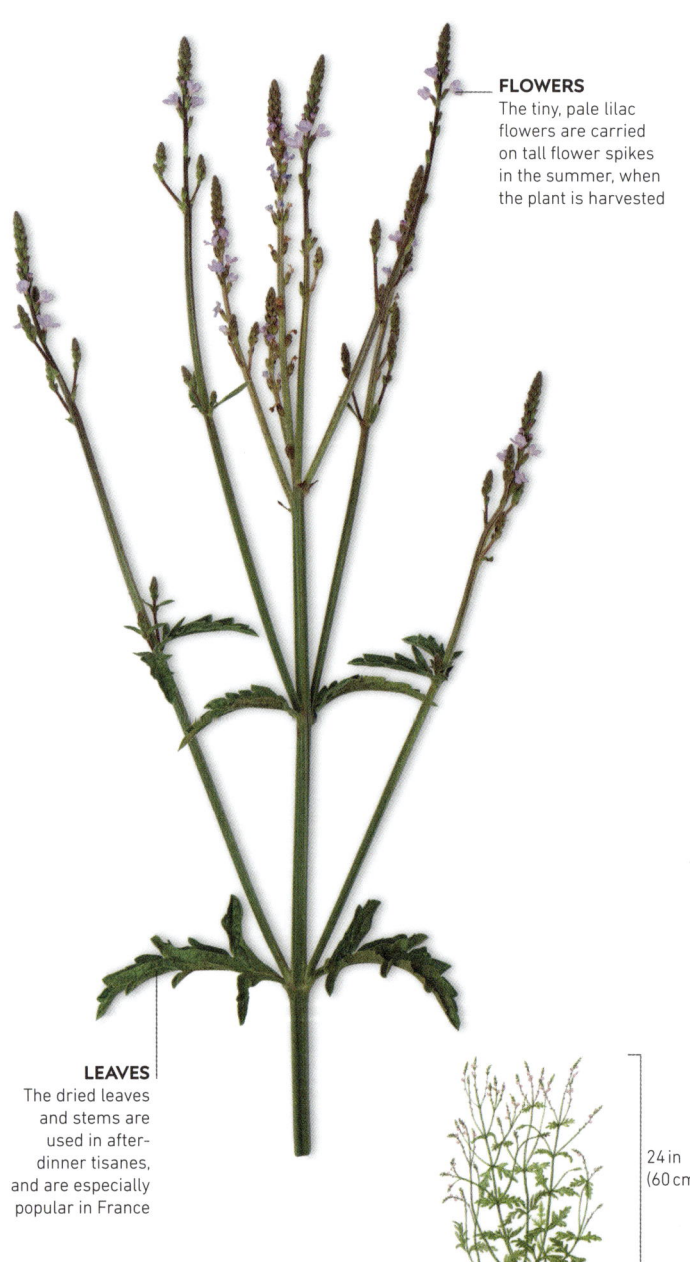

FLOWERS
The tiny, pale lilac flowers are carried on tall flower spikes in the summer, when the plant is harvested

LEAVES
The dried leaves and stems are used in after-dinner tisanes, and are especially popular in France

GROWTH HABIT
Straggly perennial with oval leaves and long flower stems; spread 24 in (60 cm).

24 in (60 cm)

Once regarded as a cure-all, and sacred to the ancient Greeks, Romans, and Druids, vervain—which grows throughout much of Europe, Asia, and North Africa—is associated with a wealth of folklore and was once used in fortune-telling. Today it is a favorite after-dinner "tisane" to stimulate the digestion, and is also used to ease headaches, nervous tension, and depression.

PARTS USED Aerial parts
MAIN CONSTITUENTS Volatile oil (incl. citral), bitter iridoids (incl. verbenin and verbenalin), alkaloids, tannins
ACTIONS Relaxant tonic, galactagogue, diaphoretic, nervine, sedative, pectoral, antispasmodic, hepatic restorative, laxative, uterine stimulant, cholagogue

HOW TO USE

TINCTURE Take 40–80 drops (2–4 ml) 3 times daily for nervous exhaustion, stress, anxiety, or depression; as a liver stimulant for sluggish digestion, toxic conditions, or jaundice; and with other urinary herbs for stones and excess uric acid.
INFUSION Drink 1 cup (1–3 tsp aerial parts per cup water) 3 times daily as a digestive stimulant, or in feverish conditions; take 1 cup at night for insomnia.
CREAM/OINTMENT Use on eczema, wounds, and running sores or for painful neuralgia.
FLOWER REMEDY Dilute 2 drops in 2 tsp (10 ml) of water in a dropper bottle and take in drop doses as required for mental stress and over exertion with related insomnia and an inability to relax.

HOW TO SOURCE

GROW Prefers a sunny site in well-drained soil, but tolerates other conditions. Sow the seeds in a seed bed in spring or fall and transplant (24 in/60 cm apart) when established, or propagate by division in late spring. Self-seeds in the right conditions.
FORAGE An inconspicuous plant that is easily missed, it can be found growing wild, mainly in hedges and dry grassy areas, throughout its native region and elsewhere. Collect the aerial parts while flowering in summer.
HARVEST Traditionally collected when the plant is in flower.

CAUTION Avoid during pregnancy. May cause vomiting if taken in excess.

Viburnum opulus
CRAMP BARK

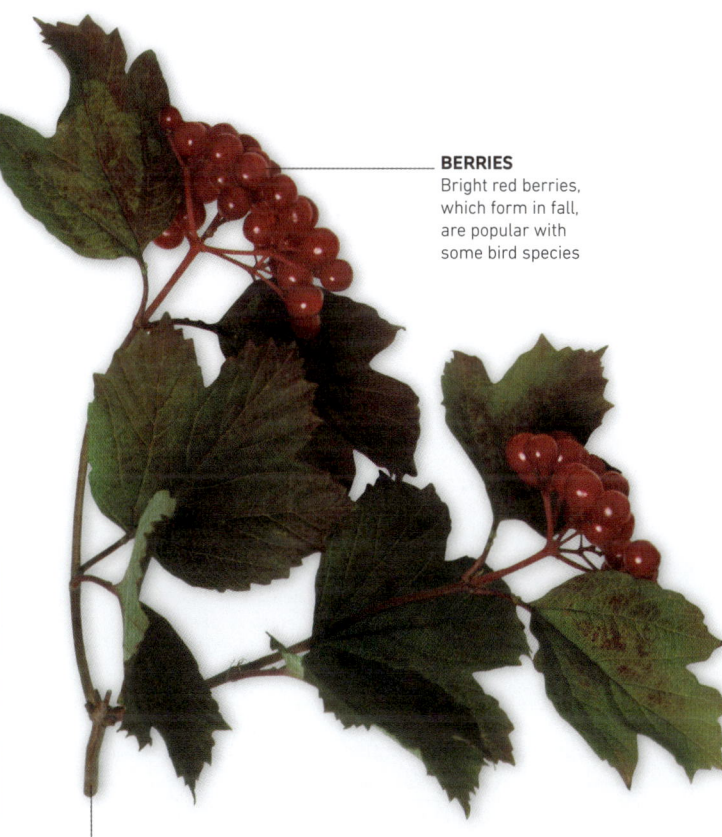

BERRIES
Bright red berries, which form in fall, are popular with some bird species

BARK
Harvested from branches in spring and summer, the bark can be used in both internal and external preparations, to ease muscle cramps

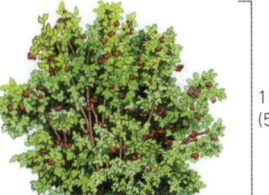

GROWTH HABIT
Vigorous, bushy shrub with lace-capped white flowers in spring; spread 12 ft (4 m).

15 ft (5 m)

As with many plants, the common name of this herb aptly describes its properties. It is effective at treating cramping and spasmodic pains affecting both smooth and skeletal muscles— so, for example, it is a useful treatment for colic as well as for leg cramps. Native to Europe, northern Asia, and North America, the shrub is an attractive and popular garden plant.

PARTS USED Bark
MAIN CONSTITUENTS Bitter (viburnin), valeric acid, tannins, coumarins, saponins
ACTIONS Antispasmodic, sedative, astringent, muscle relaxant, cardiac tonic, sedative, anti-inflammatory

HOW TO USE

TINCTURE Take 1 tsp (5 ml) 3 times daily as a relaxant for nervous or muscular tension, or for colicky pains affecting the digestive tract or urinary system. Add 20 drops (1 ml) to remedies for IBS or combine with rhubarb root for constipation.
DECOCTION Infuse (p.176) 2 tsp in 1 cup of water. Bring to a boil and simmer gently. Take ½–1 cup every 3–4 hours for period pain or colic. Can also be used with other remedies for excessive menstrual bleeding.
CREAM/LOTION Use regularly for muscle cramps, including night cramps in the legs, or for shoulder tension.
MASSAGE RUB Use the macerated oil as a basis for massage rubs for muscular aches and pains associated with cramps and spasm. Add 10 drops of lavender, thyme, or rosemary essential oil to 1 tsp (5 ml) of the macerated oil.

HOW TO SOURCE

GROW Prefers moist yet well-drained soil in sun or dappled shade, and can be a useful addition to a hedge or woodland garden. Propagate by softwood cuttings in summer, or plant seed as soon as it is ripe and over-winter in a cold frame or unheated greenhouse.
FORAGE May be found growing in woodlands in Europe or North America. As always when collecting bark, it is important not to damage the bush. Only harvest a small amount from each shrub.
HARVEST Bark from the branches is collected in spring and summer when the plant is flowering.

CAUTION Avoid during pregnancy except under professional supervision.

Viola tricolor
HEARTSEASE

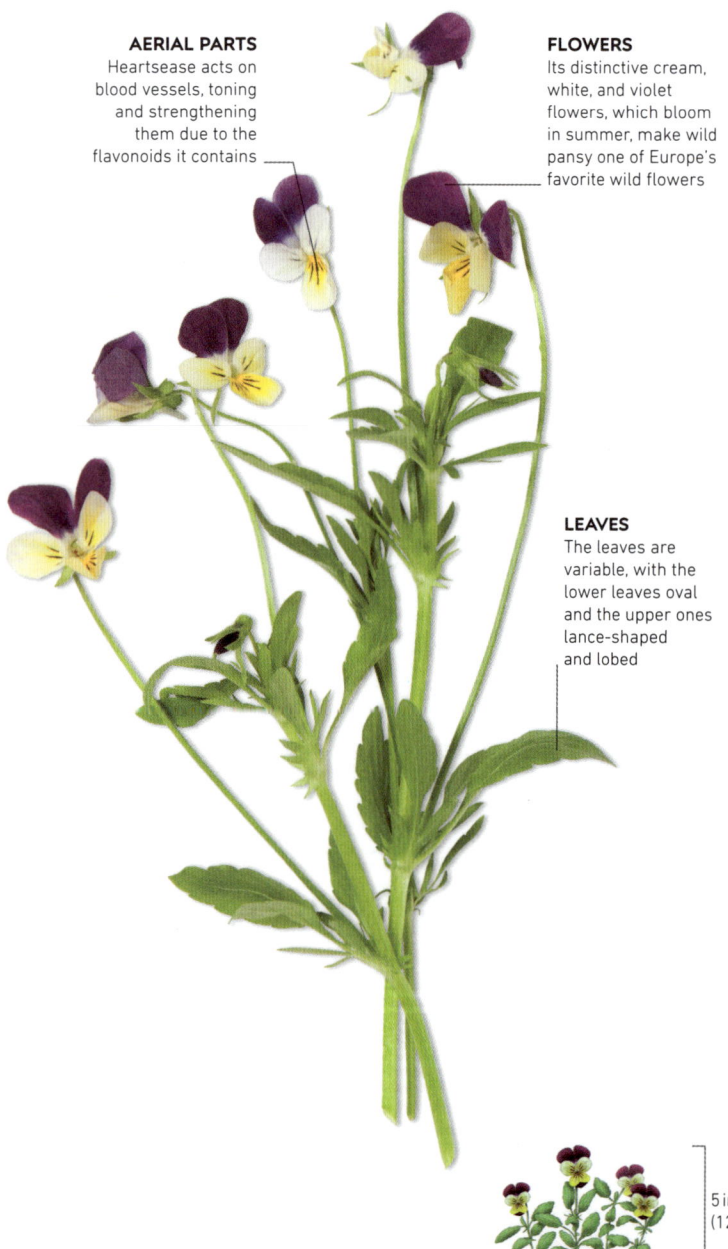

AERIAL PARTS
Heartsease acts on blood vessels, toning and strengthening them due to the flavonoids it contains

FLOWERS
Its distinctive cream, white, and violet flowers, which bloom in summer, make wild pansy one of Europe's favorite wild flowers

LEAVES
The leaves are variable, with the lower leaves oval and the upper ones lance-shaped and lobed

5 in
(12 cm)

GROWTH HABIT
Tufted annual, biennial, or short-lived perennial, with a spread of 15 in (38 cm).

The name "heartsease" is reputedly derived from its use in medieval love potions, although it was also once used for heart problems. Also known as wild pansy, the herb is native to Europe, North Africa, and temperate regions of Asia. Today it is mainly used for skin disorders and coughs, as well as making an attractive garnish in cooking.

PARTS USED Aerial parts
MAIN CONSTITUENTS Saponin, salicylates, flavonoids (incl. rutin), volatile oil, mucilage
ACTIONS Expectorant, anti-inflammatory, diuretic, antirheumatic, laxative, stabilizes capillary membranes

HOW TO USE

CREAM/OINTMENT Use regularly for skin rashes, eczema, diaper rash, or cradle cap.
INFUSION Drink 1 cup (1 tsp herb per cup of boiling water) 3 times daily as a cleansing remedy for toxic conditions, or as a gentle stimulant for the circulation and immune system in rheumatic disorders, chronic skin conditions, urinary infections, and chronic infections.
WASH Use 1 cup of above infusion (p.176) to bathe diaper rash, cradle cap, weeping sores, varicose ulcers, or oozing insect bites.
SYRUP Add 1 lb (450 g) of honey or sugar to 2 cups of strained infusion, bring to a boil, and simmer gently for 5–10 minutes to form a syrup. Use in 1 tsp (5 ml) doses to soothe bronchitis and asthma.
TINCTURE Take 1 tsp (5 ml) in a little water 3 times daily for capillary fragility, urinary disorders, or skin disorders

HOW TO SOURCE

GROW Prefers moist but well-drained soil in full sun or dappled shade. Sow seeds in seed trays in a cold frame in summer or in spring when ripe; transplant to final positions when large enough to handle. Alternatively, take basal cuttings in spring or divide established clumps in fall.
FORAGE Found in grassy places, such as meadows and waste ground. Gather in summer while flowering. The flowers are edible and can be added to salads or used to garnish pasta dishes.
HARVEST Collect all the aerial parts in summer.

CAUTION Very high doses may cause nausea due to the saponin content.

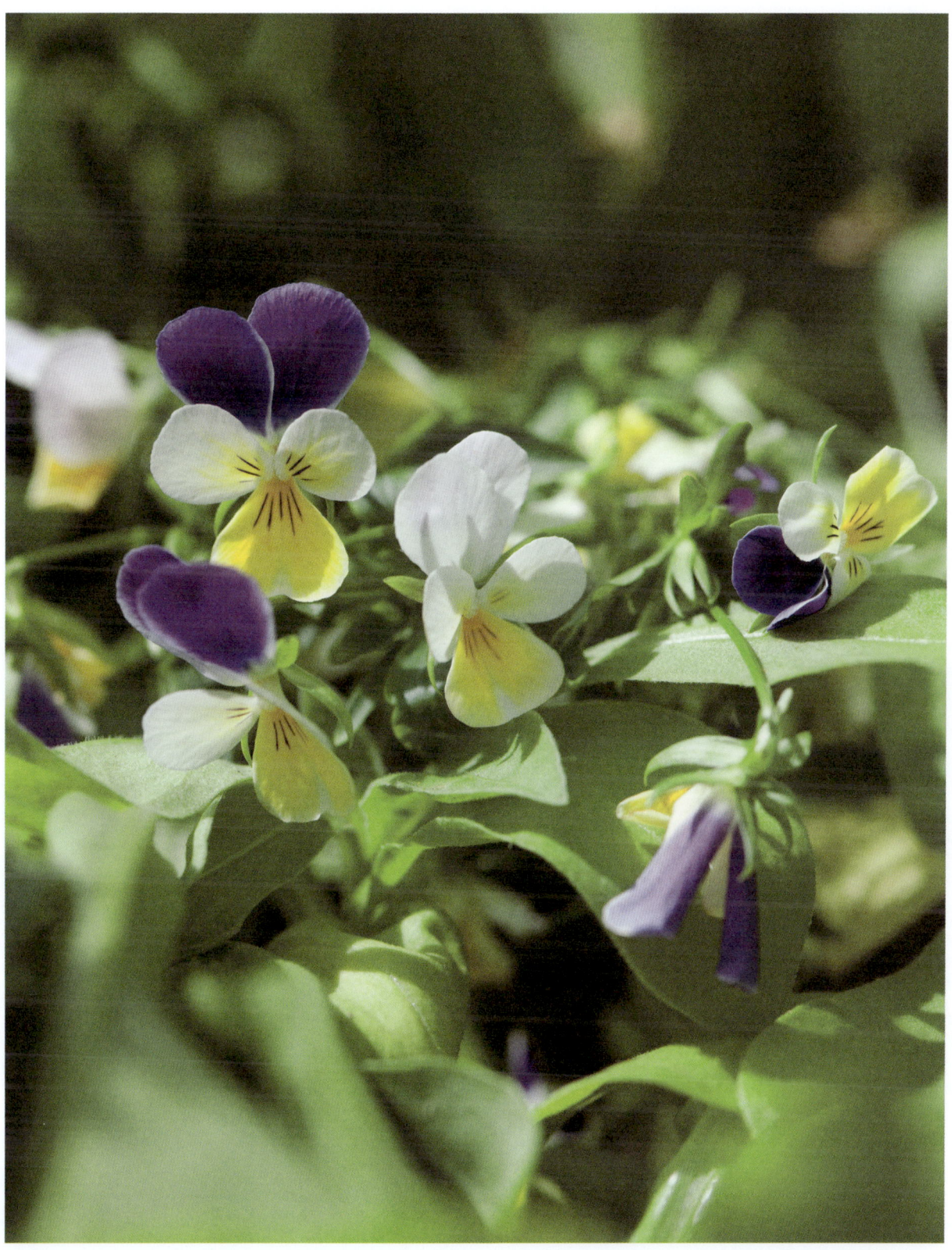

Viscum album
MISTLETOE

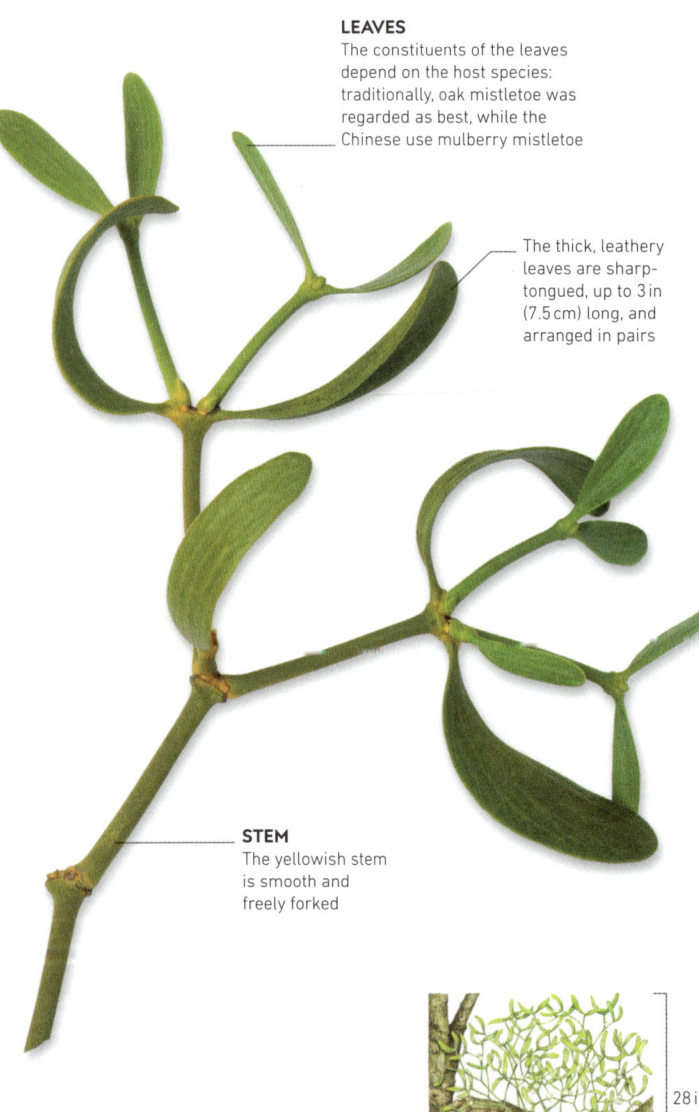

LEAVES
The constituents of the leaves depend on the host species: traditionally, oak mistletoe was regarded as best, while the Chinese use mulberry mistletoe

The thick, leathery leaves are sharp-tongued, up to 3 in (7.5 cm) long, and arranged in pairs

STEM
The yellowish stem is smooth and freely forked

GROWTH HABIT
Bushy parasitic that grows on various trees; flowers appear in fall and fruits in winter.

28 in (70 cm)

Traditionally associated with fertility rites, and significant in Norse legend as the only plant capable of killing the Norse god Baldur, mistletoe has been use as a cancer treatment since the days of the Druids. Some modern research has confirmed this action, although its most common use is to lower high blood pressure. It is native to Europe and northern Asia.

PARTS USED Leaves, branches, berries
MAIN CONSTITUENTS Alkaloids, glycoproteins, viscotoxin, flavonoids, acetylcholine, polysaccharides (berries)
ACTIONS Hypotensive, sedative, anti-inflammatory, diuretic, immune tonic

HOW TO USE

NB Use only under medical supervision
INFUSION Drink ½–1 cup (1–2 tsp leaves per cup boiling water) 3 times daily for high blood pressure, petit mal, or to assist with withdrawal in benzodiazepine addiction. Combine with skullcap, valerian, or betony (*Stachys officinalis*) for nervous disorders. Take ½ cup of a half-strength infusion 3 times daily for panic attacks or headaches.
TINCTURE Best made from the fresh plant; take 10 drops 3 times a day to lower blood pressure.
FLUID EXTRACT Consult an herbalist for usage to strengthen the immune system during treatments for cancer, including after surgery and during radiotherapy.
BERRY EXTRACTS Used in anthroposophical medicine to treat cancer.

HOW TO SOURCE

GROW Encourage mistletoe to grow on garden trees by making a small incision in the bark and crushing freshly gathered ripe berries into the cut. The berries are ripe in late winter/early spring. Collect berries only from the same type of tree (i.e. mistletoe berries from an oak tree will usually only grow on another oak). Once established, the plant is spread to other parts of the tree by birds.
FORAGE Often found growing high up on deciduous trees, it can easily be seen in winter; use pruning shears on an extendable pole to cut the stems in fall.
HARVEST Gather leaves and branches in late fall and ripe berries in late winter.

CAUTION Avoid during pregnancy. Can be toxic (especially the berries); take only under professional supervision.

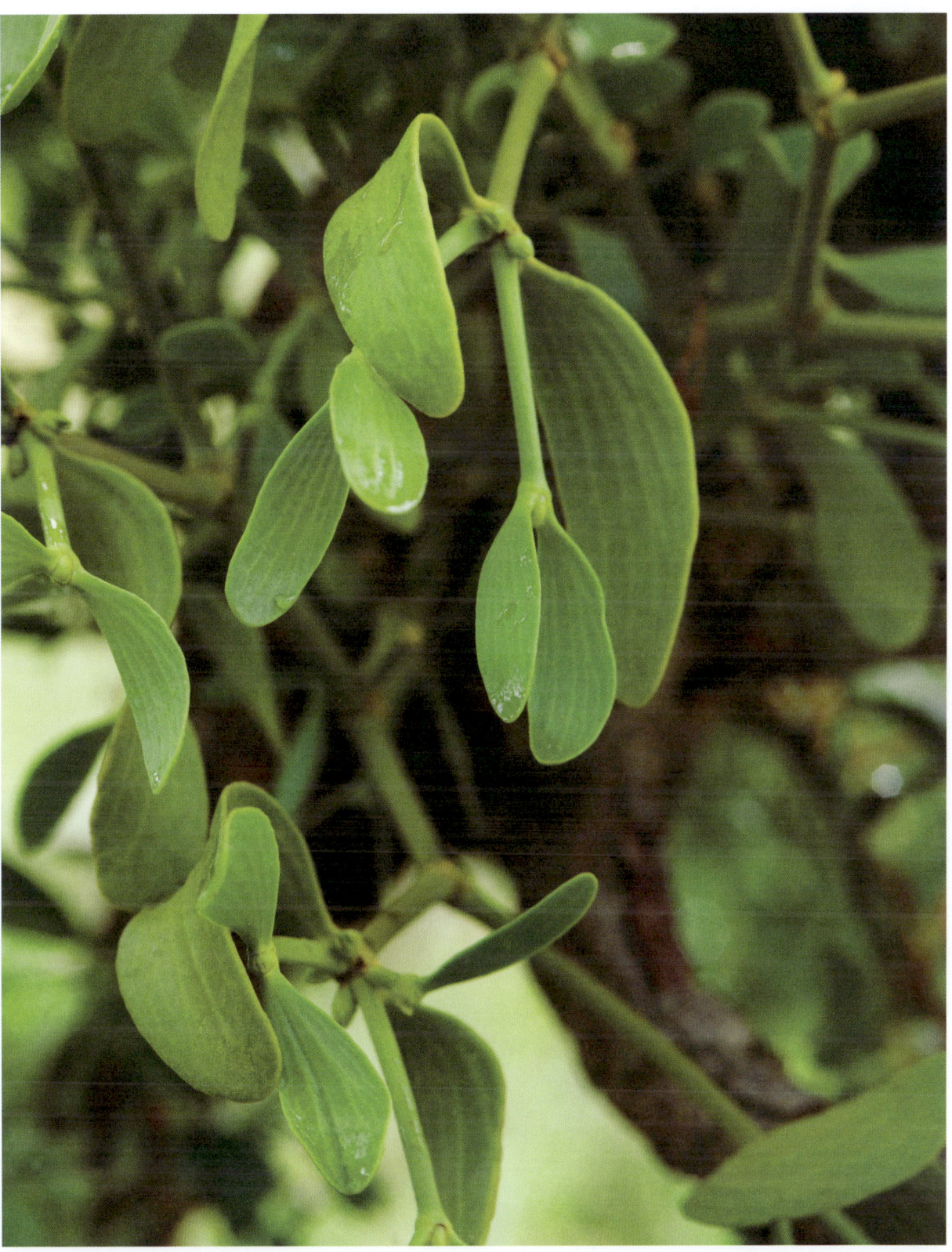

Vitex agnus-castus
AGNUS CASTUS

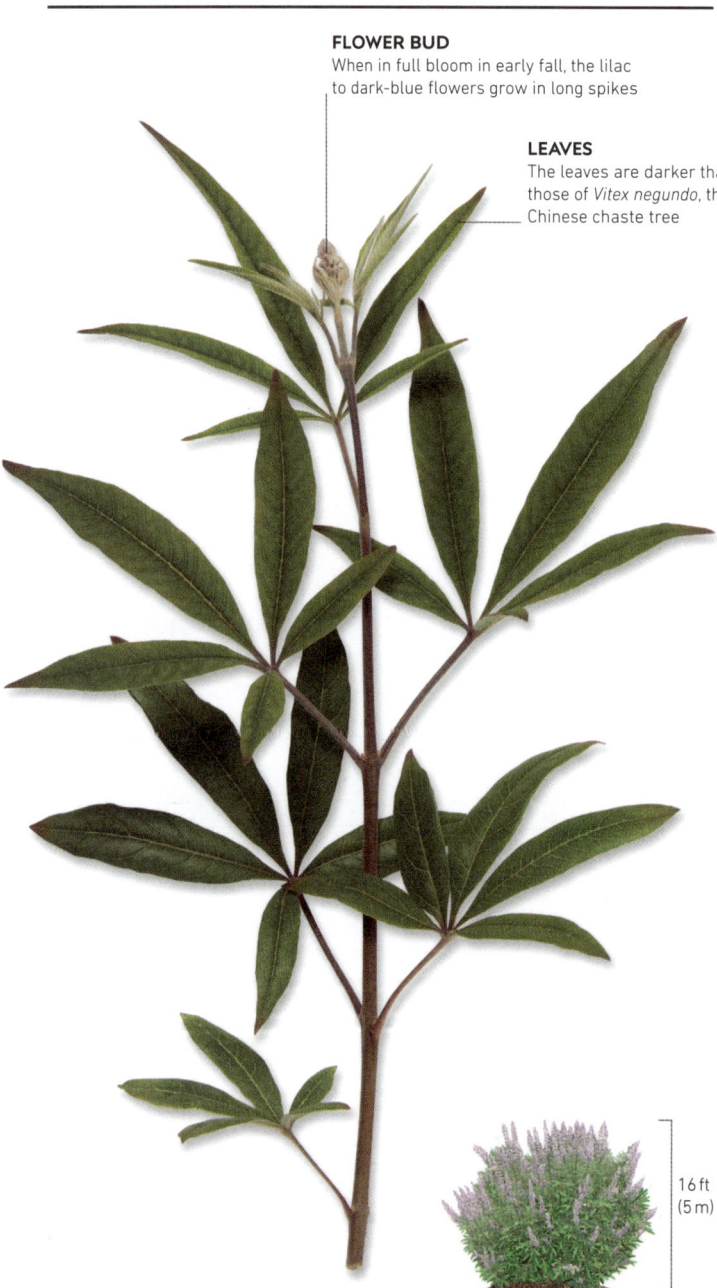

FLOWER BUD
When in full bloom in early fall, the lilac to dark-blue flowers grow in long spikes

LEAVES
The leaves are darker than those of *Vitex negundo*, the Chinese chaste tree

GROWTH HABIT
Spreading shrub or small tree with pale lilac flowers in early fall; spread 6–25 ft (2–8 m).

16 ft (5 m)

Native to the Mediterranean region, agnus castus was known as the "chaste tree," while its berries were called "monk's pepper"—a reference to their medieval use as an anaphrodisiac to reduce the libido of celibate monks. The herb has the opposite effect on women, stimulating the production of female hormones, and is used for a wide range of gynecological problems.

PARTS USED Fruit
MAIN CONSTITUENTS Iridoid glycosides (incl. aucubin and agnuside), volatile oil (incl. cineol), flavonoids, alkaloids (incl. viticine), bitter, fatty acids
ACTIONS Hormone regulator, progesterogenic, galactagogue

HOW TO USE

TINCTURE Take up to 40 drops (2 ml) first thing in the morning during the second half of a menstrual cycle to stimulate hormone production in irregular menstrual cycles or PMS. It is easy to overdose, so start with a low dose and gradually increase the amount if there are no side effects (see below). It will also ease migraine or acne related to the menstrual cycle.
TABLETS/ CAPSULES Readily available commercially; follow the dosage directions on the package and take to ease PMS.

HOW TO SOURCE

GROW Prefers well-drained soil in full sun and a warm site. Sow seeds in a cold frame in fall or spring; transplant to 4 in (10 cm) pots when large enough to handle. Alternatively, take semi-ripe cuttings in summer. Grow until well established before planting in permanent positions. Protect from cold, dry winds and severe winters. Prune in spring while still dormant.
FORAGE Generally cultivated, but can be found growing wild in southern Europe and naturalized in other subtropical regions. Can be confused with the Chinese chaste tree (*Vitex negundo*), which has paler leaves and flowers and is native to India and China. Does not always set seed to form berries in cooler climates.
HARVEST Gather ripe berries in fall.

CAUTION Excess can cause formication—a sensation like ants crawling over the skin. Do not use if taking progesterone drugs. Avoid during pregnancy except under professional supervision.

Withania somnifera
ASHWAGANDHA

Also known as Indian ginseng, ashwagandha is found in the drier regions of India and the Middle East. The name translates as "that which has the smell of a horse" and the plant is traditionally associated with the strength and sexual energy of a stallion. Traditionally used as a tonic, modern research has shown it to have significant antitumor activity.

PARTS USED Root, leaves
MAIN CONSTITUENTS Alkaloids (incl. anaferine and isopelietierine), steroidal lactones (incl. withanolides and withaferins), saponins, iron
ACTIONS Tonic, nervine, sedative, adaptogen, anti-inflammatory, antitumor

HOW TO USE
POWDER/CAPSULES Take 250 mg–1 g of powdered root or capsule equivalent 3 times daily as a restorative tonic for over-work, exhaustion, sleep problems, and debility caused by chronic disease. Regular use can also help in degenerative disorders such as arthritis.
FLUID EXTRACT Take 40–80 drops (2–4 ml) in water 3 times daily as an energy tonic, a calming remedy for insomnia, to nourish the blood in anemia, or for stress or debility.
DECOCTION Take ½–1 cup of a decoction made from 1 tsp of dried root and 4 fl oz (120 ml) of milk or water simmered for 15 minutes for stress or exhaustion.

HOW TO SOURCE
GROW Prefers dry, stony soil in full sun. Sow seeds in spring in seed trays and transplant to 3 in (7.5 cm) pots when the seedlings are large enough to handle. Alternatively, propagate by heeled greenwood cuttings in late spring. Rarely seen cultivated in the West.
FORAGE Unlikely to be found growing wild outside its native region.
HARVEST The leaves are collected in spring and the root is dug in fall.

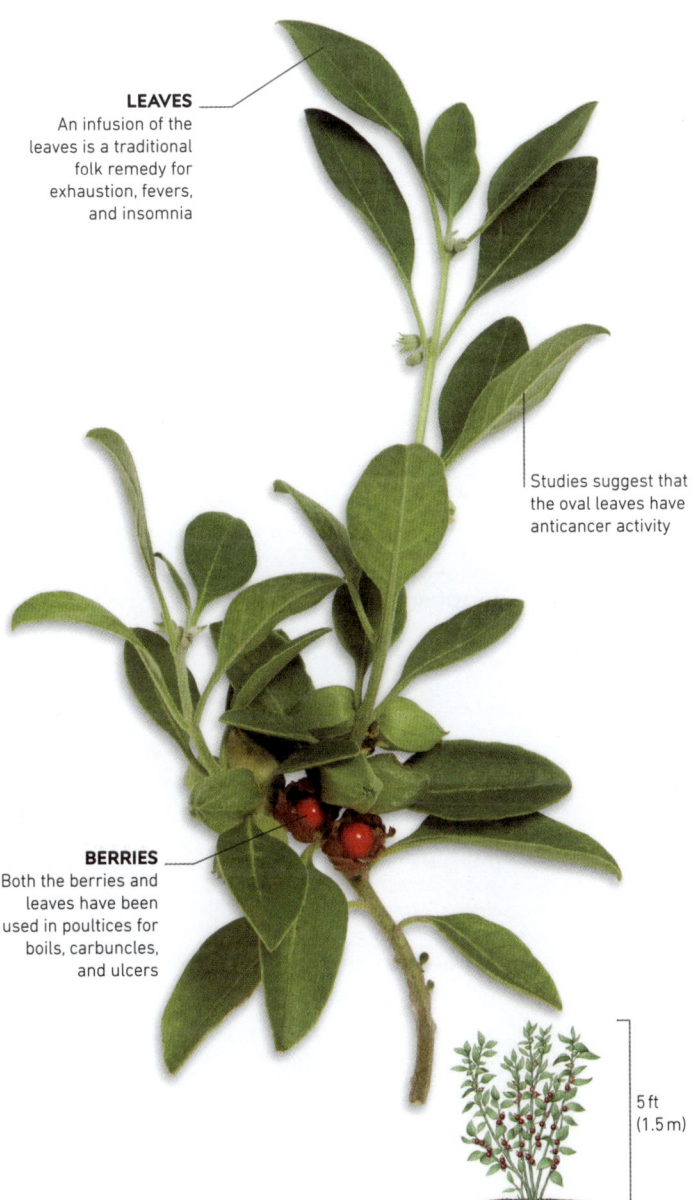

LEAVES
An infusion of the leaves is a traditional folk remedy for exhaustion, fevers, and insomnia

Studies suggest that the oval leaves have anticancer activity

BERRIES
Both the berries and leaves have been used in poultices for boils, carbuncles, and ulcers

5 ft
(1.5 m)

GROWTH HABIT
Upright evergreen shrub with inconspicuous yellow flowers; spread 3 ft (1 m).

CAUTION Avoid during pregnancy.

Zea mays
CORN SILK

Cultivated for 4,000 years both as a cereal crop and for fodder, maize was originally grown by the Aztecs and Mayans in South America and is now the continent's most widely grown crop. Corn silk, used medicinally, consists of the brown whiskery parts of the styles and stigmas that can be seen at the top of the cobs, and is mainly used for urinary disorders.

PARTS USED Styles and stigmas (corn silk), maize meal
MAIN CONSTITUENTS Allantoin, saponins, flavonoids, mucilage, volatile oil, vitamins C and K, potassium
ACTIONS Diuretic, urinary demulcent, mild stimulant

HOW TO USE

INFUSION Generally regarded as more effective than the tincture. Drink 1 cup (2 tsp herb per cup boiling water) up to 6 times daily for cystitis, urethritis, benign prostate gland enlargement, urinary retention, or urinary gravel.
TEA Combine 1 tsp each of dried corn silk and agrimony with 1 cup of boiling water, infuse for 15 minutes, and strain. Give to children with bed-wetting problems; consult an herbalist for advice on dosage.
TINCTURE Take 1–2 tsp (5–10 ml) 3 times daily for acute or chronic inflammation of the urinary system.
POULTICE Mix 2 tsp of powdered maize meal with a little water into a paste, spread on gauze, and use as a poultice for ulcers and boils.

HOW TO SOURCE

GROW Prefers moist but well-drained soil in full sun. Sow seeds directly in spring when the ground is not too wet. Can be grown in gardens with the ripe cobs used as a food.
FORAGE Maize is widely cultivated worldwide and corn silk can be gleaned from standing crops just before harvest, as long as landowners do not object. Snip the brown whiskery parts of the styles and stigmas from the cob with scissors.
HARVEST The corn silk is harvested with the ripe cobs in summer, then separated and dried.

FLOWER
The male inflorescence is called a tassel and is made up of many small flowers, while the female forms the cob and only the stigma can be seen

LEAVES
The leaves form at nodes on the stem, and can grow up to 3 ft (1 m) in length and up to 4 in (10 cm) wide. The ears of corn are produced under the leaf and close to the stem

28 in (70 cm)

GROWTH HABIT
Annual cereal crop. Each plant has a spread of 18–24 in (45–60 cm).

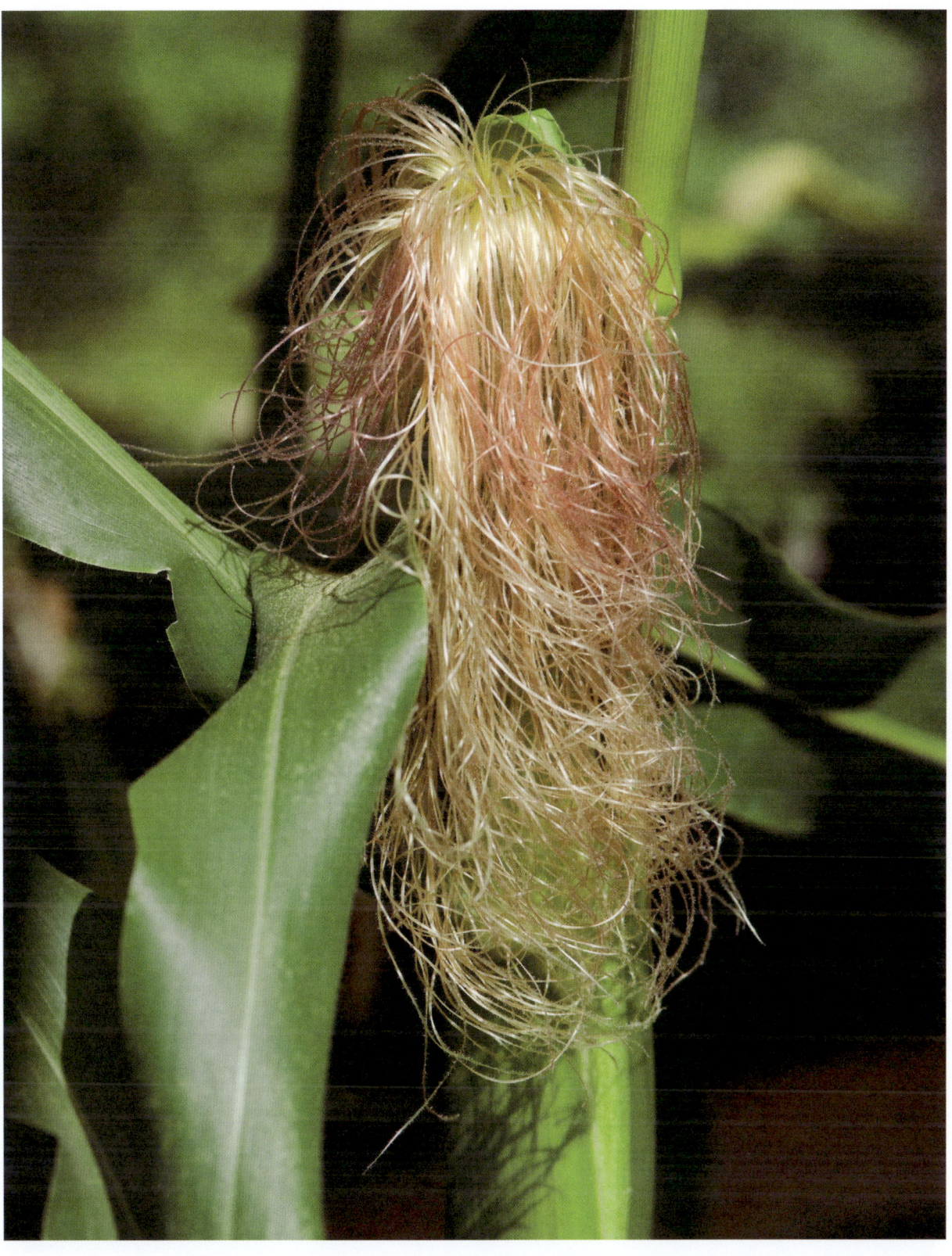

Zingiber officinale
GINGER

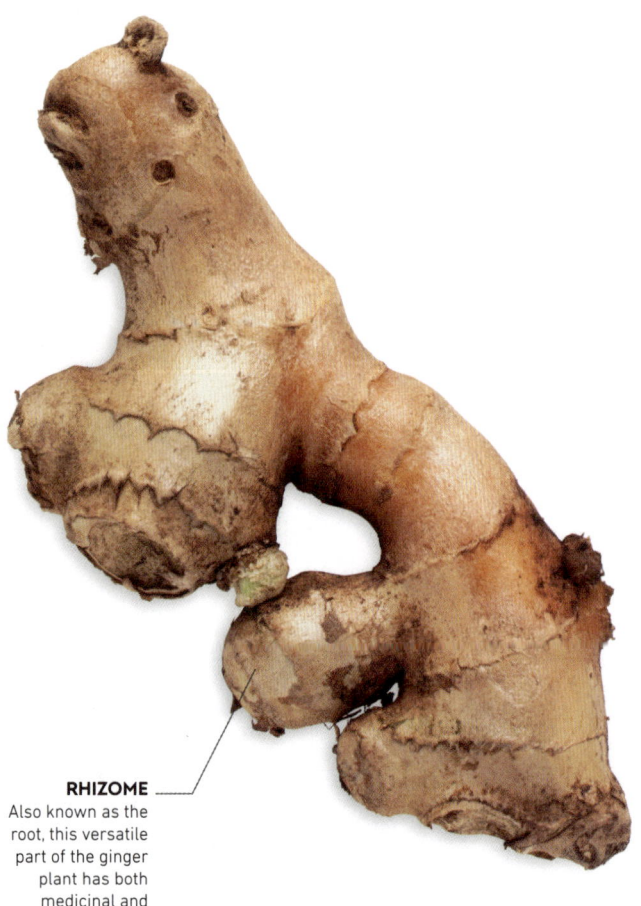

RHIZOME
Also known as the
root, this versatile
part of the ginger
plant has both
medicinal and
culinary uses

Part of the same family as cardamom and turmeric, ginger has been used both as a medicine and as a spice since ancient times. First recorded in Chinese medical literature around 2,000 years ago, this versatile plant has long been used across India, Africa, and Europe. It is often used to treat digestive and inflammatory disorders.

PARTS USED Rhizome (root)
MAIN CONSTITUENTS Volatile oils, phenols, saponins, resins, trace amounts of salicylate vitamins and minerals
MAIN ACTIONS Anti-emetic, antiseptic, carminative, spasmolytic, peripheral circulatory stimulant, anti-inflammatory, diaphoretic

HOW TO USE
INFUSION Grate or chop 1–2 in (3–5 cm) pieces of freshly peeled ginger root and combine with hot water. Take 1 cup 3 times a day to reduce feverish symptoms associated with colds and flu.
DECOCTION Take 1 cup of a standard decoction of the root (p.176) 2–3 times daily for inflammation, cold extremities, period pains, or digestive problems such as nausea.
TINCTURE Take 20–40 drops (2–4 ml) in a little hot water 3 times a day to help reduce inflammation and improve circulation.
POWDER Add ½–1½ tsp (1–3 g) 2–3 times a day to food. Add to onions and garlic at the start of cooking.
FRESH GRATED GINGER Eat 1½–2 tsp (3–4 g) in cooked food each day to reduce digestive discomfort.

HOW TO SOURCE
GROW Propagate indoors by planting a piece od the rhizome into moist, fertile potting soil with good drainage, leaving the "eye bud" pointing out of the soil. The plant will be fully grown within 8–10 months.
FORAGE Unlikely to be found growing in the wild.
HARVEST Dig up the root in the fall.

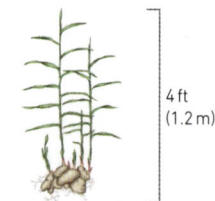

4 ft
(1.2 m)

GROWTH HABIT
Flowering plant with
long, thin leaves and
yellow–green flowers.

CAUTION Do not use if taking blood-thinning medication, or if suffering from peptic ulcers or gallstones.

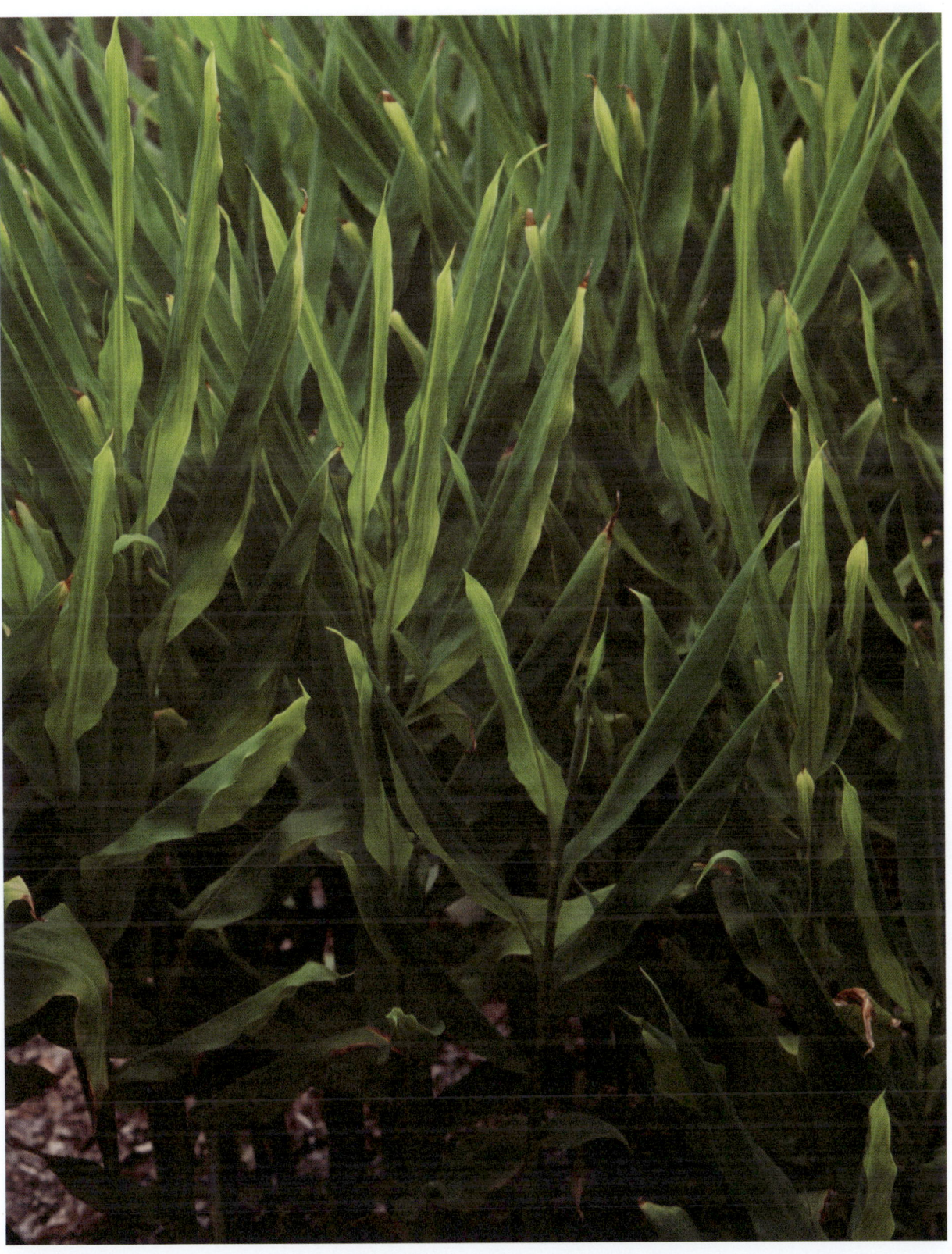

USE HERBS

Discover more than 150 recipes for effective
homemade herbal remedies to help you heal
from the inside and on the outside.

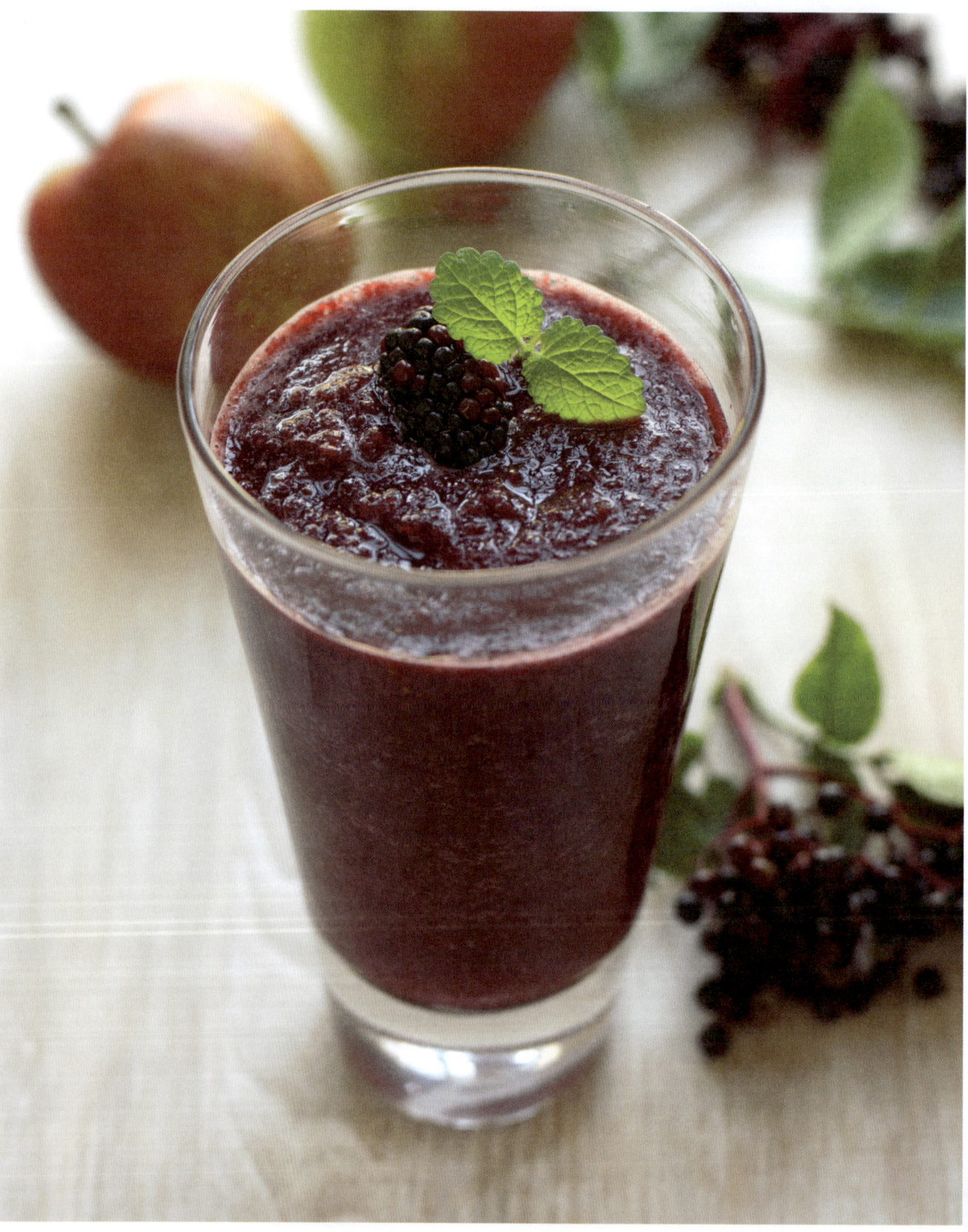

HEAL FROM THE INSIDE

HERB BASICS

INFUSIONS

Often referred to as herbal teas, infusions are the best way to harness the properties of the softer, green, or flowering parts of a plant. A standard therapeutic infusion is 1 heaped tsp of a single dried herb or 2 tsp of a mixture of dried herbs (for fresh herbs use double the amount) to 6fl oz (175ml) boiling water, but see individual herb entries in the A-Z (pp.34–171) for specific dosage instructions.

INGREDIENTS
1 heaped tsp dried herb, or
   2 tsp chopped fresh herb
6fl oz (175ml) boiling water

METHOD
1 Place the chopped herbs in a cup or teapot, and pour the boiling water over the herbs.
2 Leave to steep for 10 minutes, preferably covered to avoid the loss of volatile oils in the steam. Strain the infusion before use.

DECOCTIONS

To use the woodier parts of a plant, make a decoction. A standard decoction is 1 tsp dried herb or 2 tsp fresh herb to 175ml (6fl oz) water, but see individual herb entries for specific dosage instructions. Use a steel or enameled cast iron pan if possible, as aluminum can react with anything cooked in it and could taint the decoction. This recipe makes three cups.

INGREDIENTS
1 tsp (½oz/15g) dried herb
   or mixture of herbs, or
   2 tsp (1oz/30g) fresh herbs
1¼ pints (750ml) cold water

METHOD
1 Place the chopped herbs in a saucepan, and pour in the water.
2 Cover the pan with a lid and bring to a boil, then simmer gently for 15–20 minutes.
3 Strain the decoction and divide into 3 doses for use that day.

MACERATED OILS

This is the quickest, most practical method of making a macerated or infused oil, and is known as the "heat" method. Adjust the quantities below to make a larger or smaller amount of oil; there should be enough oil to completely cover the chopped herbs in the bowl.

INGREDIENTS
3½oz (100g) dried herbs or
   10oz (300g) finely chopped
   fresh herbs
16fl oz (500ml) vegetable oil,
   such as organic sunflower
   or olive oil

METHOD
1 Place the finely chopped herbs in a heatproof bowl,and add the oil to completely cover the herbs.
2 Place the bowl over a pan of boiling water on the stove, cover the bowl, and heat gently for 2 hours. Top up the water as needed.
3 Strain the mixture and repeat by adding fresh herbs to the oil and warming again for 1 hour.
4 Strain the oil, pour into a sterilized dark glass bottle (p.210), and label with the name and date.
5 If using fresh herbs, let the oil stand for a few hours after straining to allow water from the herbs to sink to the bottom. Pour off the oil into the sterilized bottle and discard any water. Store in a cool place and use within 3 months.

TINCTURES

The medicinal properties of herbs can be extracted using a mixture of alcohol and herbs to give a preparation called a tincture. The alcohol acts as a preservative, making this an excellent way to store herbs out of season; a tincture will keep for up to 12 months.

Volume for volume, tinctures are much stronger than infusions, decoctions, or macerates, so should be used in smaller quantities. See individual herb entries in the A–Z (pp.34–171) for specific dosage instructions. Tinctures may vary in strength (eg. 1:3 or 1:5), so always follow the dosage instructions on the bottle when buying. Dosages in the A–Z are based on a 1:5 tincture unless otherwise specified. These quantities makes an approximately 1:5 tincture.

INGREDIENTS

7oz (200g) dried herb (fresh herbs will need to be dried prior to use, in order to reduce the water content of the tincture)

1¾ pints (1 liter) 80 proof vodka

METHOD

1 Chop the herbs finely, and place in a large, sterilized, sealable jar (p.210).
2 Immerse the herbs completely in the alcohol.
3 Seal the jar and store for 2 weeks away from direct sunlight, shaking occasionally.
4 Strain the mixture through a muslin cloth and then filter through an unbleached coffee filter.
5 Pour into a sterilized dark glass bottle (p.210). Label clearly with the name and date, and store in a cool, dark place.

IMPORTANT SAFETY INFORMATION

HERB SAFETY

Herbs and herbal remedies should be treated with respect. Individual herb entries in the A–Z (pp.34–171) give cautionary notes for each herb. Follow the method, dosage, and usage instructions closely.

ESSENTIAL OIL SAFETY

Essential oils contain the active ingredients of a plant in a highly concentrated form, and should always be diluted in vegetable base oil before use. A typical dilution for a massage oil is 2 percent combined essential oils to 98 percent base oil. Essential oils must be diluted before adding to a bath, e.g. 5 drops of essential oil in 1 tbsp (15 ml) of vegetable oil or milk. They should never be taken internally without professional recommendation, and children under two should not be treated with essential oils. Some essential oils, such as basil and sage, should be avoided during pregnancy; consult an aromatherapist before using any essential oils at this time. Do not take essential oils if also taking homeopathic medication.

SOAP SAFETY

Soap-making requires accurate measuring and is potentially dangerous. The soap recipes in this book are not to be attempted by children. Buy 100 percent sodium hydroxide (caustic soda) and always wear protective plastic gloves and goggles. When you first make a soap, it is extremely alkaline because of the caustic soda and has a very high pH value that drops over several weeks as the soap dries out. Test its pH value (pH testing kits are widely available) to see if it is too alkaline to use. It will eventually drop to a pH of 10–10.5, which is normal for soap but can still be an irritant to sensitive skin.

MAKING JUICES AND SMOOTHIES

These juice recipes provide an instant means of detoxing and revitalizing your body, while the smoothies are a healthy yet tasty way to combine fruits, seeds, grains, and nuts to provide vitamins, minerals, phytonutrients (from fruit), essential fatty acids, and protein (from seeds).

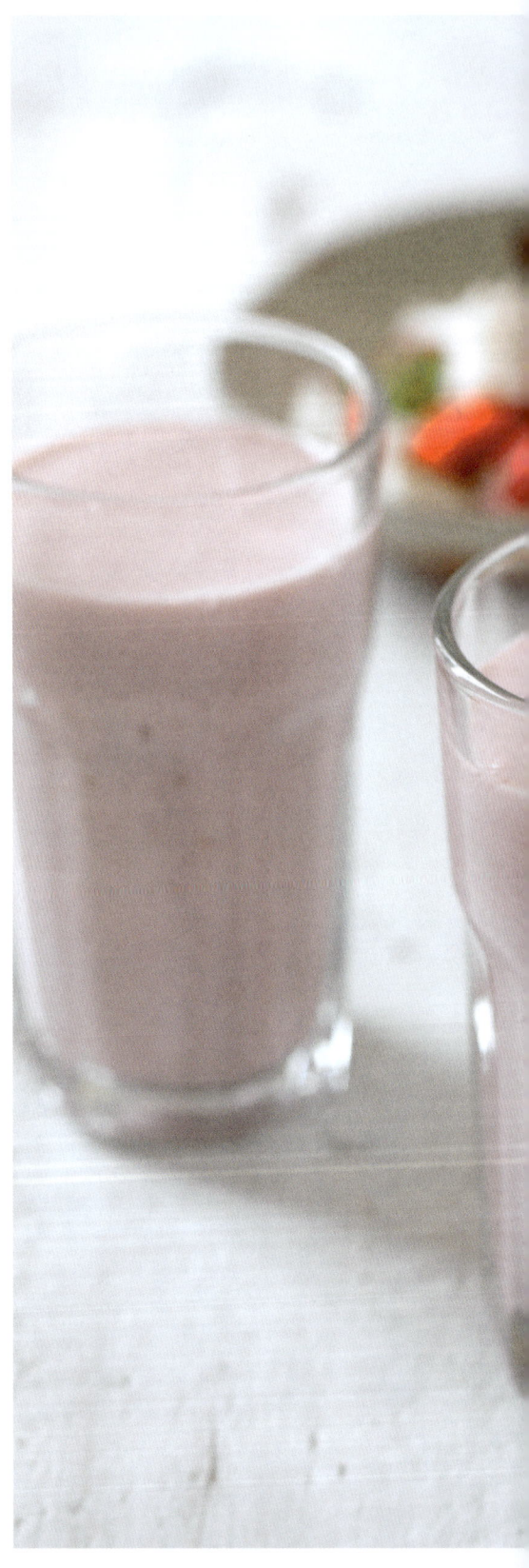

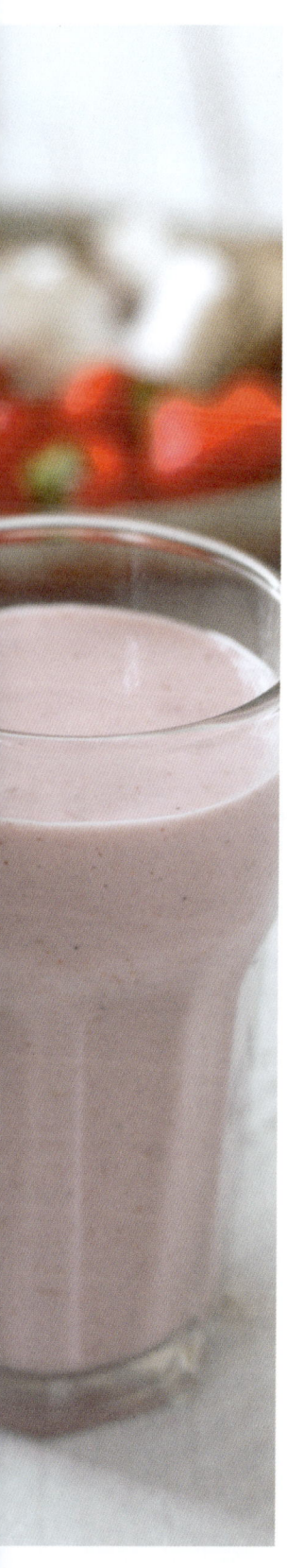

STRAWBERRY AND MACADAMIA SMOOTHIE

ACTS AS A MALE TONIC

INGREDIENTS
½ vanilla bean
⅓ cup (50g) raw macadamia nuts
pulp of 1 young medium-sized coconut
1¾ cup (250g) fresh strawberries
a little of the coconut juice (optional)

MAKES 4 SERVINGS

This healthy twist on strawberries and cream uses coconut pulp and macadamia nuts. Macadamia nut oil is a rich source of monounsaturated fatty acids, which are reputed to lower cholesterol, while coconut pulp helps to clear the effects of summer heat in the body, quenches the thirst, and is a male reproductive tonic.

METHOD
1 Slit the vanilla bean open with a sharp knife, then scrape out the seeds.
2 Place the nuts and the coconut pulp in a blender or food processor.
3 Add the strawberries and vanilla seeds. Pulse all the ingredients to give a smooth, silky texture. If the smoothie seems very thick, add enough coconut juice to give it a better texture. Pour into 4 glasses and serve.

GOJI BERRY AND PINE NUT SMOOTHIE

INGREDIENTS
⅓ cup (50g) almonds
½ cup (50g) goji berries (fresh or dried)
⅛ cup (20g) pine nuts
1 tsp flaxseed oil
2–3 leaves of fresh peppermint
1½–1⅔ cups (350–400ml) mineral water (start with less water and adjust to a consistency and thickness you like)

MAKES 2 SERVINGS

Goji berries provide many amino acids and trace minerals—in particular germanium, a trace mineral thought to have anti-cancer properties. Not surprisingly, they have become known as a "superfood." The berries are also a rich source of carotenoids, including zeaxanthin (which strengthens eyesight) and vitamins C, B complex, and vitamin E.

METHOD
1 To sprout the almonds, soak them in cold water for half an hour, then rinse in a colander under running water. Place in a large bowl, cover with water, and leave overnight to soak. The next day, pop the skins off, place the almonds in a clean bowl, cover with mineral water, and refrigerate for up to 24 hours before draining.
2 Wash the goji berries and, if dried, soak them for few hours in a bowl of mineral water (allow enough space for the berries to expand and sufficient water—⅔ cup/150ml of water should be enough—for the fruit to remain submerged). Drain the berries.
3 Place all ingredients in a blender or food processor and blend with the mineral water to give a smooth, silky texture. If the consistency is a bit too thick, add a little more water and blend.

BLACK CURRANT BOOSTER SMOOTHIE

INGREDIENTS
½ cup (50g) fresh black currants (or used dried and soak first)
¼ cup (50g) roasted barley (p.240)
4 tsp agave syrup
4 tsp coconut oil
1 cup (250ml) rice milk (unsweetened)
A little mineral water

MAKES 2 SERVINGS

Black currants are rich in vitamin C, rutin, and other flavonoids. Their high essential fatty acid levels may help treat inflammatory conditions and manage pain, as well as regulate the circulatory system and enhance the immune system. Use warm rice milk and add a little more roasted barley and some nuts to turn this smoothie into a nourishing breakfast in winter.

METHOD
Put all the ingredients except the mineral water in a blender or food processor and blend until smooth. Add enough mineral water to ensure the smoothie is of a pourable consistency.

SOUR CHERRY AND CACAO SMOOTHIE

INGREDIENTS
⅓ cup (50g) sour cherries, stoned if fresh, or dried
1⅓ cup (300ml) rice or almond milk
4 tsp cacao (raw cocoa) powder
4 tsp hemp seeds, shelled
4 tsp flaxseed oil

MAKES 2 SERVINGS

This smoothie is ideal before or after exercising and for long-distance runners, as the anti-inflammatory properties of cherries aid quicker muscle recovery and pain relief. Sour cherries are also a source of natural melatonin, a potent antioxidant with immune system-modulating properties. If eaten regularly, they may even help regulate the body's natural sleep patterns.

METHOD

1 If using dried sour cherries, soak them for few hours in ⅔ cup (150ml) of mineral water.

2 Combine half the rice or almond milk with the rest of the ingredients in a blender or food processor and blend to a smooth, silky, pourable consistency. Add the rest of the milk in stages until the texture of the smoothie is to your liking.

ALMOND AND ROSE SMOOTHIE

INGREDIENTS
⅓ cup (50g) almonds
1½–1⅔ cups (350–400ml) mineral water
2½ tbsp rose syrup
4 tsp almond oil
1 drop rose otto (optional)
8 damask rose petals (optional)

MAKES 2 SERVINGS

Almonds are a great food for strengthening the heart and blood vessels. They contain nutrients such as magnesium, potassium, copper, selenium, manganese, and vitamin E, which is known for its antioxidant activity. Almonds are also reported to lower cholesterol levels, while rose creates a sense of relaxed well-being.

METHOD

1 To sprout the almonds, soak them in cold water for half an hour, then rinse in a colander under running water. Place in a large bowl, cover with water, and leave overnight to soak. The next day, pop the skins off, place the almonds in a clean bowl, cover with filtered or bottled mineral water, and refrigerate for up to 24 hours before draining. Discard the soaking water.

2 Combine half the mineral water with the rest of the ingredients in a blender or food processor and blend to a smooth, silky, pourable consistency. Add the rest of the water in stages until the texture of the smoothie is to your liking.

PISTACHIO AND AVOCADO SMOOTHIE

INGREDIENTS
½ cup (50g) pistachios (plus a few for decoration)
1 small avocado, pitted, peeled, and quartered
1 tsp hemp seed oil
2 tsp flaxseed oil
juice of ½ lemon
fresh juice of 6 celery ribs
freshly ground black pepper, to taste
pinch of salt
3–4 fresh basil leaves
a little mineral water

MAKES 2 SERVINGS

Pistachios are revered in Ayurvedic and Middle Eastern traditions as a tonic for the whole body. In traditional Chinese medicine, they are believed to positively influence the liver and especially the kidneys. The addition of avocado, hemp seed oil, and flaxseed oil add body and a rich blend of omega oils to this smoothie.

METHOD
1 Put all the ingredients except the mineral water into a blender or food processor and blend until smooth. Add enough mineral water to ensure the smoothie is of a pourable consistency.
2 Serve in glasses, with a sprinkle of finely chopped pistachios on top of each.

MACA AND MANGO SMOOTHIE

INGREDIENTS
2 large ripe mangoes
2 tsp maca root powder
2 tsp hemp seeds, shelled
2 tsp flaxseeds
2 tsp coconut oil
juice of 1 lemon
4 fresh peppermint leaves
a little mineral water (optional)

MAKES 2 SERVINGS

Maca root (*Lepidium meyenii*) does not taste tremendously interesting, but it has a reputation for invigorating the body and enhancing sexual stamina. Peruvians consider it to be a superfood. Coconut oil, flaxseeds, and hemp seeds all provide essential fatty acids, while fresh ripe mango provides body and flavor.

METHOD
Place all the ingredients in a blender or food processor and blend to a smooth, silky texture. Dilute with mineral water as desired, if necessary.

PLUM AND FENNEL SMOOTHIE

DETOXES

INGREDIENTS
9–10 large, dark plums
1 cup mineral water
½ tsp fennel seeds
2 tbsp flaxseeds, soaked
2 tbsp shelled hemp seeds,
   soaked

MAKES 2 SERVINGS

All the ingredients in this smoothie have a natural laxative quality. This is a good drink to take not only for occasional constipation, but also as a part of a more extensive detox regime. If you prefer a very smooth texture without chunks, use a teaspoon each of flaxseed and hemp seed oils instead of the soaked seeds.

METHOD
1 Stew the plums first: put them in a saucepan with the mineral water, add the fennel seeds, and bring to a boil. Put the lid on and simmer over low heat for 10–12 minutes. Allow to cool.
2 Transfer to a blender or food processor, add the remaining seeds (or oils, if using), and blend to a smooth consistency.

POWER BERRY SMOOTHIE

NOURISHES BLOOD

REJUVENATES,
REVITALIZES

INGREDIENTS
2 tbsp fresh raspberries
2 tbsp fresh blackberries
2 tbsp fresh blueberries
2 tbsp fresh black currants
2 tsp acai berry powder
1¼ pints (800ml) lemongrass
   infusion, cold (p.176)
a little mineral water
   (optional)
a dash of maple syrup or a
   pinch of stevia powder
   (optional)

MAKES 2 SERVINGS

These fragrantly sweet but subtly tart fresh berries are a powerhouse of phytonutrients with antioxidant, antimicrobial, and anticarcinogenic properties. Their seed oil contains exceptionally high levels of vitamins E and A and omega-3 and omega-6 fatty acids, and they also protect the heart and nourish the liver.

METHOD
1 Place the fresh berries and acai berry powder in a blender or food processor, add the lemongrass infusion, and blend to a smooth, silky texture.
2 If necessary, add a little mineral water to achieve a consistency you like. Ensure that most of the seeds from the fruit have been ground down so that they release their oils. Add the maple syrup or stevia powder to sweeten only if needed.

EARLY AUTUMN RAMBLER'S DELIGHT

INGREDIENTS

3½ apples, peeled, cored, and chopped

⅓ pear peeled, cored, and chopped

12 ripe elderberries, rinsed, with all stems removed

20 ripe blackberries, rinsed

MAKES 2 SERVINGS

This is a great way to use freshly picked elderberries and blackberries, which contain high levels of antioxidants that help to fight free-radical damage and enhance the immune system. Blackberries are extremely high in phenolic compounds, which are known to be health-promoting, antiviral, and antibacterial, while elderberries contain potassium and vitamins C and E.

METHOD

1 Place all the ingredients into a blender or a food processor and blend until smooth.

2 Divide between two glasses and top with elderberry and elderflower syrup (p.204) to enhance the antiviral content of the smoothie.

NOTE: Unripe, raw elderberries and elder bark should be avoided, so make sure you use completely ripe elderberries with no stem attached to make this smoothie.

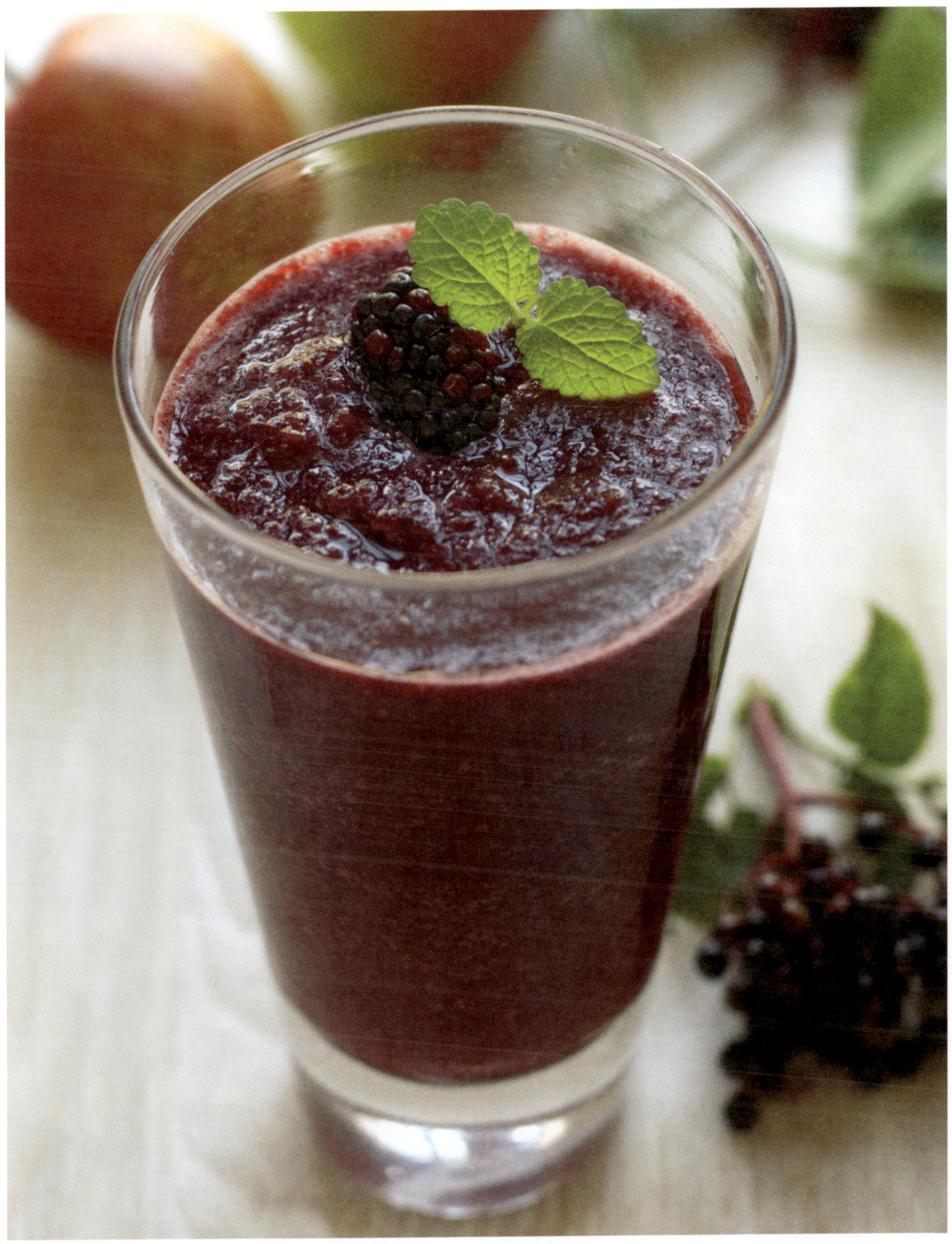

GARDEN GREENS JUICE

MAKES 2 SERVINGS

If you have a vegetable garden, a great way to use up any excess produce is to serve it as refreshing, detoxifying drinks. Zucchini, cucumber, and celery ribs all provide a mild base to which you can add fragrant kale leaves, sour chard, and spinach. The marjoram added to this juice aids digestion and alleviates abdominal distension and gas.

METHOD
Wash and juice all the vegetables and herbs, and mix thoroughly. Add the lemon juice to taste if you wish or, if you prefer a more powerful lemon flavor, add an eighth of a lemon (organic is preferable) and mix well until blended.

DETOXES

INGREDIENTS
2 handfuls of kale leaves
2 Swiss chard leaves
1 large handful of spinach leaves
½ cucumber
1 small zucchini
3 celery ribs
2 dandelion leaves (large)
2 stems fresh marjoram
a dash of lemon juice (optional)

RED PEPPER AND SPROUTED SEED JUICE

MAKES 2 SERVINGS

This fragrant, spicy juice is a great way to start the day. Chile stimulates the body, particularly the circulation; strengthens the digestive system; alleviates indigestion; and provides a sense of vigor and warmth, which is beneficial in winter. It also causes the body to perspire, and therefore cool down, which can help during periods of hot weather.

METHOD
Juice all the ingredients and mix thoroughly.

STIMULATES DIGESTION

STIMULATES CIRCULATION

INGREDIENTS
1 red bell pepper, seeded and cut into quarters
¾oz (20g) sprouted alfalfa seeds
¾oz (20g) sprouted red clover seeds
¼oz (10g) sprouted broccoli seeds
½ cucumber
2–3 fresh mint leaves
½ small fresh red chile, seeded

GINGER AND FENNEL JUICE

INGREDIENTS
1 large fennel bulb
½in (1cm) cube fresh ginger, peeled
2 celery ribs
½ small cucumber
½ small zucchini
1 stem fresh basil

MAKES 2 SERVINGS

Fennel bulb, celery, cucumber, and zucchini have a cooling, anti-inflammatory effect on the body, and are beneficial for inflammatory conditions in the stomach, lungs, throat, skin, and vagina. They are also diuretic and work to purify the skin and moisten the lungs. Ginger and basil are included to add fragrance, remove any bloated feelings, and improve digestion.

METHOD
Juice all the ingredients, mix well, and drink immediately.

FENNEL AND BROCCOLI SPROUT JUICE

INGREDIENTS
1 large fennel bulb
1½oz (45g) sprouted broccoli seeds
1½oz (45g) sprouted alfalfa seeds
1 large carrot
2 celery ribs
2–3 fresh mint leaves
dash of lemon juice

MAKES 2 SERVINGS

This juice aims to expel body waste by increasing urination and clearing the bowels to eliminate putrefactive bacteria. Broccoli sprouts are also beneficial for inflammatory eye conditions, while carrots, fennel, and alfalfa seeds are alkaline-forming and help clear acidic conditions, thus helping rheumatism.

METHOD
Juice all the ingredients, add the lemon juice to taste, and mix well.

BUCKWHEAT GREENS AND PEA SHOOT JUICE

INGREDIENTS

2 tbsp young buckwheat greens, finely chopped

4 tbsp fresh pea shoots

2 zucchini

1 cucumber

2 tbsp fresh marjoram leaves

a dash of lemon juice

¾ cup (200ml) mineral water

MAKES 2 SERVINGS

Pea shoots and buckwheat greens are excellent sources of enzymes, vitamins, and chlorophyll. Buckwheat also contains rutin (4–6 percent), which strengthens the capillaries (rutin belongs to a group of plant compounds called bioflavonoids—powerful antioxidants that fight free radicals) and is useful for reducing varicose veins and hemorrhoids.

METHOD

Juice all ingredients, add the mineral water and lemon juice to taste, and mix well.

TOMATO SALSA JUICE

INGREDIENTS

5 ripe tomatoes

½ cucumber

1 small clove of garlic

½ fresh red chile, seeded

1 stem fresh basil leaves

2 ribs celery

1 tsp extra virgin olive oil

salt, to taste

1 red bell pepper, seeded (optional)

MAKES 2 SERVINGS

This is a great juice to make when you feel like something substantial and savory, but have no time to make a cooked meal. Basil has a reputation for restoring the vital spirits, quickening the brain, and awakening joy and courage. It also enhances digestion, clears respiratory congestion and phlegm, and lifts depression.

METHOD

Juice all the vegetables and herbs, add the olive oil, season to taste with a little salt if you wish, and mix well. If you prefer your juice red, add 1 seeded red bell pepper to the vegetables and herbs when you juice them.

ARTICHOKE LEAF AND FENNEL JUICE

DETOXES

COMBATS NEGATIVE EMOTIONS

INGREDIENTS

1 tsp artichoke leaves
   (from a globe artichoke
   plant), finely chopped
1 medium fennel bulb
4 fresh dandelion leaves
4 celery ribs
½ zucchini

MAKES 2 SERVINGS

The liver needs help every now and then to eliminate wastes from the body. Artichoke leaves, which have a strong, bitter taste, contain cynarin, a compound that stimulates the liver to release these toxic substances and which also improves liver function. Fennel, dandelion leaves, celery ribs, and zucchini also enhance the elimination of waste through the kidneys.

METHOD

Juice all the ingredients, mix thoroughly, and drink. If you find the juice overly bitter, dilute it with some mineral water until it tastes palatable.

SUNFLOWER GREENS AND WHEATGRASS JUICE

DETOXES

REJUVENATES, REVITALIZES

INGREDIENTS

3½oz (100g) sunflower
   greens
3½oz (100g) wheatgrass
   blades
1¼ cups (300ml) or more
   mineral water to dilute
   to taste

MAKES 2 SERVINGS

The juice from wheatgrass and sunflower greens (young plants) is a natural aid that is often used in the treatment of degenerative diseases and to help slow cellular deterioration and relieve inflammation. Its high chlorophyll content also helps detoxify the liver, cleansing and energizing the body.

METHOD

Juice the sunflower greens and wheatgrass, blend well, and add enough mineral water to dilute the flavor of the juice and give it a palatable taste.

MAKING TEAS

The recipes for the tea blends provided here allow you to explore the wonderful flavors of plants, with subtle nurturing and healing qualities in a single cup. All the plants mentioned here can be used either fresh or dry—and may inspire you to grow your own healing teas in your garden.

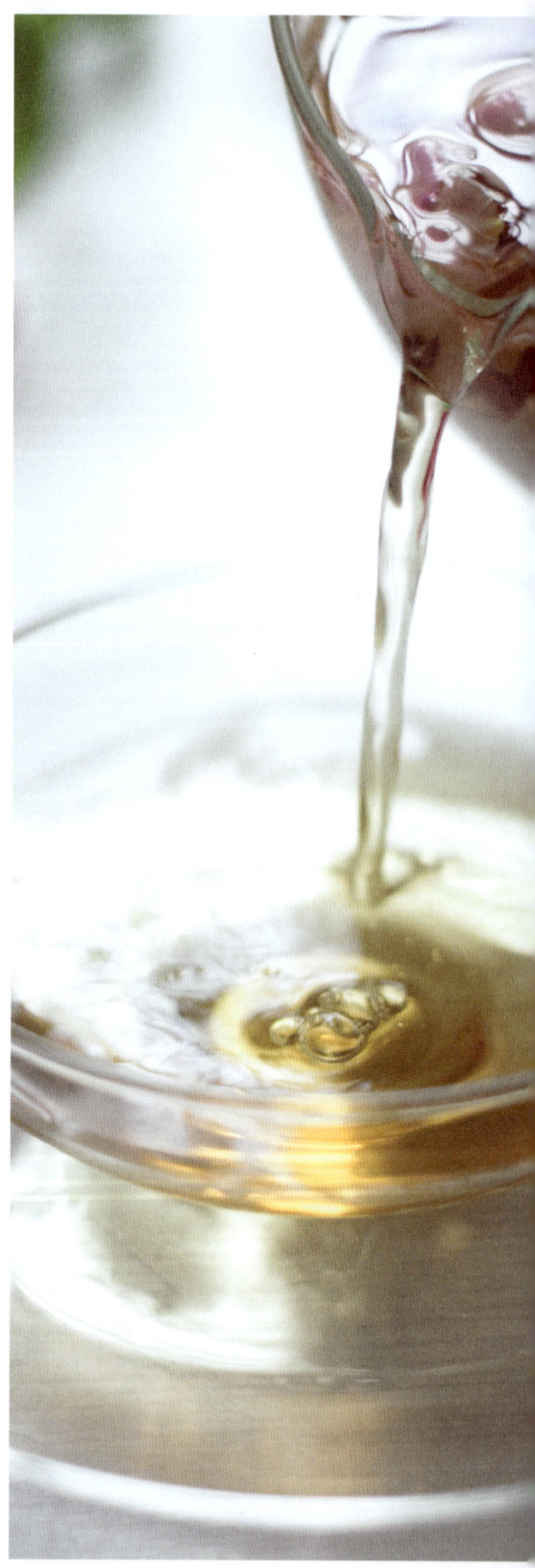

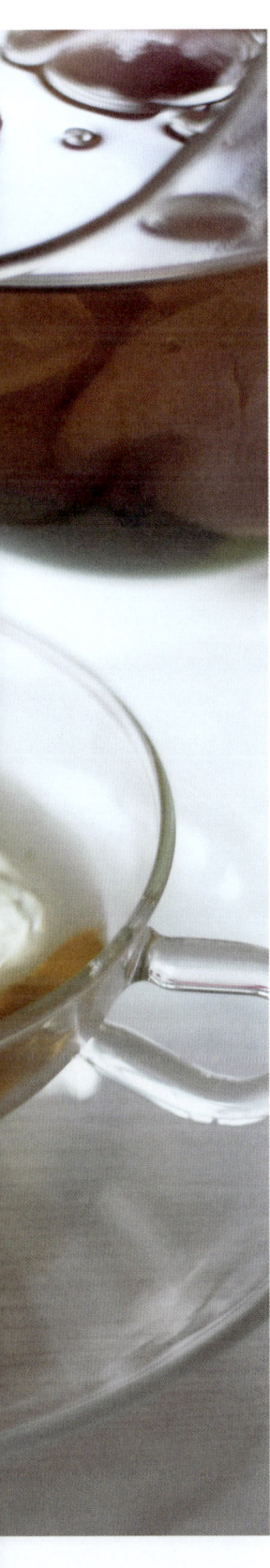

LEMON BALM AND ROSE TEA

ENHANCES MOOD

INGREDIENTS
16 leaves of fresh lemon
  balm (the soft flowering
  tops can also be used), or
  1 tbsp dried lemon balm
petals from 2 rose heads, or
  2 tbsp dried rose petals

MAKES 2–3 SERVINGS

This herbal tea contains a fusion of
empowering yet relaxing lemon balm and
mood-enhancing, sensual rose petals to make
the ultimate summer refreshment. It can be
enjoyed hot or cold, and is best drunk slightly
bitter. For the best results, pick fresh lemon
balm leaves and fresh perfumed rose petals
from the damask rose (*Rosa* x *damascena*) or
French rose (*Rosa gallica*).

METHOD
1 Place the fresh lemon balm leaves and rose petals in
a large teapot. If using dried lemon balm and rose petals,
spoon them into the teapot instead.
2 Boil 16fl oz (500ml) of water, allow to cool for
5 minutes, then pour it into the teapot. Allow to infuse
for 5 minutes and then serve. More water can be added
later if needed to reinfuse the leaves and rose petals.

JASMINE AND LEMONGRASS TEA

ALLEVIATES ANXIETY

REVIVES PASSION

REVIVES PASSION

INGREDIENTS
1 stem lemongrass, chopped
1 tbsp jasmine flowers
a dash of lime juice

MAKES 2 SERVINGS

Both jasmine flowers and lemongrass help relax the mind, alleviate anxiety, improve communication, and revive passion. For the best flavor, buy fresh lemongrass from your local specialty foods store or a supermarket.

METHOD
1 Place the chopped lemongrass in a teapot and add the jasmine flowers and lime juice.
2 Dilute ¾ cup of boiled water with ¼ cup of cold water so that the temperature of the hot water is approximately 158°F (70°C).
3 Pour the water into the teapot, allow the aroma to develop, and serve. In hot weather, this tea can be served chilled.

GOJI BERRY AND DAMIANA TEA

ENHANCES SEXUAL EXPRESSION

ENHANCES SEXUAL EXPRESSION

INGREDIENTS
1 tbsp goji berries, fresh or
    dried
1 tsp damiana
½ tsp licorice root

MAKES 2 SERVINGS

Damiana has a distinctive fragrance and flavor. It lifts depression, relieves anxiety, alleviates fatigue, and enhances reproductive energy. Goji berries also improve fertility, strengthen the heart, improve disease resistance, and alleviate menopausal symptoms. Licorice is a tonic that is restorative to the adrenal glands and alleviates fatigue.

METHOD
Place all the ingredients in a teapot, cover with 1¼ cups of boiling water, allow to stand for 10–15 minutes, then serve. The infusion can also be left to cool and served as a cold drink.

Note: This tea is not suitable for use during pregnancy.

ROSE HIP AND BILBERRY TEA

INGREDIENTS

1 tbsp rose hip shells, fresh
  or dried
1 tbsp bilberries, fresh
  or dried
1 tsp orange rind
1 tsp goji berries, fresh
  or dried

MAKES 2 SERVINGS

Rose hip helps to maintain healthy collagen in the skin;
bilberries enhance blood perfusion to give skin a rosy,
plumped complexion; and bilberries and goji berries are
anti-inflammatory. These fruits are also known to be
powerful antioxidants, while orange rind harmonizes the
digestive system and helps improve the absorption of
nutrients. This tea is also delicious served cold.

METHOD

Place all ingredients in a teapot and cover with 1¼ cups of
boiling water. Allow to infuse for 10–15 minutes, strain, and serve.
(After straining, all the ingredients can be added to oatmeal
and eaten.)

CHRYSANTHEMUM AND ELDERFLOWER TEA

INGREDIENTS

½ tbsp chrysanthemum
  flowers (*Chrysanthemum
  morifolium*)
½ tbsp elderflowers
½ tbsp peppermint
½ tbsp nettle leaves

MAKES 2 SERVINGS

This is a good tea to drink to alleviate symptoms of hay
fever or to ward off colds or flu. All the ingredients reduce
sweating, defend the body from pathogenic influences,
have anti-allergic activity, and calm allergic reactions—
especially to pollen and dust. Chrysanthemum also cools
the body, neutralizes toxins, improves and brightens the
eyes, and protects against liver damage.

METHOD

Place all the ingredients in a teapot, cover with 1¼ cups of boiling
water, allow to infuse, and serve. Drink 3–4 cups a day during the
hay fever season.

CHAMOMILE AND FENNEL TEA

INGREDIENTS
1 tsp chamomile flowers
1 tsp fennel seeds
1 tsp meadowsweet
1 tsp marshmallow root,
   finely chopped
1 tsp yarrow

MAKES 3 SERVINGS

This is a soothing, anti-inflammatory infusion of herbs that are well known for their beneficial effect on an unsettled, bloated, or acidic digestive system. It will encourage better food assimilation, help regulate the bowels, and improve an over-acidic system.

METHOD
1 Put the herbs in a large teapot.
2 Boil 16fl oz (500ml) of water, and add to the teapot. Allow to infuse for 5 minutes and serve. Drink 1 cup of the infusion 2–3 times a day.

NOTE: This tea is not suitable for use during pregnancy.

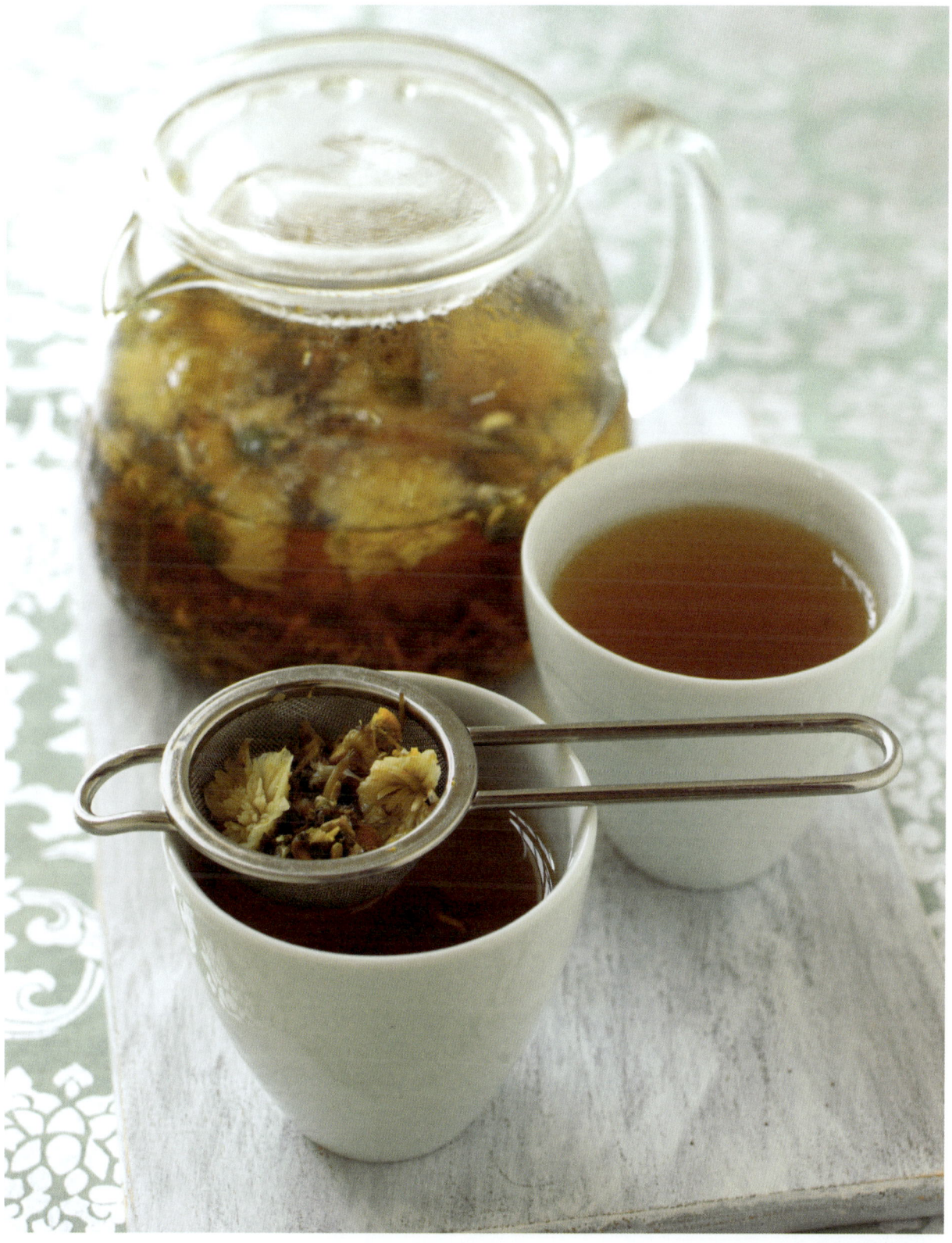

DANDELION AND BURDOCK TEA

SOOTHES INFLAMED SKIN

STIMULATES LIVER
AND KIDNEY

INGREDIENTS
1 tsp dandelion leaves
1 tsp burdock leaves
1 tsp cleavers herb
1 tsp red clover flowers

MAKES 3–4 SERVINGS

This classic blend of herbs helps clear up blemished skin. It treats eczema and acne by gently invigorating the liver and kidneys to remove accumulated waste, while its anti-inflammatory activity helps improve skin eruptions on the head, neck, and upper body. It is also appropriate for anyone who wishes to detox.

METHOD
Place all the ingredients in a teapot, pour in 2 cups of boiling water, allow to infuse for 10–15 minutes, and serve. Drink hot or cold through the day.

Note: This tea is not suitable for use during pregnancy.

YARROW AND CALENDULA TEA

RELIEVES PMS

HARMONIZES EMOTIONS

IMPROVES CIRCULATION

INGREDIENTS
1 tsp yarrow
1 tsp marigold flowers
1 tsp lady's mantle
1 tsp vervain
1 tsp raspberry leaf

MAKES 3–4 SERVINGS

These herbs all benefit the female body. Yarrow and calendula (marigold) relieve blood and energy stagnation in the abdomen and improve blood circulation to the womb. Vervain invigorates the liver, releases tension, and relaxes the mind. Lady's mantle, an astringent, relieves congestion through urination. Raspberry leaf will help relieve period pains.

METHOD
Place all the ingredients in a teapot, pour in 2 cups of boiling water, allow to infuse for 10–15 minutes, and serve. Drink hot or cold through the day. Take 2–4 cups with the onset of pain, and reassess with your health professional if the pain persists.

Note: This tea is not suitable for use during pregnancy.

SKULLCAP AND ORANGE FLOWER TEA

INGREDIENTS
1 tsp skullcap
1 tsp orange flowers
1 tsp St John's wort
1 tsp wood betony
1 tsp lemon balm

MAKES 3–4 SERVINGS

Herbal teas such as this can help you relax and begin to put things into perspective—especially if you are suffering from feelings of depression. Skullcap, St. John's wort, wood betony, lemon balm, and orange flower are all known to help ease tensions, relax the body and mind, and lift the spirits.

METHOD
Place all the ingredients in a teapot, pour in 2 cups of boiling water, allow to infuse for 10–15 minutes, and serve. Drink hot or cold through the day.

Note: This tea is not suitable for use during pregnancy.

BLACKBERRY AND WILD STRAWBERRY TEA

INGREDIENTS
2 tsp blackberry leaves
1 tsp wild strawberry leaves
1 tsp raspberry leaves
1 tsp black currant leaves

MAKES 3–4 SERVINGS

The leaves of these fruits are well known for their ability to heal, as well as for their revitalizing and rejuvenating qualities. Their ability to cleanse the body of the excesses of winter is remarkable. Use fresh leaves to make this tea in the spring, and harvest and dry some for use during the winter months.

METHOD
Place all the ingredients in a teapot, pour in 2 cups of boiling water, allow to infuse for 10–15 minutes, and serve. Drink hot or cold through the day.

Note: This tea is not suitable for use during pregnancy.

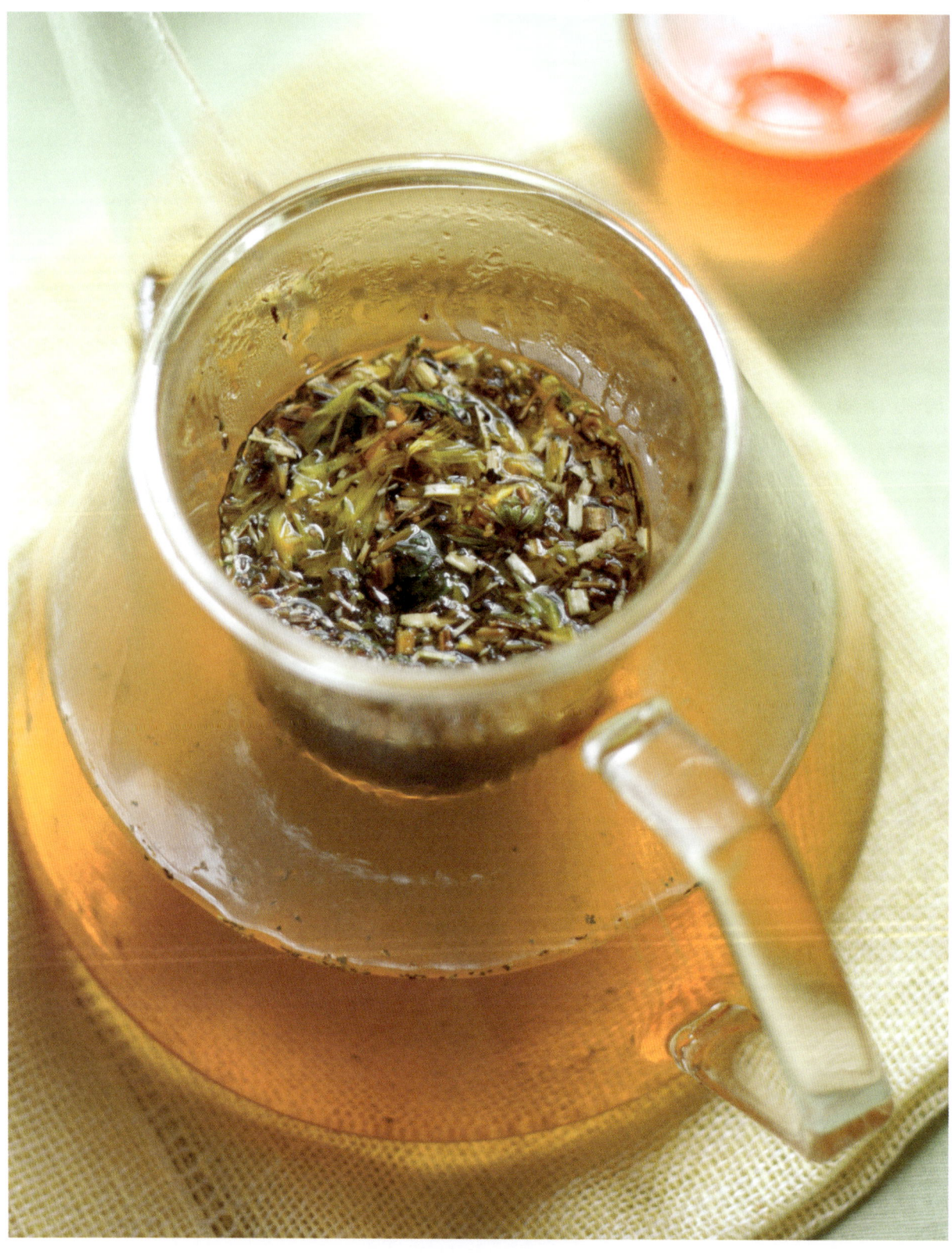

PEPPERMINT AND CALENDULA INFUSION

INGREDIENTS
1 tsp peppermint leaves
1 tsp calendula flowers
1 tsp motherwort
1 tsp vervain
rose petal syrup (p.210)
   to sweeten

MAKES 4 SERVINGS

This infusion works for premenstrual tension and period pains. Peppermint releases tension and calms the mind. Motherwort and vervain are used to treat menstrual irregularities, have a relaxing effect on the nervous system, and relieve tension and pain. Calendula aids the other herbs in nurturing the womb, and roses have a healing influence.

METHOD
1 Put all the herbs into a large teapot.
2 Boil 1 pint (600ml) of boiling water, and pour over the herbs. Allow to infuse for 20 minutes, then strain the liquid through a tea strainer into a clean jug. Drink 1 mug of the infusion 2–3 times a day, either hot or at room temperature.

NOTE: This tea is not suitable for use during pregnancy.

"THIS BLEND OF HERBS WORKS WELL WHETHER IT IS MADE FROM FRESH PLANT MATERIAL OR FROM DRY, AND IS BEST DRUNK SLIGHTLY BITTER"

HAWTHORN FLOWER AND LAVENDER TEA

INGREDIENTS
1 tsp hawthorn flowers
1 tsp lavender
1 tsp rosebuds
1 tsp orange flowers
1 tsp jasmine

MAKES 3–4 SERVINGS

There are some heartaches, such as overwhelming emotions, sense of loss, and lack of self-worth, that only the soft and enlightened fragrance of flowers can soothe. Hawthorn "lightens the heart," lavender relaxes the mind, rose eases a broken heart, and orange flower and jasmine encourage a desire to make things better and start anew.

METHOD
Place all the ingredients in a teapot, pour in 2 cups (500ml) of boiling water, allow to infuse for 10–15 minutes, and serve. Drink hot or cold throughout the day.

NETTLE AND CLEAVERS TEA

INGREDIENTS
2 tsp nettle leaves
2 tsp cleavers

MAKES 2 SERVINGS

This is a great tea for gentle cleansing at any time of the year. In spring, fresh nettles and cleavers can be juiced and drunk to cleanse and nourish the body. Cleavers help reduce fluid retention in the skin, reduce puffiness under the eyes, and improve the complexion. Nettles also nourish the blood and cleanse the body through increased urination.

METHOD
Place the ingredients in a teapot, pour in 1¼ cup (300ml) of boiling water, allow to infuse for 10–15 minutes, and serve. Drink hot or cold throughout the day.

MULLEIN AND MARSHMALLOW TEA

INGREDIENTS
1 tsp mullein leaves
1 tsp marshmallow leaves
1 tsp ribwort plantain

MAKES 2 SERVINGS

Mullein leaves and flowers and marshmallow leaves, flowers, and roots all provide mucilaginous, anti-inflammatory protection for the respiratory and urinary system. This tea can also be used to treat dry coughs, nervous coughs, dry lungs, and inflamed bronchial tubes. Marshmallow leaf and plantain leaf also soothe an inflamed urinary tract.

METHOD
Place all the ingredients in a teapot, pour in 1¼ cup (300ml) of boiling water, allow to infuse for 10–15 minutes, and serve. Drink hot or cold throughout the day.

HORSETAIL AND CORN SILK TEA

ACTS AS A DIURETIC

ACTS AS A DIURETIC

INGREDIENTS
2 tsp horsetail
2 tsp corn silk
2 tsp dandelion leaves
2 tsp cleavers
2 tsp ribwort plantain leaves

MAKES 5–6 SERVINGS

This refreshing and cleansing tea is especially good for reducing occasional inflammatory conditions in the urinary system, such as cystitis, caused by nonspecific microorganisms. These herbs not only increase urination, they also cool irritation and soothe inflammation of the urinary system, and contain potassium.

METHOD
Place all the ingredients in a teapot, pour in 1 pint (600ml) of boiling water, allow to infuse for 10–15 minutes, and serve. Drink hot or cold throughout the day.

MAKING CORDIALS AND SYRUPS

Fruit cordials and syrups help increase energy levels and nourish the body. The natural benefits of the plants in these cordial and syrup recipes are aided by sugar and honey, which help alleviate dry coughs, sore throats, and general irritations of the respiratory system.

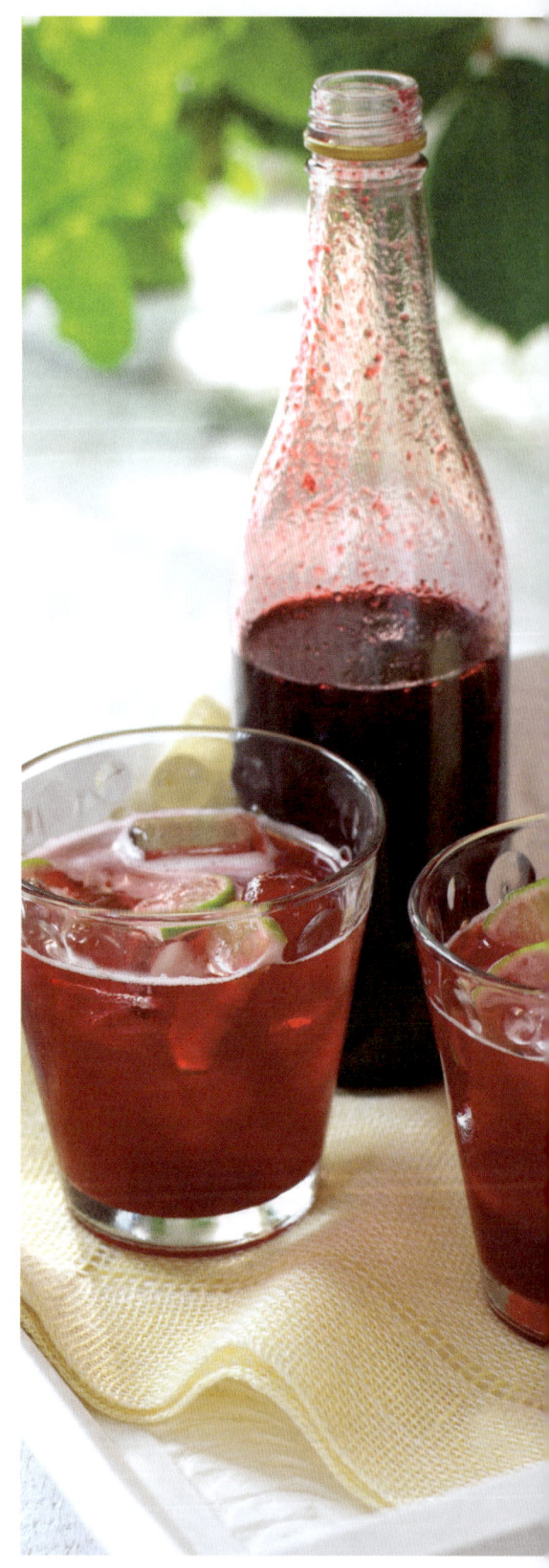

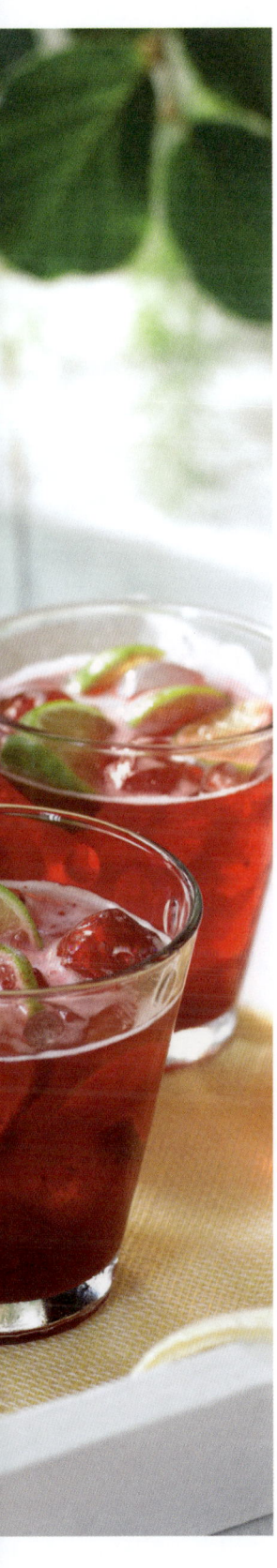

BLACKBERRY AND LIME CORDIAL

SOOTHES A SORE THROAT

REJUVENATES

INGREDIENTS
2¼lb (1kg) fresh
    blackberries
juice of 4 limes
1 pint (600ml) water
1¾ cup (350g) superfine
    sugar

MAKES 16FL OZ (500ML)

Blackberries are packed with antioxidants and are used in many recipes as a traditional remedy for colds and sore throats. This cordial also benefits from the antiseptic and refreshing taste of limes, which help detoxify and cool the body.

METHOD

1 Over low heat, simmer the blackberries and lime juice in the water in a saucepan for approximately 15 minutes.
2 Leave to cool for 10 minutes or so, then push the mixture through a sieve and discard the pulp and pips. Pour the strained juice into a clean saucepan, and add the sugar. Stir over low heat until the sugar has dissolved, and then simmer for about 5 minutes until the mixture is syrupy.
3 Pour into sterilized bottles (p.210) seal, refrigerate, and use within a few days. Dilute to taste with fizzy or still mineral water and fresh mint or lime slices to make a refreshing drink.

ELDERBERRY AND ELDERFLOWER CORDIAL

INGREDIENTS

1¾oz (50g) fresh or dried
  elderflowers
¾ cup (100g) elderberries
  (if using dried, rehydrate
  in water first)
1 small cinnamon stick
1 tsp anise seed
1 tbsp fresh ginger, grated
1 quart (1 liter) water
2 cups (400g) sugar
juice of ½ lemon

MAKES 2 CUPS

This is a useful winter tonic: elderflowers, elderberries, and fresh ginger enhance the body's defense mechanisms that ward off seasonal colds and flu, anise seed gently clears the lungs, and ginger and cinnamon bring warmth to the body. Sugar moistens the respiratory passages and alleviates the dry cough often caused by central heating.

METHOD

1 Place all the ingredients except the sugar and lemon juice in a saucepan, cover, and simmer over low heat for 25–30 minutes.
2 Strain the liquid into a measuring jug. Decant 2 cups into a saucepan and add the sugar. (Any extra liquid can be drunk as a tea.)
3 Stir gently over low heat to dissolve the sugar. When all the sugar has dissolved, add the lemon juice and simmer gently for another 10–15 minutes with the lid off. Then bring it to a boil for 2–3 minutes and remove from the heat.
4 Pour into a sterilized (p.210) 1 pint (600ml) glass bottle while still hot, seal, label with a list of the ingredients, and date. Keep refrigerated and use within 3–4 weeks.
5 Add a tablespoon of the cordial to a cup of cold or hot water, or drizzle on pancakes or breakfast cereals.

SWEET VIOLET AND GINGER HONEY

INGREDIENTS

¾oz (20g) fresh violet leaves and flowers (or use viola, or heartsease, if not available)

1oz (30g) fresh ginger

¾oz (20g) fresh plantain leaves

1oz (30g) fresh houttuynia leaves

2¼ cups (500g) honey

MAKES 1¾–2¼ CUPS (400–500G)

This syrupy extract of fresh violets, ginger, plantain, and houttuynia should be made in spring when all these ingredients are growing fresh in the garden. Violets, plantain, and houttuynia are all good expectorants with strong anti-inflammatory actions. Fresh ginger is diaphoretic. Houttuynia, with its orangelike flavor, adds to the gingery taste.

METHOD

1 Carefully harvest the fresh leaves and flowers and wash and air-dry them.

2 Finely chop them, place in a clean jar, and cover completely with honey. Mix thoroughly to ensure all the herbs are well covered. Add extra honey if necessary.

3 Leave in a warm place for 5 days, then strain the honey through a clean piece of cheesecloth and decant it into a smaller sterilized jar (p.210). Discard the strained herbs.

4 Seal the jar, label with a list of all the ingredients, and date.

5 The honey makes a great drink mixed either with cold or hot water. It will only keep for a few weeks.

LEMON BALM AND HONEY PUREE

MAKES ½ CUP (125G)

This puree, which uses fresh, young, juicy lemon balm leaves, is best prepared in late spring before the plant becomes somewhat woody and the leaves less juicy. It works well as a sweetener for other herbal infusions or summer cocktails, and can be served as a hot or cold drink by adding one or two teaspoons of the puree to boiling or chilled water.

METHOD

1 Place the leaves in a blender or food processor, add the honey and lemon juice, and blend until you get a smooth, green puree.
2 Dilute with water and drink. The puree will last for a week or two if kept refrigerated.

RELAXES

INGREDIENTS
¾oz (20g) fresh lemon balm
   leaves
½ cup (100ml) honey
Juice of ½ lemon

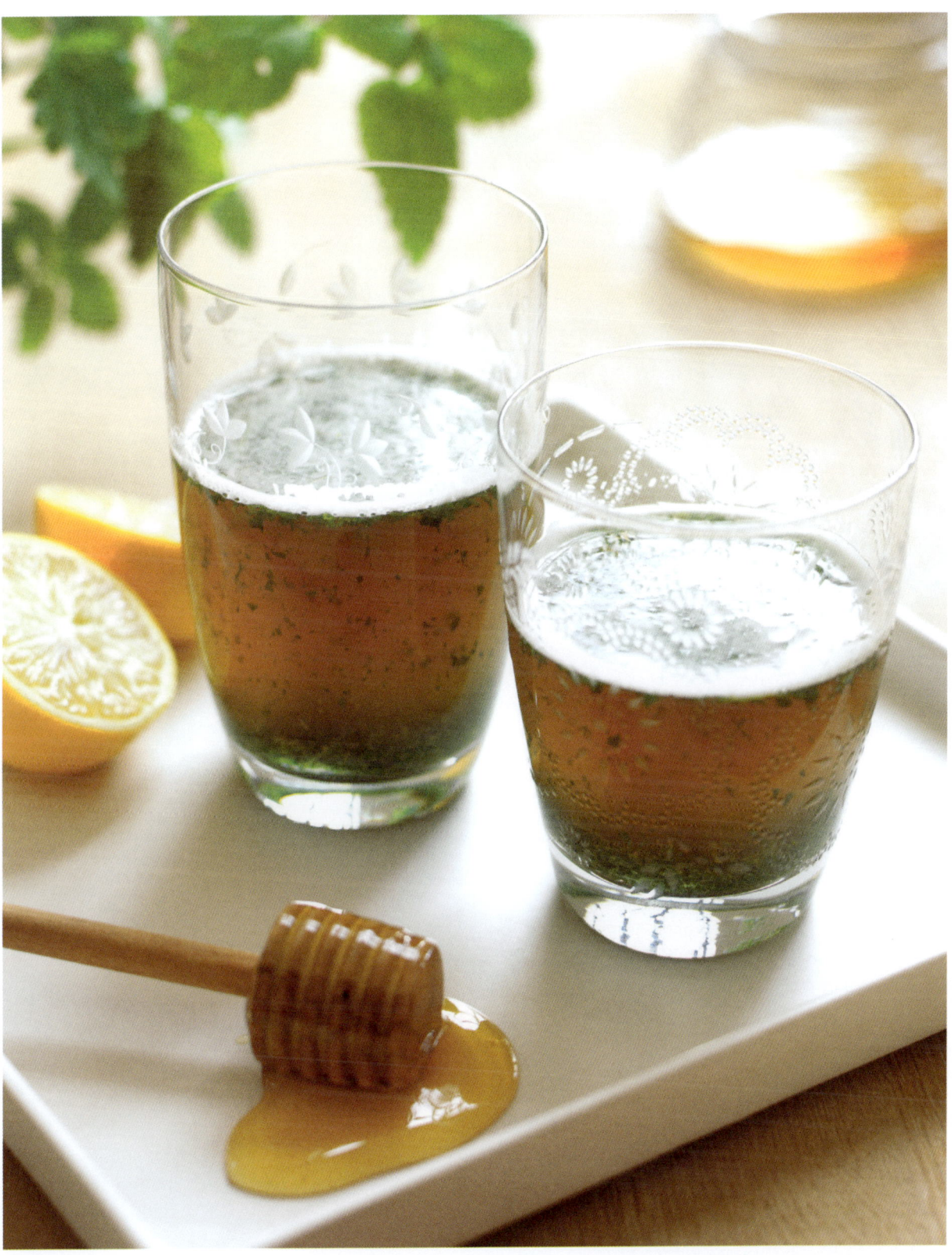

ROSE HIP SYRUP

INMPROVES JOINT HEALTH

NOURISHES SKIN

INGREDIENTS
1lb 2oz (500g) fresh rose
 hips
2½ cups (600ml) water
2 cups (400g) sugar

MAKES ABOUT 2 CUPS

This syrup is for beautiful skin and healthy joints. Rose hips contain vitamins A, B₁, B₂, and a high concentration of vitamin C, and are known for their anti-inflammatory activity in helping reduce muscle and joint stiffness and arthritic pain. They also have antiscorbutic, antihemorrhagic, diuretic, and skin-regenerating properties, and help maintain healthy collagen.

METHOD
1 Pick the rose hips when they are at their best; traditionally they are picked after the first few fall frosts.
2 Slice the fruit in half and scoop out the seeds and hairs with a small spoon (rose hip fruit is full of these small hairs, which can irritate sensitive skin, so it is advisable to wear gloves to do this job). Wash the cleaned halves under running water to further remove the little hairs from the fruit.
3 Place the fruit in a saucepan, add the water, and simmer, uncovered, over low heat for 20–30 minutes until the fruit is soft and the water has reduced slightly.
4 Strain the mixture and decant the liquid into a clean saucepan. Discard the fruit. Add the sugar to the strained liquid and allow it to dissolve over low heat, stirring constantly.
5 Once all the sugar has dissolved, increase the heat and boil for 2–3 minutes. Decant the syrup into a sterilized bottle (p.210). Seal and label with the name and date. Keep refrigerated and use within 6 weeks.

MULLEIN AND ANISEED SYRUP

MAKES ¾ CUP

A mild expectorant to soothe winter coughs, this syrup uses tinctures of mullein, marshmallow root, thyme, and anise seed, combined with the anti-inflammatory action of plantain and licorice, to soothe inflammation and relieve coughs. Manuka honey helps to moisten and soothe inflamed air passageways, and makes the tinctures more palatable. This is also a quick way to make a syrup.

METHOD

Blend the tinctures and honey, mix thoroughly, and pour into a sterilized (p.210) 9fl oz (250ml) amber glass bottle. Seal, label with all the ingredients, and date.

Note: This syrup is not suitable for use during pregnancy. Persistent coughs must always be investigated in consultation with your medical professional.

ACTS AS AN EXPECTORANT

INGREDIENTS

4 tsp mullein leaf tincture
4 tsp marshmallow
  root tincture
1 tbsp anise seed tincture
1 tbsp thyme tincture
4 tsp plantain tincture
2 tsp licorice root tincture
½ cup (100ml) manuka
  honey

ROSE PETAL SYRUP

RELAXES

RELIEVES PERIOD PAIN

INGREDIENTS
1¼ cup (225g) granulated
   sugar
1¼ cup (300ml) water
juice of 1 lemon, strained
juice of 1 orange, strained
3½oz (100g) dried rose
   petals or 10 fresh
   rose heads

MAKES APPROXIMATELY 16FL OZ (500ML)

This fragrant syrup can be served as a sweetener for herbal infusions, poured over pancakes and ice cream, or as a cordial diluted with water. The dark-colored, perfumed rose petals of the damask rose (*Rosa* x *damascena*) or French rose (*Rosa gallica*) are best for this recipe. Keeping the temperature low is the key to making a successful syrup.

METHOD
1 Dissolve the sugar in the water in a small saucepan over low heat, and do not allow it to boil, as this will make the mixture cloudy. Add the strained lemon and orange juices, turn the heat down and simmer over low heat for 5 minutes.
2 Over the next 15 minutes, add the rose petals, a tablespoon at a time, and stir thoroughly before adding more. Remove from the heat, allow to cool, and strain. Pour into a sterilized glass bottle, seal, and label. Keep refrigerated and use within 6 weeks.

Note: To sterilize a glass jar or bottle, wash it and its lid in hot water, drain upside down, and put into a cool oven (275°F/140°C) for 15 minutes.

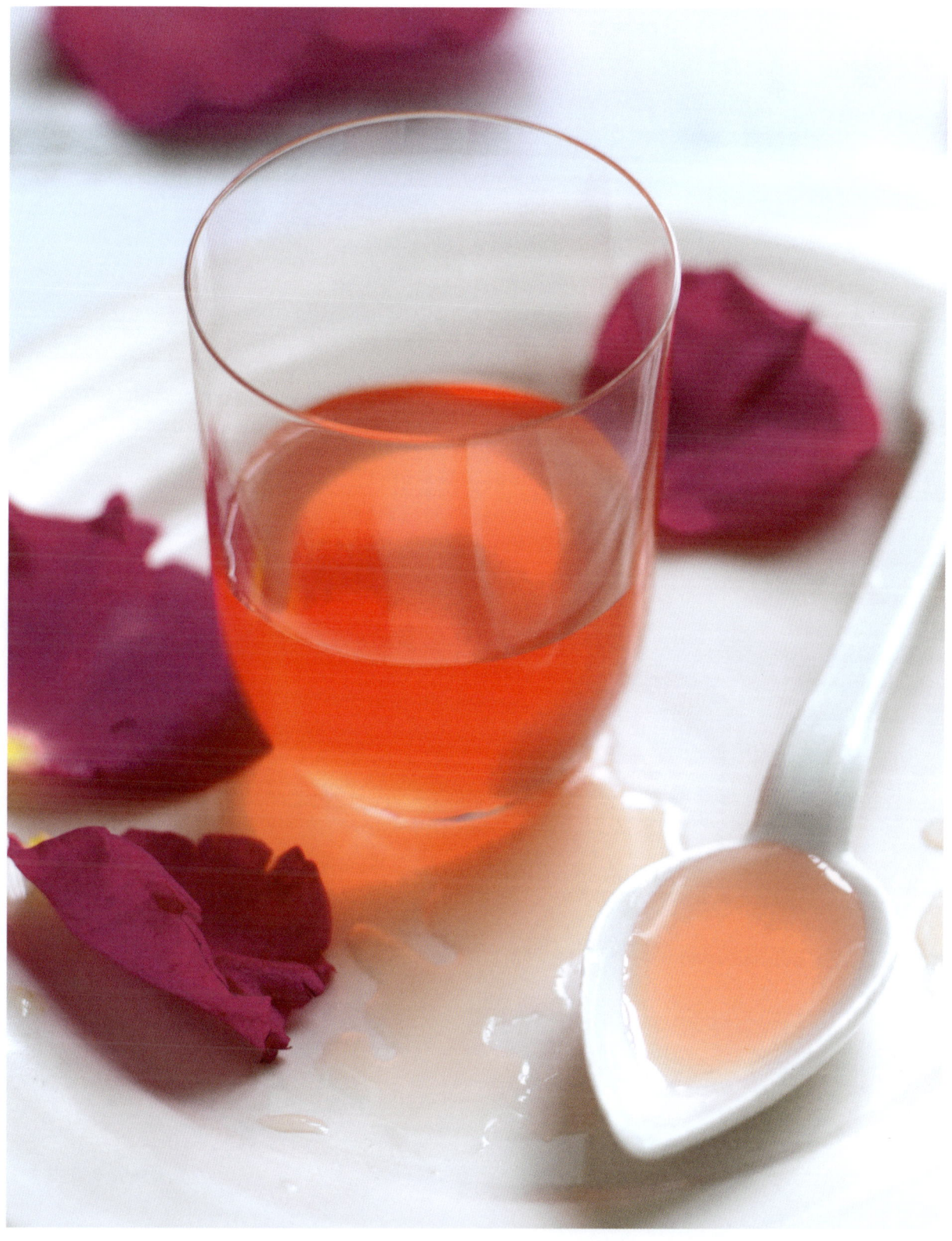

SOUR CHERRY SYRUP

QUICKENS MUSCLE
RECOVERY

REGULATES SLEEP

INGREDIENTS
1¾ cups (400ml) sour cherry
   juice, freshly pressed
   (see intro)
1¼ cups (250g) sugar

MAKES APPROX 2 CUPS

Long-distance runners take cherry juice concentrates
before and after exercising, as the anti-inflammatory
properties of cherries aid quicker muscle recovery and
pain release. Sour cherries also help preserve a youthful
appearance, benefit liver function, and regulate sleep
patterns. Approximately 200 cherries (1lb 5oz/660g)
produce 1¾ cups of cherry juice; simply pit the fruits
then blend in a blender and push the mixture through
a sieve to extract the juice.

METHOD
1 Pour the juice into a saucepan, add the sugar, and heat gently.
Dissolve the sugar in the juice, stirring constantly, then simmer for
20 minutes over low heat.
2 Strain the syrup and bottle in a sterilized glass bottle (p.210) with
a tight-fitting lid. Keep refrigerated and use within a few weeks.
3 Drink diluted with cold or hot mineral water.

ECHINACEA AND THYME SYRUP

INGREDIENTS

¾oz (20g) fresh thyme

¾oz (20g) fresh ribwort
   plantain leaves

¾oz (20g) fresh echinacea
   root, stem, and young
   green leaves

¼oz (10g) fresh ginger,
   grated

¼oz (10g) fresh garlic,
   peeled and crushed

¼oz (10g) fresh elecampane
   root

1 whole fresh red chile,
   finely chopped

1¾ cup (400ml) good-quality
   vodka

½ cup (100ml) manuka
   honey

MAKES APPROX 2 CUPS

When used regularly, this great all-year-round tonic
helps the body develop a natural resistance to viruses
and other pathogens. Take it also at the onset of a cold,
as it keeps the body warm and protected. Prepare the
syrup in late spring, when ribwort and thyme are
growing vigorously, and when fresh echinacea
and elecampane can also be harvested.

METHOD

1 Wash all the herb ingredients once they have been harvested.
Allow to dry, then chop them finely.

2 Place all the ingredients except the vodka and honey in a large
glass jar with a lid. Pour in the vodka, close the lid tightly, and
shake a few times. Label the jar with the ingredients and the date.
Place the jar in a dark cabinet and shake it at least once a day
for 3 weeks.

3 Strain the contents of the jar through a piece of cheesecloth into
a measuring jug. Decant the manuka honey into a bowl and gently
pour in the tincture, stirring continuously with a whisk until the
honey and tincture are well blended.

4 Pour the syrup into a 16fl oz (500ml) amber glass bottle with a lid,
and label with the ingredients and the original starting date.

5 Take 1 teaspoon 2–3 times a day, or up to 6 teaspoons a day at the
onset of a cold.

Note: This syrup is not suitable for use during pregnancy.

MAKING TINCTURES

Tinctures are concentrated, alcohol-based extracts of plant materials, and are much more portable and long-lasting than herbal teas. These recipes enable you to produce simple extracts and further explore the benefits of medicinal herbs.

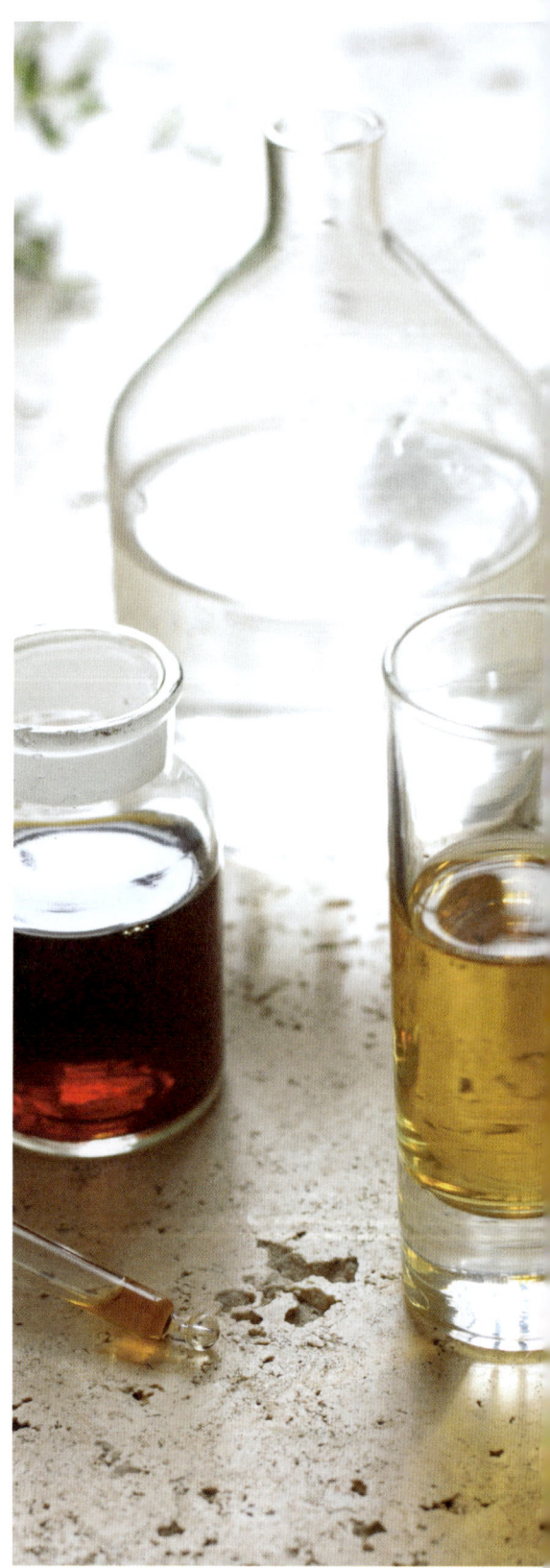

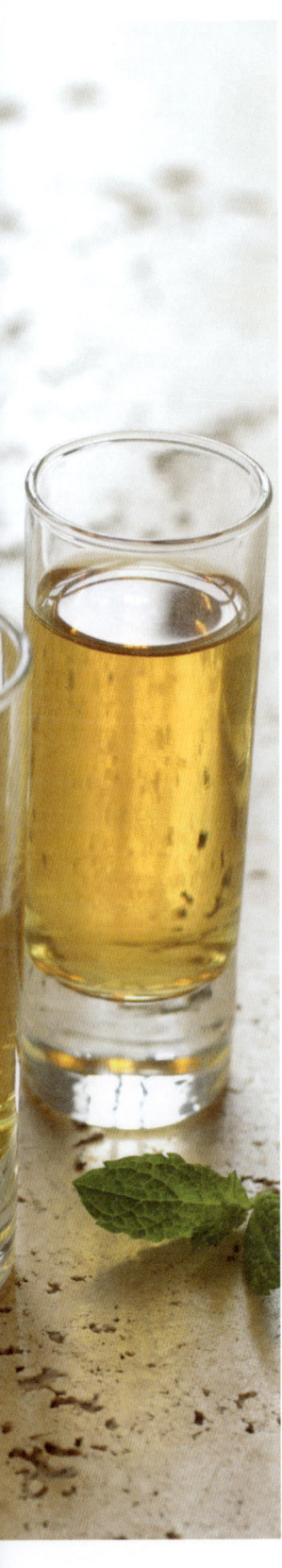

PEPPERMINT AND THYME TINCTURE

MAKES APPROX 2 CUPS (500ML)

This tincture tastes good enough to serve as an aperitif. It aids digestion and benefits the activity of the large intestine, and helps expel gas and soothe a nervous stomach.

CALMS A NERVOUS GUT

INGREDIENTS
scant 1oz (25g) peppermint
½oz (15g) thyme
scant 1oz (25g) chamomile
¾oz (20g) yarrow
½oz (15g) licorice root
2 cups (500ml) good-quality
    vodka

METHOD
1 Place all the ingredients except the vodka in a large jar.
2 Cover with the vodka, stir, and make sure all the ingredients are well immersed. Seal the jar tightly and place it in a dark cabinet. Give the jar a few good shakes every day for 3 weeks.
3 Strain the contents of the jar through a piece of cheesecloth into a measuring jug. Discard the ingredients in the cheesecloth and pour the liquid into an amber glass bottle. Label the tincture bottle with the names of all the ingredients and the date.
4 Take 1 tsp in a glass of warm or cold water and sip before or after meals. Use within 6 months.

Note: This tincture is not suitable for use during pregnancy.

ELDERBERRY AND LICORICE TINCTURE

INGREDIENTS

scant 1oz (25g) elderberries
scant 1oz (25g) echinacea
  root
¼oz (10g) licorice root
¼oz (10g) ginger root, grated
¼oz (10g) cinnamon stick,
  broken into small pieces
¾oz (20g) peppermint
1¾ cup (400ml) good-quality
  vodka

MAKES 1¼–1¾ CUP (300–350ML)

In fall, winter, and early spring, most of us require something to nurture our immunity, defend us from external pathogenic influences (rampant cold and flu viruses), stimulate our blood, warm our body, and keep our strength up. These plants are known to do just that. This blend may also be taken to shorten the duration of a cold or flu.

METHOD

1 Ensure that all the dried ingredients are finely chopped, but not powdered.
2 Place all the ingredients except the vodka into a large glass jar with a secure-fitting lid. Pour in the vodka, close the lid tightly, and shake a few times.
3 Label the jar with all the ingredients and the date. Place the jar in a dark cabinet and shake it at least once every day for 3 weeks.
4 Strain the contents of the jar through a piece of cheesecloth into a measuring jug. Discard the ingredients in the cheesecloth and pour the tincture into an appropriately sized (12–14fl oz/350–400ml) sterilized amber glass bottle (p.210). Seal the bottle.
5 Label with all the ingredients and the original starting date. Start by taking a few drops each day and build up to 1 teaspoon 2–3 times a day. Use within 6 months.

Note: This tincture is not suitable for use during pregnancy.

LIME FLOWER AND HAWTHORN BERRY TINCTURE

INGREDIENTS
¾oz (20g) lime flowers
¾oz (20g) hawthorn berries
¾oz (20g) yarrow
¾oz (20g) lemon balm
¾oz (20g) cramp bark
1¾ cup (400ml) good-quality
   vodka

MAKES 1¼–1½ CUP (300–350ML)

This heart tonic is good for relieving nervous palpitations and discomfort due to stress and anxiety. Hawthorn berries and lemon balm have heart-strengthening and nourishing qualities, while lime flowers and lemon balm relax the mind and improve sleep patterns. Yarrow and cramp bark relax the blood vessels, enabling a better supply of blood to the heart, and also lower blood pressure.

METHOD
1 Ensure that all the dried ingredients are finely chopped, but not powdered.
2 Place all the ingredients except the vodka into a large glass jar with a secure-fitting lid. Pour in the vodka, close the lid tightly, and shake a few times.
3 Label the jar with all the ingredients and the date. Place the jar in a dark cabinet and shake it at least once every day for 3 weeks.
4 Strain the contents of the jar through a piece of cheesecloth into a measuring jug. Discard the ingredients in the cheesecloth and pour the tincture into an appropriately sized (12–14fl oz/350–400ml) sterilized amber glass bottle (p.210). Seal the bottle.
5 Label with all the ingredients and the original starting date. Start by taking a few drops each day and build up to 1 teaspoon 2–3 times a day. Use within 6 months.

Note: This tincture is not suitable for use during pregnancy or if taking prescribed medication.

PASSIONFLOWER AND CHAMOMILE TINCTURE

INGREDIENTS
¾oz (20g) passionflower
¾oz (20g) chamomile
¾oz (20g) valerian root
¼ cup (30g) sour cherries, fresh or dried
1¾ cup (400ml) good-quality vodka

MAKES 1¼–1½ CUP (300–350ML)

All of these ingredients are known to regulate sleep patterns in their own way; when mixed together, they complement each other and work in synergy. Valerian is a sedative, while sour cherries are said to regulate the body's natural sleep pattern, improve sleep efficiency, and decrease the time it takes to fall asleep.

METHOD
1 Ensure that all the dried ingredients are finely chopped, but not powdered.
2 Place all the ingredients except the vodka into a large glass jar with a secure-fitting lid. Pour in the vodka, close the lid tightly, and shake a few times.
3 Label the jar with all the ingredients and the date. Place the jar in a dark cabinet and shake it at least once every day for 3 weeks.
4 Strain the contents of the jar through a piece of cheesecloth into a measuring jug. Discard the ingredients in the cheesecloth and pour the tincture into an appropriately sized (12–14fl oz/350–400ml) sterilized amber glass bottle (p.210). Seal the bottle.
5 Label with all the ingredients and the original starting date. Start by taking a few drops each day and build up to 1 teaspoon in the late afternoon and another before going to bed. Use within 6 months.

Note: The best approach with this tincture is to ascertain the lowest beneficial dose and stick with it. More is not necessarily better; it is all about building an affinity with the ingredients.

CHASTE BERRY AND DANG GUI TINCTURE

INGREDIENTS
¾oz (20g) chaste berry (also called Vitex agnus-castus)

¾oz (20g) Chinese angelica (dang gui) (*Angelica sinensis*)

¾oz (20g) motherwort

¾oz (20g) black haw root bark (*Viburnum prunifolium*)

¾oz (20g) chamomile

1¾ cup (400ml) good-quality vodka

MAKES 1¼–1½ CUP (300–350ML)

This blend of herbs eases premenstrual tension and menstrual pain. Dang gui (also known as Chinese angelica) enhances the flow of blood and, with chaste berry, balances the hormones. These herbs alleviate blood and fluid congestion in the pelvic region to relieve pain and harmonize the heart, mind, and emotions. They also alleviate anxiety, irritability, and mild forms of depression associated with hormonal changes.

METHOD
1 Ensure that all the dried ingredients are finely chopped, but not powdered.
2 Place all the ingredients except the vodka into a large glass jar with a secure-fitting lid. Pour in the vodka, close the lid tightly, and shake a few times.
3 Label the jar with all the ingredients and the date. Place the jar in a dark cabinet and shake it at least once every day for 3 weeks.
4 Strain the contents of the jar through a piece of cheesecloth into a measuring jug. Discard the ingredients in the cheesecloth and pour the tincture into an appropriately sized (12–14fl oz/350–400ml) sterilized amber glass bottle (p.210). Seal the bottle.
5 Label with all the ingredients and the original starting date. Start by taking a few drops each day and build up to 1 teaspoon 2–3 times a day. Use within 6 months.

Note: This tincture is not suitable for use during pregnancy.

GOJI BERRY AND SIBERIAN GINSENG TINCTURE

INGREDIENTS
scant 1oz (25g) goji berries
scant 1oz (25g) Siberian
ginseng (*Eleutherococcus
senticosus*)
scant 1oz (25g) oat tops or
dried oats
¾oz (20g) schisandra berries
⅛oz (5g) licorice root
1¾ cup (400ml) good-quality
vodka

MAKES 1¼–1½ CUP (300–350ML)

This tincture enhances the body's natural defenses
and improves mental concentration, physical endurance,
and a sense of well-being. It does this by energizing the
body, especially the liver and the nervous, hormonal, and
immune systems. If you can't find fresh oat tops (the top
8 in [20 cm] of the plant), use the dried oats available
from supermarkets.

METHOD
1 Ensure that all the dried ingredients are finely chopped,
but not powdered.
2 Place all the ingredients except the vodka into a large glass jar
with a secure-fitting lid. Pour in the vodka, close the lid tightly, and
shake a few times.
3 Label the jar with all the ingredients and the date. Place the jar
in a dark cabinet and shake it at least once every day for
3 weeks.
4 Strain the contents of the jar through a piece of cheesecloth into a
measuring jug. Discard the ingredients in the cheesecloth and pour
the tincture into an appropriately sized (12–14fl oz/350–400ml)
sterilized amber glass bottle (p.210). Seal the bottle.
5 Label with all the ingredients and the original starting date. Start
by taking a few drops each day and build up to 1 teaspoon 2–3 times
a day. Use within 6 months.

Note: This tincture is not suitable for use during pregnancy.

RED CLOVER AND CLEAVERS TINCTURE

SOOTHES INFLAMED
SKIN

INGREDIENTS
½oz (15g) red clover
½oz (15g) cleavers
¾oz (20g) viola (heartsease)
¾oz (20g) violet leaves (*Viola odorata*)
¾oz (20g) mahonia root (*Mahonia aquifolium*), finely chopped
¾oz (20g) gotu kola
1¾ cup (400ml) good-quality vodka

MAKES 1¼–1½ CUP (300–350ML)

These herbs are all used for acute and chronic skin inflammation, including acne, eczema, psoriasis, and other skin conditions. They help detoxify the body and eliminate waste via the urine, and have a laxative effect. They also stimulate the gall bladder and liver.

METHOD
1 Ensure that all the dried ingredients are finely chopped, but not powdered.
2 Place all the ingredients except the vodka into a large glass jar with a secure-fitting lid. Pour in the vodka, close the lid tightly, and shake a few times.
3 Label the jar with all the ingredients and the date. Place the jar in a dark cabinet and shake it at least once every day for 3 weeks.
4 Strain the contents of the jar through a piece of cheesecloth into a measuring jug. Discard the ingredients in the cheesecloth and pour the tincture into an appropriately sized (12–14fl oz/350–400ml) sterilized amber glass bottle (p210). Seal the bottle.
5 Label with all the ingredients and the original starting date. Start by taking a few drops each day and build up to 1 teaspoon 2–3 times a day. Use within 6 months.

Notes: This tincture is not suitable for use during pregnancy. Serious skin conditions always require professional advice.

ECHINACEA AND ELDERBERRY WINTER GUARD TINCTURE

INGREDIENTS

¾oz (20g) fresh ginger

2¾oz (80g) echinacea root, fresh or dried

¾oz (20g) thyme leaves, fresh or dried

2 garlic cloves (optional)

1 fresh chile with seeds (optional)

½ cup (80g) elderberries, fresh or dried

2 cups (500ml) good-quality vodka

MAKES 1 MONTH'S SUPPLY

This tincture is a delicious way of strengthening your immune system against winter ailments. It warms the body, expelling the cold, and strengthens nonspecific immunity. Fresh ginger is both warming and antimicrobial, while thyme, garlic, and chile fortify antimicrobial and diaphoretic action. Echinacea root is well known for reducing the risk of catching colds and flu.

METHOD

1 Slice the fresh ginger and echinacea thinly, pull the fresh thyme leaves from their stems, and mince the garlic and chile (if using them).

2 Gently squeeze the elderberries. Place all the ingredients in a large jar with a securely fitting lid. Cover with the vodka, mix thoroughly, and make sure all the ingredients are completely immersed.

3 Close the top tightly and place the jar in a dark cabinet. Check it every day, shaking the jar a few times. After 6 weeks, open the jar, strain the ingredients through cheesecloth, collect the liquid in a sterilized amber glass bottle (p.210), label with the names of all the ingredients, and date.

4 Take 1 tsp (5ml) 2–3 times a day in a cup of hot or cold water (the tincture can be used throughout the fall, winter, and early spring).

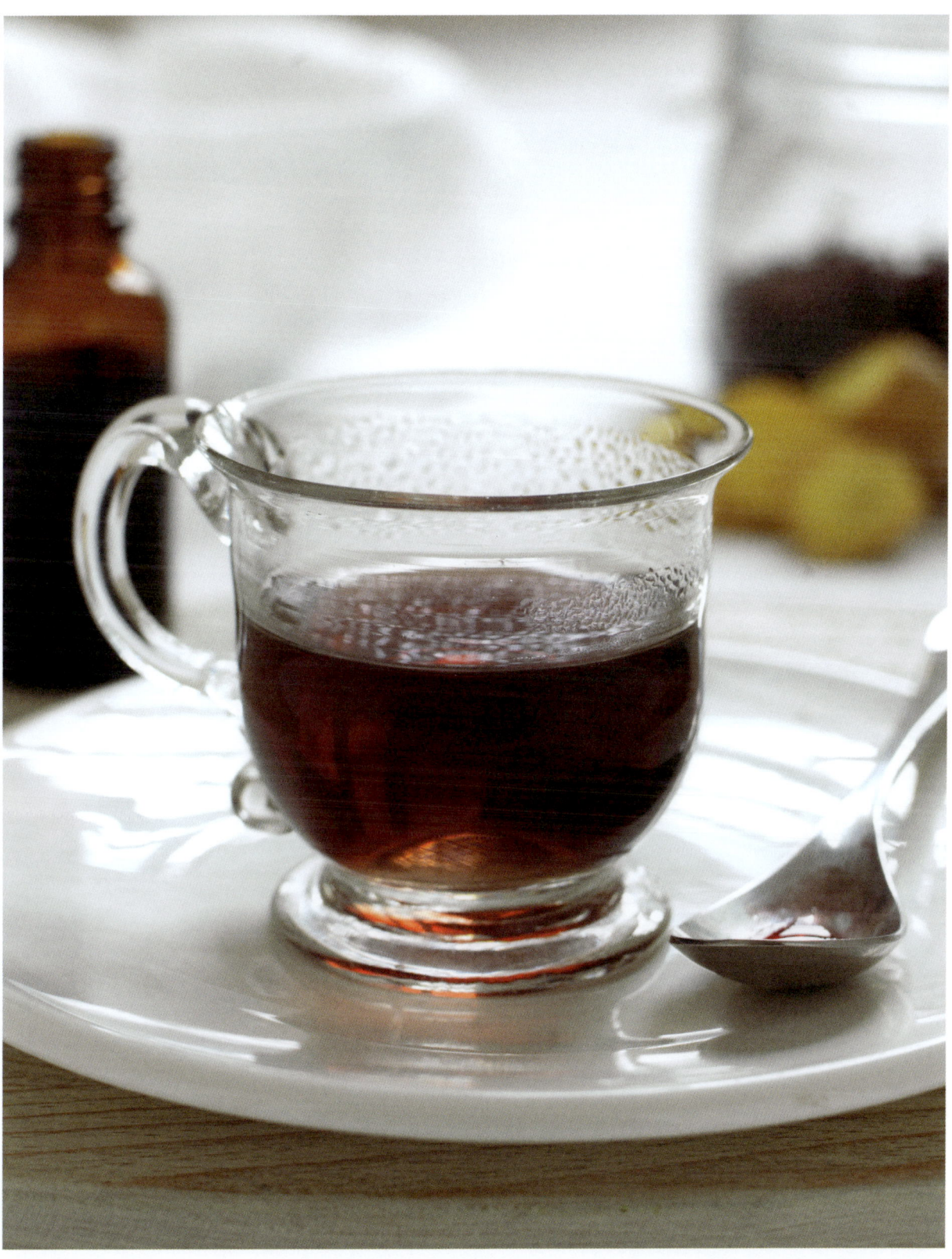

DANDELION AND BURDOCK TINCTURE

INGREDIENTS

¾oz (20g) dandelion root
¾oz (20g) burdock root
¾oz (20g) schisandra berries
¼oz (10g) artichoke leaves
¾oz (20g) milk thistle
¼oz (10g) gentian root
  (*Gentiana lutea*)
1¾ cup (400ml) good-quality
  vodka

MAKES 1¼–1½ CUP (300–350ML)

The toxic environment many of us now live in puts enormous strain on the liver, so good liver health is more important than ever before. This tincture of bitter herbs stimulates the liver to metabolize toxic residues, and influences the rest of the digestive system. It also improves blood circulation and helps make you feel calmer and less irritable.

METHOD

1 Ensure that all the dried ingredients are finely chopped, but not powdered.
2 Place all the ingredients except the vodka into a large glass jar with a secure-fitting lid. Pour in the vodka, close the lid tightly, and shake a few times.
3 Label the jar with all the ingredients and the date. Place the jar in a dark cabinet and shake it at least once every day for 3 weeks.
4 Strain the contents of the jar through a piece of cheesecloth into a measuring jug. Discard the ingredients in the cheesecloth and pour the tincture into an appropriately sized (12–14fl oz/350–400ml) sterilized amber glass bottle (p.210). Seal the bottle.
5 Label with all the ingredients and the original starting date. Start by taking a few drops each day and build up to 1 teaspoon 2–3 times a day. Use within 6 months.

Note: This tincture is not suitable for use during pregnancy.

CRAMP BARK AND VALERIAN TINCTURE

RELIEVES MINOR PAIN

RELIEVES PERIOD PAINS

INGREDIENTS
scant 1oz (25g) cramp bark
scant 1oz (25g) valerian root
¾oz (20g) passionflower
¾oz (20g) chamomile
1¾ cup (400ml) good-quality
   vodka

MAKES 1¼–1½ CUP (300–350ML)

This blend relieves broad-spectrum spasmodic pain due to stress, including discomfort associated with irritability, disturbed sleep, and nervous indigestion. Cramp bark helps relieve smooth muscle spasms, valerian and passionflower provide a mild sedative effect and relieve irritability, and chamomile has an anti-inflammatory and antispasmodic effect.

METHOD

1 Ensure that all the dried ingredients are finely chopped, but not powdered.

2 Place all the ingredients except the vodka into a large glass jar with a secure-fitting lid. Pour in the vodka, close the lid tightly, and shake a few times.

3 Label the jar with all the ingredients and the date. Place the jar in a dark cabinet and shake it at least once every day for 3 weeks.

4 Strain the contents of the jar through a piece of cheesecloth into a measuring jug. Discard the ingredients in the cheesecloth and pour the tincture into an appropriately sized (12–14fl oz/350–400ml) sterilized amber glass bottle (p.210). Seal the bottle.

5 Label with all the ingredients and the original starting date. Start by taking a few drops each day and build up to 1 teaspoon 2–3 times a day. Use within 6 months.

Note: This tincture is not suitable for use during pregnancy.

BLACK COHOSH AND SAGE TINCTURE

INGREDIENTS
¾oz (20g) black cohosh root
½oz (15g) chaste berry
¼oz (10g) sage
¾oz (20g) schisandra berries
½oz (15g) motherwort
¾oz (20g) skullcap
1¾ cup (400ml) good-quality
   vodka

MAKES 1¼–1½ CUP (300–350ML)

Herbs can be a great help for perimenopausal and menopausal women. Chaste berry regulates hormonal levels, black cohosh is known as a uterine tonic and a relaxant, and sage and schisandra berries alleviate perspiration. Skullcap is a relaxant and, together with motherwort, lifts the spirits, and motherwort may also lessen the heart palpitations that often accompany hot flashes.

METHOD

1 Ensure that all the dried ingredients are finely chopped, but not powdered.
2 Place all the ingredients except the vodka into a large glass jar with a secure-fitting lid. Pour in the vodka, close the lid tightly, and shake a few times.
3 Label the jar with all the ingredients and the date. Place the jar in a dark cabinet and shake it at least once every day for 3 weeks.
4 Strain the contents of the jar through a piece of cheesecloth into a measuring jug. Discard the ingredients in the cheesecloth and pour the tincture into an appropriately sized (12–14fl oz/350–400ml) sterilized amber glass bottle (p.210). Seal the bottle.
5 Label with all the ingredients and the original starting date. Start by taking a few drops each day and build up to 1 teaspoon 2–3 times a day. Use within 6 months.

Note: This tincture is not suitable for use during pregnancy.

BIRCH LEAF AND NETTLE ROOT TINCTURE

RELIEVES URINARY TRACT INFECTIONS

RELIEVES URINARY TRACT INFECTIONS

INGREDIENTS
scant 1oz (25g) nettle root
½oz (15g) birch leaves
scant 1oz (25g) pellitory-of-the-wall (*Parietaria officinalis*)
½oz (15g) black currant leaves
¾oz (20g) white poplar, or poplar bark (*Populus tremuloides*)
1¾ cup (400ml) good-quality vodka

MAKES 1¼–1½ CUP (300–350ML)

This tincture addresses urinary dysfunctions, water congestion, fluid retention, and uric acid accumulation. It relieves the body of metabolic waste, enhances urine flow, invigorates the urinary bladder, and strengthens the urinary tract. However, care must be taken not to use it without the supervision of a medical professional if you have stones in the urinary tract.

METHOD
1 Ensure that all the dried ingredients are finely chopped, but not powdered.
2 Place all the ingredients except the vodka into a large glass jar with a secure-fitting lid. Pour in the vodka, close the lid tightly, and shake a few times.
3 Label the jar with all the ingredients and the date. Place the jar in a dark cabinet and shake it at least once every day for 3 weeks.
4 Strain the contents of the jar through a piece of cheesecloth into a measuring jug. Discard the ingredients in the cheesecloth and pour the tincture into an appropriately sized (12–14fl oz/350–400ml) sterilized amber glass bottle (p.210). Seal the bottle.
5 Label with all the ingredients and the original starting date. Start by taking a few drops each day and build up to 1 teaspoon 2–3 times a day. Use within 6 months.

Note: Consult your doctor if your symptoms are severe or if they worsen. This tincture is not suitable for use during pregnancy.

MAKING SOUPS

Soups have a history of being used as a healing aid, especially for anyone recovering from an illness. These recipes have been specially devised to include essential life-generating plant ingredients; they all taste delicious as well as doing you good.

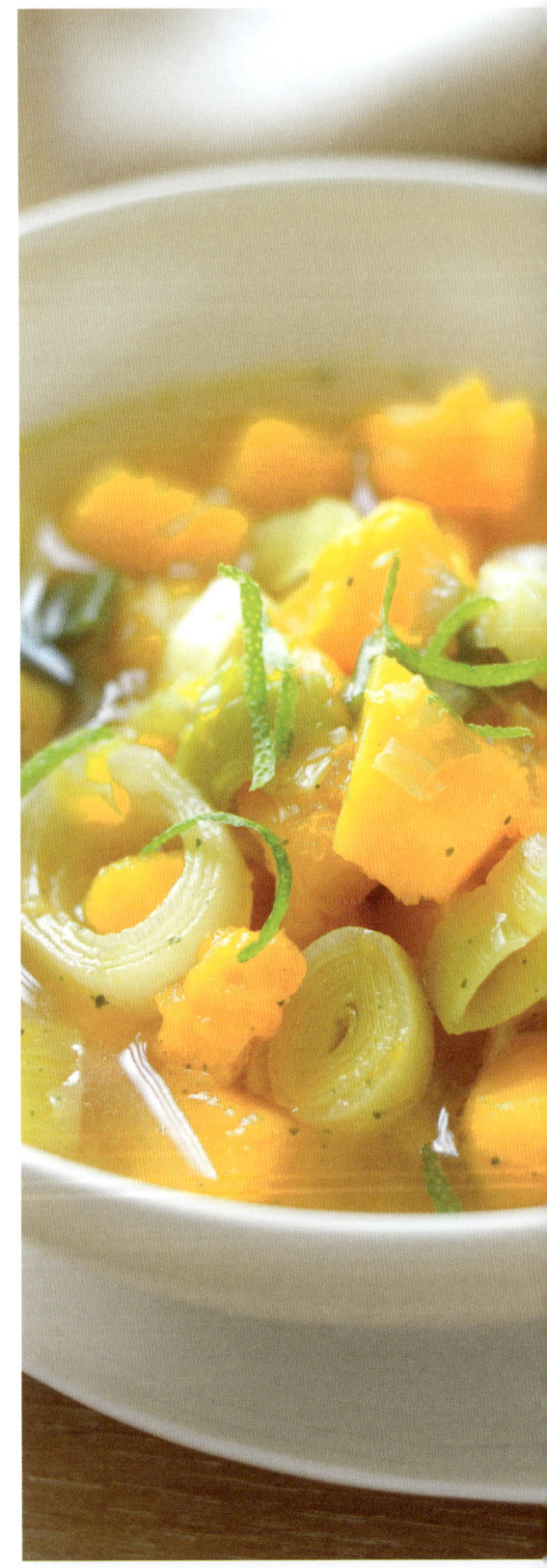

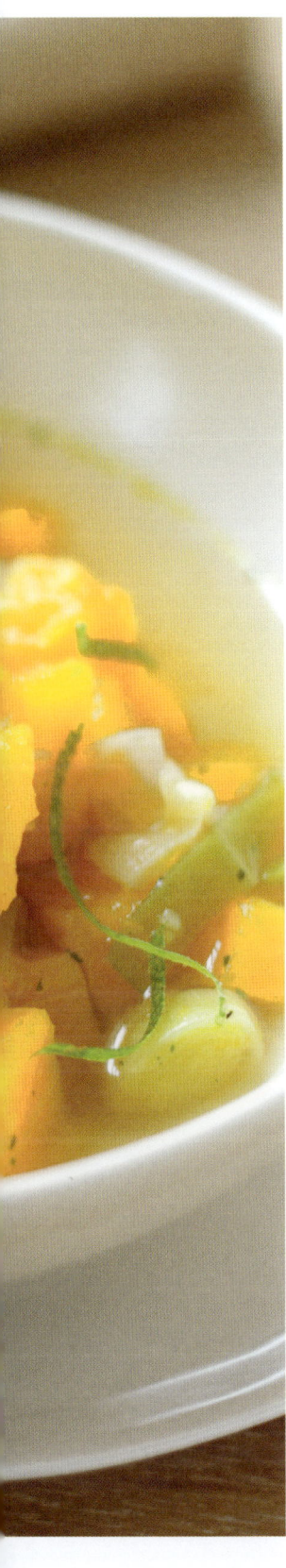

ONION SQUASH AND GINGER SOUP

WARMS AND NOURISHES

INGREDIENTS
2 tbsp olive oil
2¼lb (1kg) onion squash (or butternut squash), peeled, seeded, and cut into small chunks
1 medium-sized leek, sliced
4 garlic cloves, crushed
2 tbsp fresh ginger, grated
2¾ pints (1.5 liters) vegetable stock
lime juice and zest to taste
salt and freshly ground black pepper

MAKES 4–6 SERVINGS

This is a great warming winter soup. Ginger is famous for its healing qualities, and fresh ginger is traditionally used to ward off winter ailments: it acts as a diaphoretic, warms up the body, and helps in the elimination of cold. It also improves the digestion and assimilation of nutrients.

METHOD
1 Heat the olive oil in a saucepan, add the squash and leek, and sauté for a few minutes. Add the garlic and ginger and a splash of the stock and continue to sauté the ingredients until the leeks are soft. Add rest of the stock and bring to a boil. Simmer for approximately 10 minutes or until the squash is cooked through, but still retains some shape.
2 Remove from the heat, add the lime juice and a sprinkle of the lime zest, and season to taste with salt and pepper. The soup can be served as it is, or blended until smooth.

GREEN BEAN AND CILANTRO SOUP

INGREDIENTS

2 large potatoes, peeled and diced

2 tbsp olive oil

1 onion, finely chopped

2 carrots, scrubbed and thinly sliced

2¼lb (1kg) green beans (preferably fresh), trimmed and sliced

3 garlic cloves, chopped

1 chile pepper, seeded and finely chopped

1–2 tsp hot smoked paprika

salt and freshly ground black pepper to taste

4 tbsp fresh cilantro, finely chopped

4 tbsp half-fat crème fraîche to serve (1 tbsp per serving)

MAKES 4 SERVINGS

This soup helps balance blood-sugar levels: research has shown that bean pods contain a substance (arginine) that acts like insulin by regulating blood-sugar levels in the body, although it is weaker and acts more slowly over a prolonged period of time. Bean pods are also known to have a diuretic effect.

METHOD

1 Place the potatoes in a pot, cover with water, and bring to a boil.

2 In the meantime, heat the oil in a frying pan, add the onion, and sauté until soft. Add the carrots to the pan, stir, and continue to sauté for a few minutes. Add the beans, stir, cover the pan, turn the heat to low, and allow to sweat. Then add the chopped garlic, chile pepper, and the smoked paprika.

3 Check that the vegetables are giving off enough juices to prevent the bottom of the pan from burning; if necessary add a spoonful or two of water (the idea is that the vegetables cook in their own juices).

4 When the beans are nearly ready (soft, but chewy), add the cooked potatoes to the frying pan and add just a small amount of the water in which the potatoes were cooked.

5 Cook all the vegetables together for a few more minutes so that they combine well. Season to taste with salt and pepper.

6 Serve the soup in bowls garnished with fresh cilantro and a spoonful of crème fraîche.

BURDOCK ROOT AND CARROT SOUP

INGREDIENTS

3 shallots, finely chopped

3½oz (100g) fresh burdock root, washed and finely chopped

3 large carrots, washed and finely chopped

2 small garlic cloves, finely chopped

2 cups boiling water

salt and freshly ground black pepper

1 tbsp fresh lovage leaves, finely shredded, to garnish

a drizzle of pumpkin seed oil

MAKES 4 SERVINGS

This is a gentle, cleansing soup for the body. Burdock root is often used in the treatment of skin conditions and eczema, as well as rheumatic complaints, and is also famous as a blood purifier. It is grown commercially as a root vegetable and can be found most readily in Asian, especially Japanese, speciality stores.

METHOD

1 Place 2 tablespoons of water into a saucepan, add the shallots, and sauté for 1–2 minutes, stirring occasionally. When the shallots are soft, stir in the burdock root and carrots, keeping the pot covered and the heat turned down low so the vegetables steam in their own juices.

2 Check and stir the ingredients every few minutes and, if necessary, add a little more water. When they are sufficiently soft, add the garlic and cook for another minute. Add the boiling water and simmer for 5 minutes.

3 Pour the soup into a blender or food processor and blend until smooth and silky. Season with salt and pepper to taste and serve in individual bowls. Garnish each with shredded lovage leaves and a little pumpkin seed oil.

GOJI BERRY, MINT, AND TOMATO SOUP

INGREDIENTS

¾ cup (100g) dried goji berries

1 tbsp olive oil

3 shallots, peeled and finely chopped

2 beefsteak tomatoes, skinned and finely chopped

1 pint (600ml) vegetable stock

1 tbsp fresh mint leaves, chopped, plus extra to garnish

MAKES 4 SERVINGS

Goji has become famous through the centuries as a food that protects the body from premature aging. It is now recognized as a "superfood," being a rich source of antioxidants and a tonic that alleviates anxiety and stress; promotes a lighter, more cheerful mood; improves sleep; and increases energy and strength.

METHOD

1 Wash the berries and soak them in water for a few minutes to rehydrate them. Heat the oil in a saucepan, sauté the shallots for a few minutes, then add the tomatoes and goji berries. Stir for few minutes before adding the stock. Stir and simmer for a further 20 minutes.

2 Add the mint leaves and remove from the heat. Pour the mixture into a blender or food processor and pulse until smooth. Serve garnished with the extra mint leaves.

Note: To skin the tomatoes, cut a cross incision through the skin at the base of the tomato and place in a heatproof bowl. Pour over boiling water to cover and leave to stand for a few minutes. Remove the tomatoes from the water with a slotted spoon. The skin should now peel away easily.

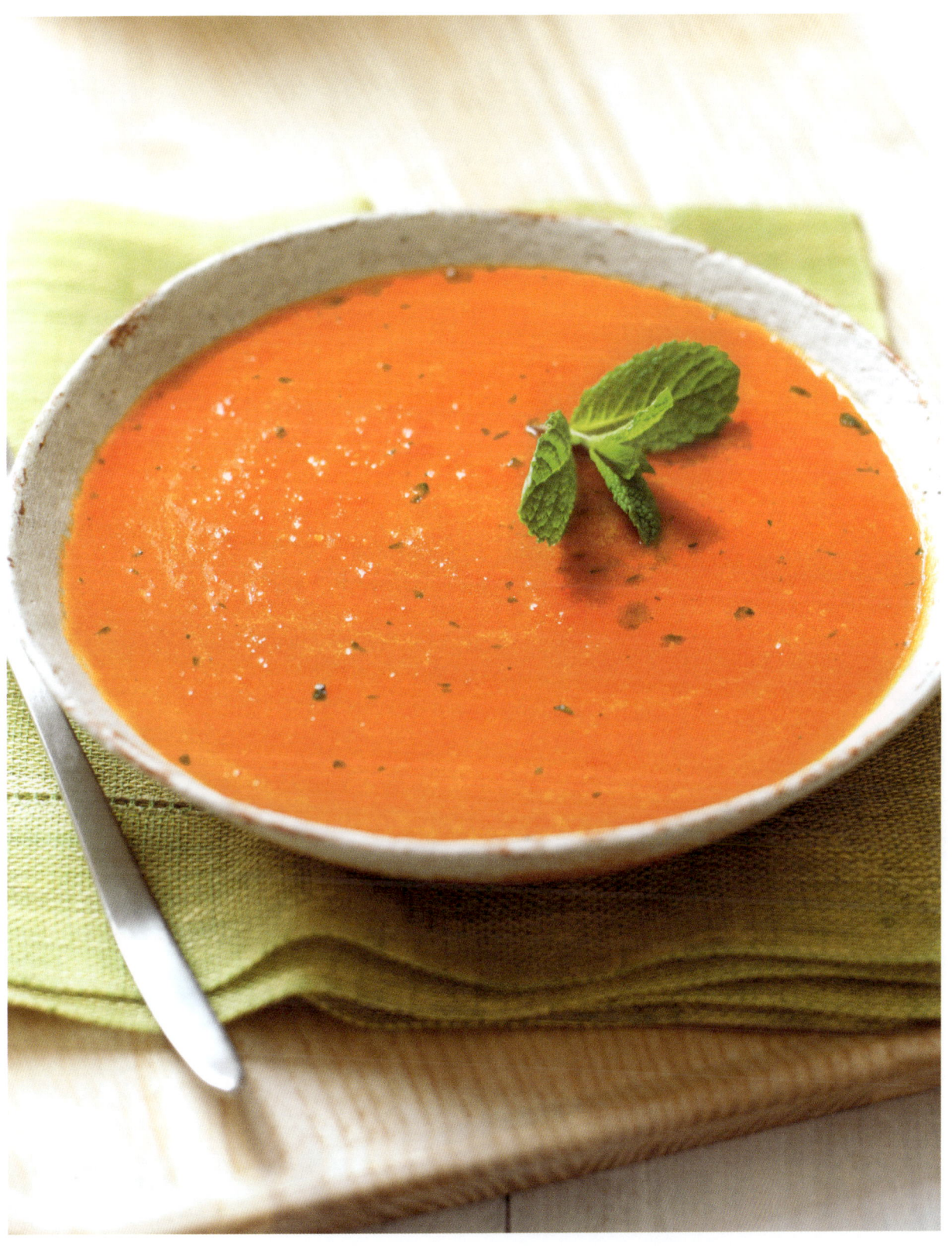

NETTLE AND SWEET POTATO SOUP

MAKES 4 SERVINGS

Nettle soup is a classic spring cleanser that has been used as a health tonic for generations in Europe; nettles are full of vitamins and minerals and purify the blood, clear toxins, lower blood pressure, and improve the quality of skin and hair. Sweet potato, which is rich in vitamin A, also helps improve digestion, remove toxins from the body, and relieve inflammation and dryness.

PURIFIES SKIN

ACTS AS A SPRINGTIME TONIC

INGREDIENTS

1 tbsp olive oil
1 medium-sized onion, or 4 shallots, chopped
1 medium-sized sweet potato, chopped into small pieces
2 garlic cloves, squeezed
1 quart (1 liter) vegetable stock
9oz (250g) young nettle leaves, washed and chopped
salt and freshly ground black pepper
2–3 tbsp barley miso paste
4 tsp half-fat crème fraîche, or plain yogurt

METHOD

1 Heat the oil in a saucepan and sauté the onions or shallots and sweet potato for 2–3 minutes. Add the garlic and stock and bring to a boil. Simmer for 20 minutes, then add the nettles and turn off the heat.

2 Pour the soup into a blender or food processor and blend until smooth.

3 Season to taste with salt and pepper and the miso paste. Serve in individual bowls, each with a swirl (1 teaspoon) of crème fraîche or yogurt.

GINSENG AND ASTRAGALUS LONGEVITY SOUP

INGREDIENTS
½oz (15g) wood ear fungus
  (hei mu er/*Auricularia
  auricula*)
½oz (15g) fresh or dried
  astragalus root
½oz (15g) fresh or dried
  ginseng root
6 shallots, trimmed with the
  skins left on
3 garlic cloves, trimmed with
  the skins left on
1 large carrot, scrubbed
1in (2.5cm) piece fresh
  ginger, thinly sliced
1½ quarts (1.5 liters) water
1¾ cups (150g) fresh shiitake
  mushrooms
1¾ cups (150g) fresh oyster
  mushrooms
1 large piece wakame
  seaweed, cut into small
  pieces, or 1 tbsp dried
¼ cup (15g) goji berries,
  pre-soaked if dried
7oz (200g) soba noodles
2–3 tbsp barley miso paste
1 handful flat-leaf parsley,
  chopped
freshly ground black pepper

MAKES 4 SERVINGS

The energizing ingredients in this soup include ginseng, which enhances energy levels and restores strength after a prolonged illness, and astragalus root, which is well known for its beneficial effect on the immune system. It strengthens the lungs, helps prevent colds, and alleviates any shortness of breath. Wood ear fungus is rich in amino acids, phosphorus, iron, and calcium.

METHOD
1 Put the fungus, astragalus root, ginseng root, shallots, garlic, whole carrot, and ginger into a large saucepan, cover with the water and bring to a boil. Simmer over very low heat for half an hour with the lid on tightly.
2 Take the pan off the heat, strain the liquid through a colander or sieve, and return it to the pan. Discard the astragalus root and ginseng. Squeeze the garlic and shallots from their skins and return them to the soup. Slice the fungus and carrot into small pieces and return them to the soup. Add the shiitake mushrooms and wakame seaweed and bring the soup back to simmering. Add the goji berries. After 10 minutes, add the soba noodles and let them cook through for 5–7 minutes.
3 Serve in individual bowls. Allow each person to add enough barley miso paste to their liking and garnish with the parsley and a grinding of black pepper.

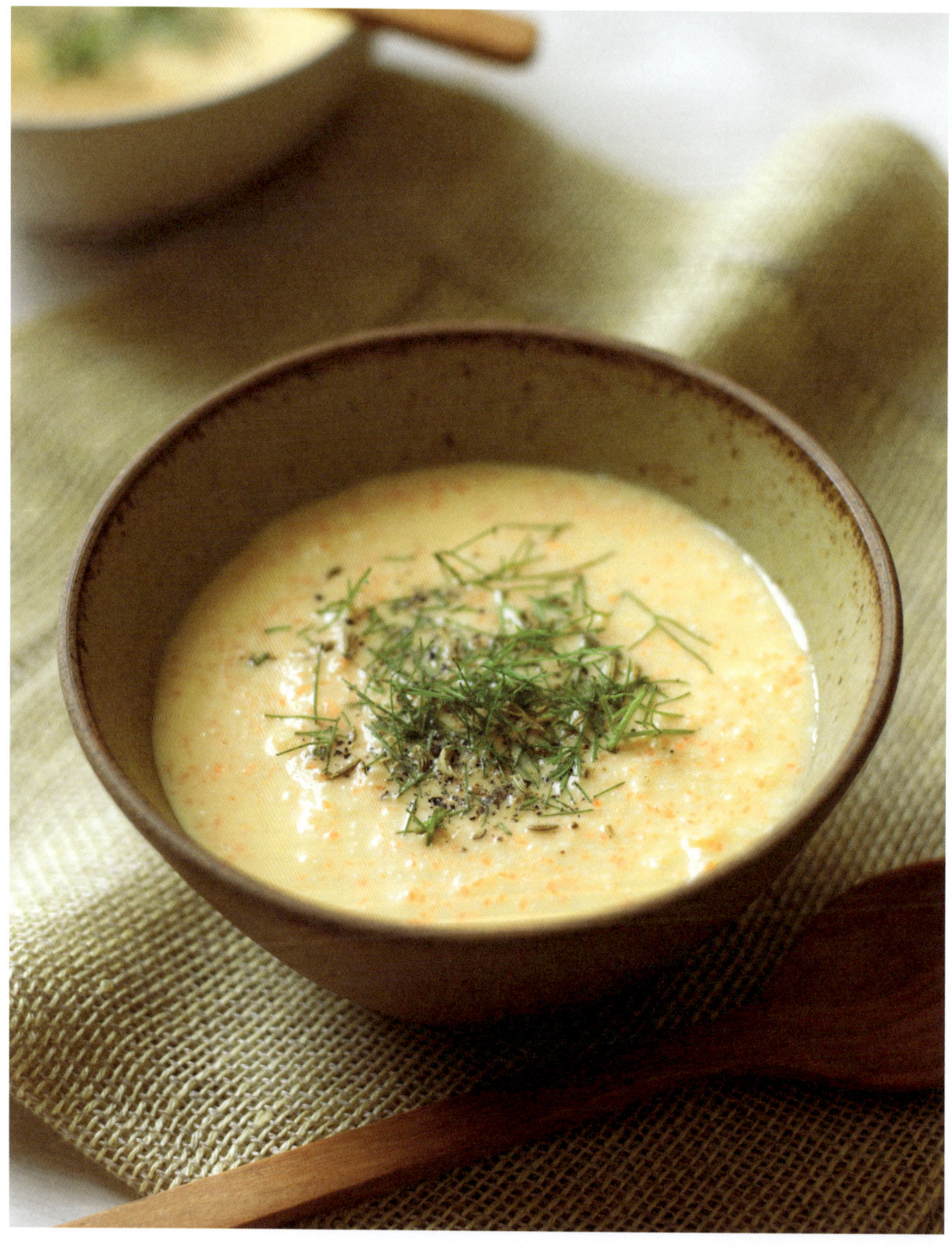

RAW CARROT AND ALMOND SOUP

MAKES 4 SERVINGS

This is a cooling soup, perfect for a hot, sunny summer lunch. Fennel is a cooling and cleansing herb with antispasmodic properties, excellent for expelling gas, gently stimulating the digestion and kidneys, and brightening the eyes. This is balanced by the addition of almonds, which are warming by nature as well as extremely nutritious.

METHOD

1 To sprout the almonds, soak them in cold water for half an hour, then rinse them in a strainer under running water. Place them in a large bowl, cover with water, and leave overnight to soak. The following day, pop the skins off the almonds and place the almonds in another clean bowl, pour in the water, and refrigerate. Allow the almonds to continue soaking for up to 24 hours.

2 Strain the almonds, reserving the almond-soaked water. Place the carrots in a blender or food processor with the garlic, the strained, soaked almonds, and 1 tablespoon of the almond-soaked water. Blend, adding the rest of the water gradually until the mixture is smooth and silky. Place in the refrigerator and leave to chill for a few hours until cool.

3 Put the fennel seeds, peppercorns, and salt into a pestle and mortar and grind to a fine powder. Then add the fernlike fennel leaves to the spices. Serve the soup in bowls, with a teaspoon of the seasoning on top.

STRENGTHENS LUNGS

INGREDIENTS

1½ cups (200g) whole almonds
2 cups (500ml) water
1¼ cups (150g) carrots, peeled and chopped
2 garlic cloves
½ tsp fennel seeds
¼ tsp black peppercorns
pinch of sea salt
1 tbsp fresh fennel leaves, finely chopped

ZUCCHINI AND SEA GREENS SOUP

INGREDIENTS

1 handful dried wakame seaweed, or any other colorful soft-leaf seaweed such as dulse

4 shallots, chopped

1 medium-sized fennel bulb, chopped

5 medium-sized zucchini, sliced

1 tbsp fresh parsley, finely chopped, plus more for garnish

2 cups water

salt and freshly ground black pepper to taste

a drizzle of pumpkin seed oil

MAKES 4 SERVINGS

This soup is healthy yet nourishing, and beneficial to the body. Zucchini is cooling by nature, as it helps build body fluids and relieve dryness, while seaweed is an excellent source of minerals. Seaweed is also known for its ability to help remove toxic waste from the body, improve kidney function, alkalize the blood, assist in weight control, and lower cholesterol.

METHOD

1 Soak the seaweed in at least 2 cups of clean water.

2 Place a tablespoon of water in a saucepan and heat. Add the chopped shallots and cook over low heat with the lid on, stirring occasionally.

3 When soft, add the fennel and zucchini. Continue to cook the vegetables with the lid on until they are tender.

4 Drain the seaweed. Place the cooked vegetables (not the seaweed) in a blender or food processor, add the chopped parsley and water, and blend until smooth. Add salt and black pepper to taste.

5 Divide the rehydrated seaweed leaves into 4 piles, pour the soup into individual bowls, and scatter the seaweed over the top of each serving. Sprinkle over the fresh parsley and a little pumpkin seed oil and serve.

SPROUTED PUY LENTIL AND TURMERIC SOUP

INGREDIENTS

1 tbsp olive oil

4 shallots, chopped

1 tsp turmeric powder

2 garlic cloves

1½ cups (100g) fresh shiitake mushrooms, sliced

2½ cups (200g) sprouted Puy lentils (see note)

1 quart (1 liter) homemade vegetable stock or cold water

juice of ½ lemon

salt and freshly ground black pepper

1 tbsp cilantro, chopped

MAKES 4 SERVINGS

The sprouted lentils in this warming fall soup are easier to digest than dried lentils and have an enhanced nutritional value, while turmeric helps improve the digestion and liver conditions such as jaundice. The soup also has anti-inflammatory properties, helping relieve swelling and pain, including rheumatic and arthritic pain.

METHOD

1 Heat the oil in a saucepan, add the chopped shallots, and sauté for 1 minute. Add the turmeric, garlic, and mushrooms and stir. Add the lentils and stock or water and bring to a boil. Simmer for 10 minutes.

2 Switch the heat off and add the lemon juice and salt and black pepper to taste. Pour the soup into individual bowls and serve garnished with the chopped cilantro.

Note: To sprout lentils, place ¾ cup of dried Puy lentils in a glass jar large enough (usually three times the volume of the lentils) for the lentils to expand while sprouting. Fasten a piece of cheesecloth over the opening of the jar, fill it with water, and leave overnight. In the morning, pour out the water, rinse the jar and lentils with clean water, and leave the jar of lentils upside down at an angle to drip-dry through the cheesecloth. In the evening, rinse the lentils again and leave to drip-dry overnight. Repeat the process twice daily until the young shoots show (2–4 days). The lentils are ready to use when the shoots are the length or more of a dried Puy lentil.

ROASTED BARLEY AND CHESTNUT SOUP

INGREDIENTS

5½oz (150g) sweet chestnuts, fresh or precooked

6 shallots, trimmed, with skin left on

4 garlic cloves with skin left on

2 large carrots, washed

1¼ cups (200g) celeriac, peeled and cubed

1in (2.5cm) piece fresh ginger, washed

2 cups (500ml) water

1½ cups (200g) shiitake mushrooms, stems removed and sliced

2 long blades wakame seaweed, chopped into small pieces, or 2 tbsp wakame flakes

3½oz (100g) roasted barley (see note)

1 tbsp barley miso

flat-leaf parsley, to garnish (optional)

MAKES 4 SERVINGS

This tonic soup makes a great nourishing lunch on a cold winter's day, as it primarily supports kidney energy. It will help warm up the whole system, and eating it once a week during the winter season is most useful for individuals suffering from aches and pains aggravated by the cold weather.

METHOD

1 If using fresh chestnuts, roast them first. Cut into the tip (apex) of each nut with a sharp knife and place them on a baking tray. Bake in the oven at 350°F (180°C) for 20–25 minutes. Take them out of the oven. Wrap each chestnut in a cloth and squeeze hard to crush the shell, then peel it all off.

2 Put the whole shallots, garlic, carrots, celeriac, and ginger into a large saucepan, cover with the water, and bring to a simmer. Cook, covered, over low heat for at least 1 hour, occasionally adding some more water if necessary.

3 Take the saucepan off the heat and strain the liquid through a colander into a clean saucepan. Pick out the garlic and shallots from the cooked vegetables and squeeze them out of their skins directly into the liquid.

4 Add the chestnuts to the soup and bring to a boil. Add the mushrooms, wakame seaweed, and roasted barley, and simmer for 15–20 minutes. Then stir in the barley miso until dissolved, remove from the heat, and serve in bowls with the parsley garnish (if using).

Note: To roast barley, soak it overnight in lukewarm water, drain, and leave to dry on a baking sheet covered with a clean dish towel. When the barley is still damp, heat a large frying pan over high heat. Turn the heat down to medium and add a quarter of the barley, stirring constantly. When the grain is golden brown and makes a gravely noise as you stir it, transfer it out of the pan and allow to cool completely on a plate. Repeat with the remaining 3 batches. Store in an airtight jar if you prepare the barley a few days before making the soup.

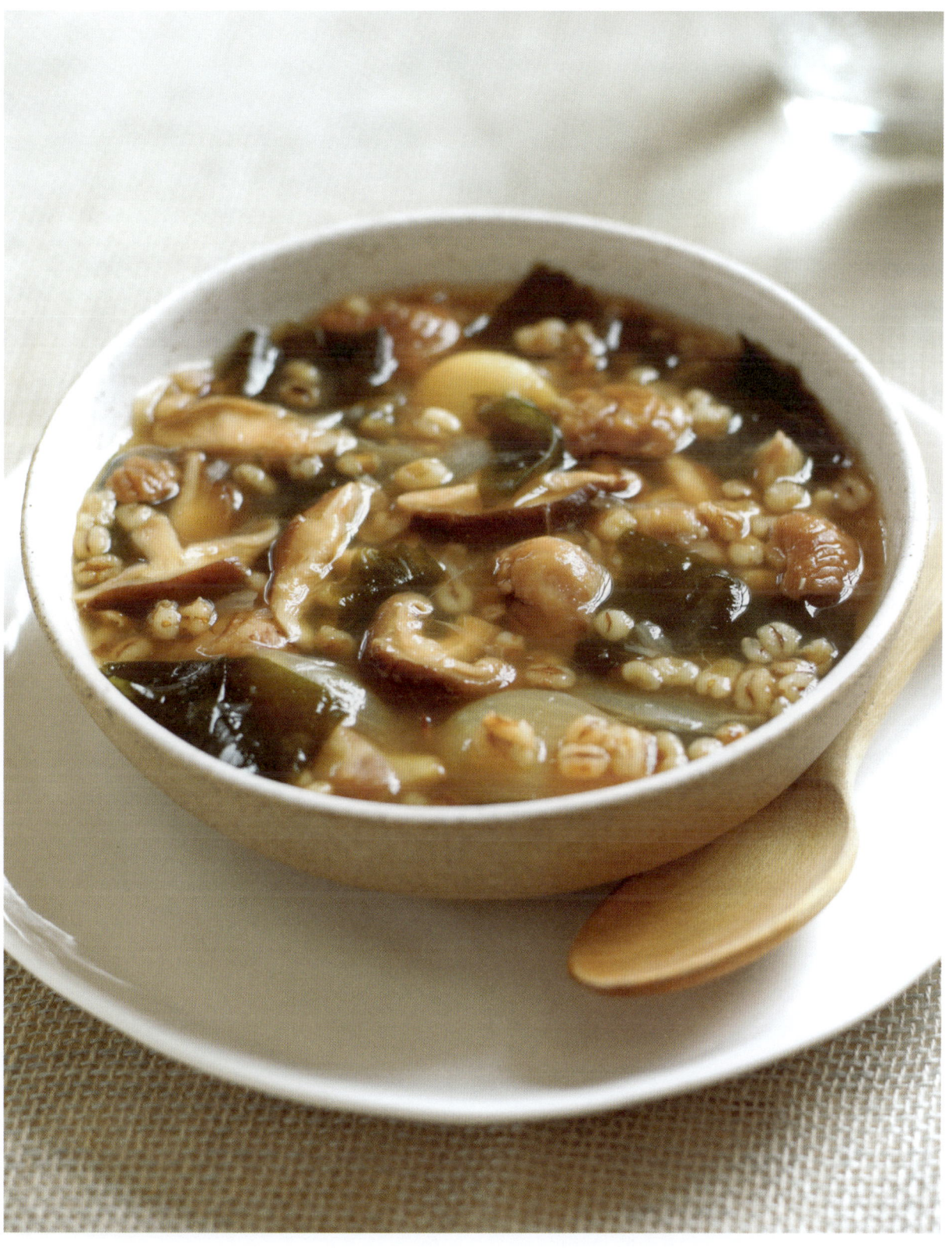

MAKING SALADS

Raw vegetables and herbs are the essence of nourishment, providing nutrients, fluids, and fiber and enhancing the elimination of wastes. These salads combine the healing qualities of fresh vegetables with phytonutrients from herbs, and bring health awareness to the eating experience.

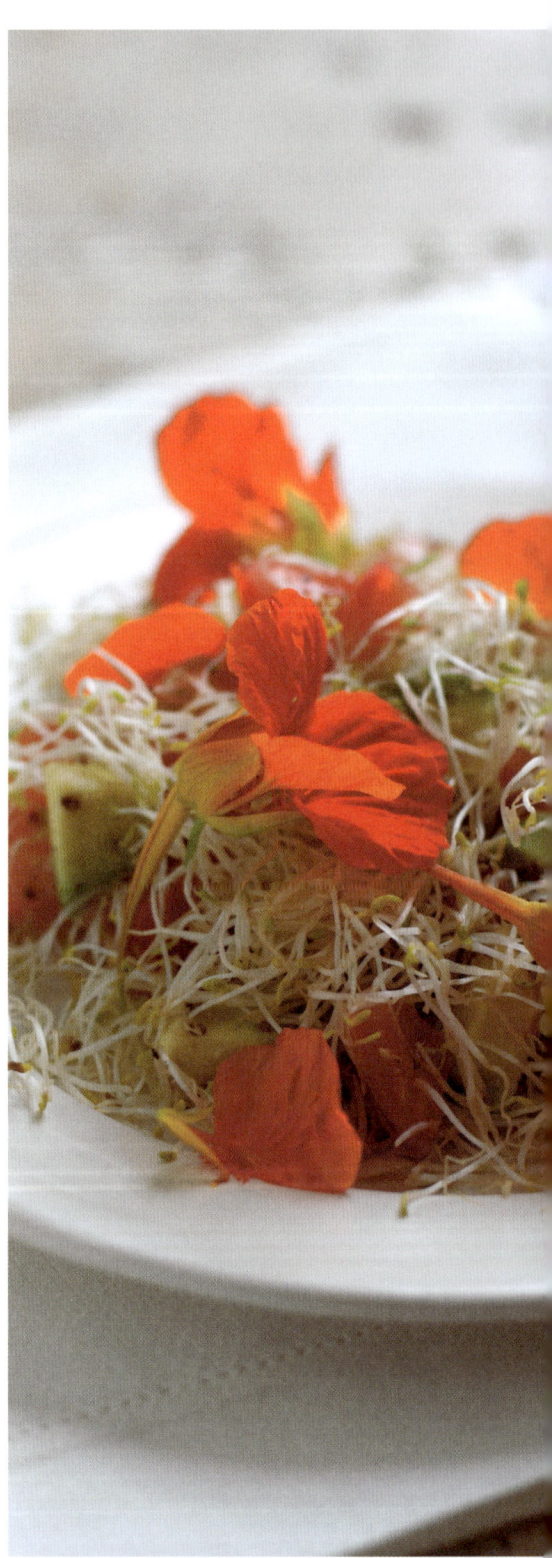

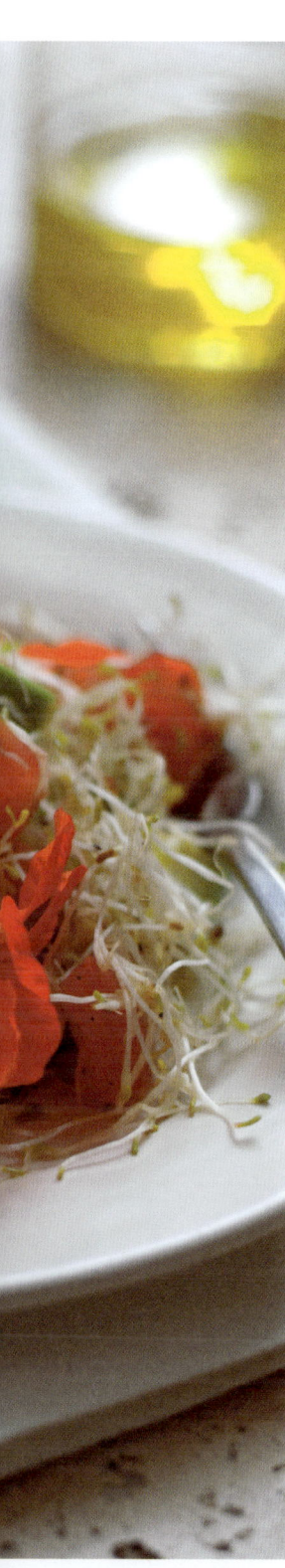

NASTURTIUM AND SPROUTED SEED SALAD

INGREDIENTS
2½oz (75g) alfalfa sprouts
1 avocado, chopped
1 large tomato, chopped
8 nasturtium flowers

FOR THE DRESSING
1 tbsp olive oil
juice of ½ lemon
¼ tsp mustard
salt and freshly ground
   black pepper, to taste

MAKES 2 SERVINGS

Sprouted seeds are a great source of fresh nutrients. Sprouts in general are a mineral-rich food; they often have diuretic and bowel-regulating properties, and are therefore important foods in a detox regime. Nasturtium flowers impart a delicately peppery taste to this salad. As a medicine, they are thought to have a beneficial influence on the lungs and kidneys.

METHOD

1 Rinse the alfalfa sprouts thoroughly in a strainer under running water, then dry them well in a salad spinner or with a clean dish towel.
2 Mix all the dressing ingredients together and blend well to create a smooth vinaigrette.
3 Place the alfalfa sprouts in a serving bowl and add the avocado and tomato. Pour in the dressing and mix thoroughly. Top the salad with the nasturtium flowers and serve.

ZUCCHINI SPAGHETTI WITH CILANTRO AND PINE NUT PESTO

PURIFIES SKIN

EASES CONSTIPATION

INGREDIENTS

1 zucchini

1 summer squash

2 tbsp fresh cilantro, finely chopped

⅓ cup (50g) pine nuts, coarsely ground

2 tsp hemp oil

2 tsp pumpkin seed oil

juice ½ lemon

salt and freshly ground pepper to taste

MAKES 2 SERVINGS

Strands of zucchini and summer squash take the place of pasta in this summer lunch dish. Zucchini has a gentle laxative effect and, when combined with omega fatty acids from hemp and pumpkin seed oils, will help nourish and clear the skin of impurities. Pine nuts add a source of protein to turn this dish into a light, but complete, meal.

METHOD

1 Put the zucchini and summer squash through a vegetable spiralizer to slice them into long threads, or "spaghetti"; if you don't have a spiralizer, slice them lengthwise as thinly as you can, or use spaghetti squash.

2 Put the cilantro in a bowl, add the pine nuts, hemp oil, and pumpkin seed oil, and mix well to make a pesto.

3 Place the zucchini and squash in a serving bowl, add the cilantro pesto, and toss the ingredients well. Add some lemon juice and salt and black pepper to taste, and serve.

RED CLOVER SPROUTS AND LEMON BALM SALAD

INGREDIENTS

1 large carrot, scrubbed
3½oz (100g) red clover sprouts
1¾oz (50g) broccoli sprouts
½ mango
1 garlic clove, peeled
3 tbsp olive oil
juice of 1 lime
salt and freshly ground black pepper, to taste
8 fresh lemon balm leaves, finely chopped

MAKES 2 SERVINGS

Red clover is often used in the treatment of premenstrual syndrome, and the flowers are a popular ingredient in natural products that help alleviate hot flashes, prevent loss of bone density, and balance hormones in menopausal women. These sprouts have the same healing properties as the mature flowers.

METHOD

1 Put the carrot through a vegetable spiralizer to slice it into long threads, or "spaghetti"; if you don't have a spiralizer, slice the carrot into thin sticks or use a vegetable peeler. Put the sprouts and carrot in a large serving bowl.

2 To make the dressing, cut the mango in half, remove the pit, and scoop out the flesh into a blender or food processor. Add the garlic, olive oil, and lime juice, and blend until smooth. Season with salt and black pepper. Pour the dressing over the vegetables, mix well, add the lemon balm leaves, and serve.

Note: You can sprout red clover and broccoli by placing 2 tablespoons of each of the seeds into a large glass jar. Pour in spring or filtered water, fasten a piece of cheesecloth on the opening of the jar, and leave overnight. Rinse the seeds the following morning by pouring out the old water, adding fresh water, then emptying that out, too. Leave the jars at an angle of 45 degrees and repeat the rinsing process every morning and evening until the sprouts are ready to eat (when they develop small green leaves, after 4–5 days). Once the seeds have sprouted, store in a glass jar with a tight-fitting lid, refrigerate, and eat within a day or two.

DANDELION AND PRIMROSE LEAF SALAD

INGREDIENTS

1oz (30g) dandelion leaves
1 tsp wild chives
¼oz (10g) daisy leaves
   (*Bellis perennis*)
¼oz (10g) yarrow leaves
¾oz (20g) primrose leaves
¼oz (10g) arugula leaves
1 head of endive
1½ tbsp flaxseed oil
1½ tbsp lemon juice
white pepper to taste
sesame salt to taste
   (see note)

MAKES 2 SERVINGS

This is an early spring-forager detox salad. Dandelion and endive are a gentle stimulant for the liver and bladder. Some of the fresh ingredients can be found growing in gardens or small woodland areas, others you may need to buy, such as arugula, chives, and endive. Arugula can also be grown from seed.

METHOD

1 Rinse all the salad leaves and dry them in a salad spinner.
2 To make the dressing, mix the flaxseed oil, lemon juice, white pepper, and sesame salt in a small bowl. When the salad leaves are dry, place them in a serving bowl, toss with sesame salt, and add the dressing.

Note: To prepare the sesame salt, soak 1 tablespoon of golden, or shelled, sesame seeds and 1 tablespoon of black sesame seeds in a bowl of water overnight. The following day, discard the water, tie up the sesame seeds in cheesecloth, and allow them to drip-dry. When dry, lightly pan-roast the seeds, adding 3 good pinches of sea salt as you go, and toss them. Then grind the seeds in a pestle and mortar or food processor and store in a sealed container until needed.

Note: Omit the yarrow leaves from this salad if you are pregnant.

EDIBLE FLOWER SALAD

INGREDIENTS

1¾oz (50g) sunflower greens (young sunflower plants)

1¾oz (50g) buckwheat greens (young buckwheat plants)

1¾oz (50g) broccoli sprouts (p.245)

1 yellow bell pepper, cut into strips

1 red bell pepper, cut into strips

1 small cucumber, cut into thin rounds

2 ripe tomatoes, cut into wedges

1 tbsp calendula petals

12 nasturtium flowers, stems removed

1 tbsp viola flowers, stems removed

1 tbsp fragrant rose petals

FOR THE DRESSING

2 tbsp fresh basil leaves

2 tbsp sesame oil

½ garlic clove, peeled

1 tbsp mirin rice wine

1 tbsp lemon or lime juice

salt and freshly ground black pepper to taste

MAKES 4 SERVINGS

This summer salad is designed to excite the senses with its abundance of summer colors and unusual tastes. It is worth noting that fresh calendula, nasturtium, viola, and rose flower petals all have unique flavors, so it is best to become accustomed to these different tastes before deciding to incorporate them into your version of this salad.

METHOD

1 Harvest the sunflower and buckwheat greens, rinse them in clean water, and dry them in a salad spinner before placing them in a salad bowl. Rinse the broccoli sprouts under running water and allow to dry off before adding them to the greens. Add the peppers, cucumber, and tomatoes to the other ingredients.

2 Add the flowers and flower petals to the salad, reserving a few of each for a garnish.

3 Blend all the ingredients for the dressing in a blender or a food processor, pour the dressing over the salad, and gently toss. Just before serving, sprinkle the remaining flowers over the top of the salad.

BROCCOLI AND ROSEMARY SALAD

INGREDIENTS

1 large head of broccoli, chopped into florets
1 small avocado, pitted and peeled
2 garlic cloves, peeled
Juice of ½ lemon
Salt and freshly ground black pepper to taste
1 sprig fresh rosemary, leaves stripped and finely chopped (or 1 tsp dried rosemary)
16 olives, pitted

MAKES 2 SERVINGS

Broccoli is an excellent source of sulfur, iron, and B vitamins; it has been credited with enhancing the body's resistance to many diseases, due in part to the important antioxidant sulforaphane. It is essential not to overcook it in order to preserve its healthy chlorophyll. Rosemary stimulates blood circulation, relieves abdominal discomfort due to weak digestion, and improves the memory.

METHOD

1 Make sure that the broccoli florets are cut to a similar size, then place them in a steamer until they are warmed through, but still firm and green.

2 Put the avocado flesh in a blender or food processor with the garlic, lemon juice, salt, and black pepper, and blend until smooth. Thoroughly combine all the ingredients, making sure the broccoli is well dressed.

3 Transfer into a serving dish, scatter the chopped rosemary over the top, and garnish with the olives.

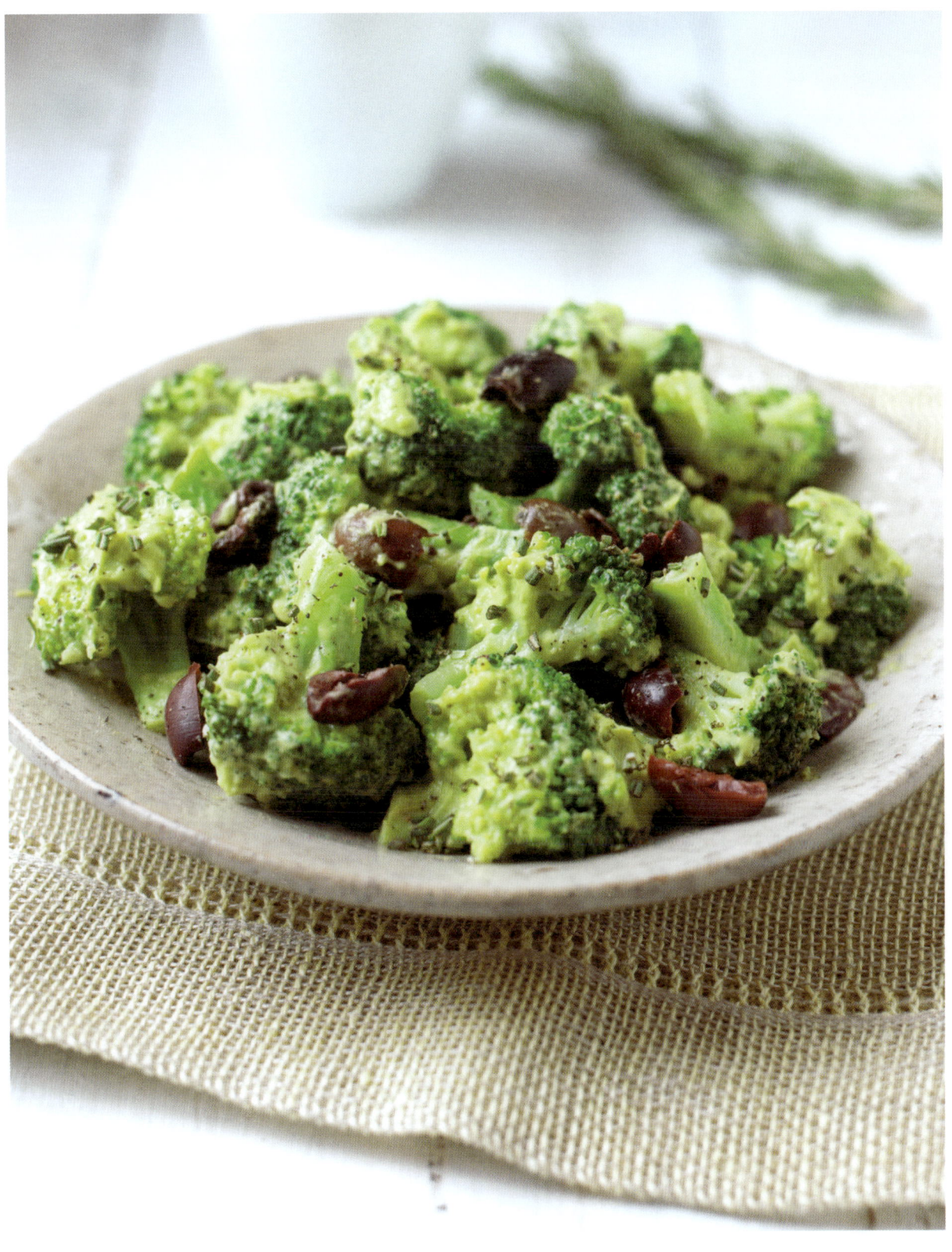

SAUERKRAUT AND AVOCADO SALAD

INGREDIENTS
2 medium white cabbages
2 tbsp salt

FOR THE SALAD
1¾oz (50g) alfalfa sprouts, washed
1 avocado, pitted, peeled, and sliced
1 tbsp pumpkin seed oil
freshly ground black pepper to taste

MAKES 2 SERVINGS

Fermented foods such as sauerkraut play an important role in enhancing intestinal health by promoting the growth of organisms that increase nutrient absorption. Cabbage also contains compounds that support colon and breast health, and has antioxidant, antibacterial, and antiviral properties. Once prepared, sauerkraut actually contains more vitamin C than fresh cabbage.

METHOD

1 To make the sauerkraut (fermented cabbage), shred the cabbage finely in a food processor, pack into a bowl, sprinkle with salt, mix thoroughly, and leave for half an hour.

2 Pound the cabbage with the end of a rolling pin until the juices start flowing. Fill a sterilized glass jar (p.210) with the salted cabbage, adding a handful at the time and pounding it down in the jar with the end of a rolling pin each time so that no air is left between the added layers ("beating in" is essential to the success of this process). Firmly compress the layers of cabbage, leaving some space at the top of the jar for the cabbage to expand (the juices may also overflow).

3 Place the jar on a plate, cover with a saucer as wide as the neck of the jar, and store in a well-ventilated, cool, but not cold, place (see note below). Check the jar and remove any residue from the top regularly. After 1 week, the cabbage will have fermented sufficiently to be eaten, and should keep for at least 2 weeks if refrigerated.

4 To make the salad, combine 1 cup of the sauerkraut with the rest of the ingredients in a salad bowl and season to taste.

Note: You can also buy ready-made sauerkraut, but it is often sterilized and your homemade version will taste much better. The ideal temperature for fermentation is 68–72°F (20–22°C). Fermentation will stop and the cabbage will spoil above 76°F (24°C) or below 55°F (13°C). If your sauerkraut develops a pinkish hue on its surface, goes dark, or is very soft and mushy, it has not fermented properly and should not be eaten.

NORI ROLLS

INGREDIENTS

2 heaping tbsp sesame seeds

5 square sheets toasted nori seaweed

1 small or ½ large papaya, peeled, seeded, and cut into thin strips

1 red bell pepper, seeded and cut into thin strips

1 chile, seeded and cut into thin strips

4in (10cm) inner white part of a leek, sliced thinly lengthwise

1 avocado, pitted, peeled, and cut into thin strips

FOR THE DRESSING

juice of 1 lime

1 garlic clove, crushed

½ tsp fresh ginger, finely grated

1 tbsp fresh cilantro, finely chopped

1 tsp light barley miso paste

½ tsp lime zest

1 tsp maple syrup

3 tbsp mineral water

MAKES 3–4 SERVINGS

Sheets of nutritious toasted nori seaweed taste delicious as part of a healthy snack, and are ideal to use as a wrap filled with fresh vegetables. These rolls make an excellent light, detoxing meal to eat on the go—a true raw food "sandwich." In this recipe, the rolls are served as a salad with a tasty dressing.

METHOD

1 First, toast the sesame seeds in a small pan over low heat for 3–4 minutes, stirring frequently, until they turn lightly golden and begin to release a nutty aroma.

2 To make the dressing, put all the dressing ingredients into a blender or food processor with 1 tablespoon of toasted sesame seeds and blend until smooth.

3 Have a small bowl of water ready. Place a sheet of nori on a sushi mat or a square of parchment paper a little longer and wider than the sheet of nori.

4 Put a small amount of each ingredient heaped on top of one another in a line ¾–1¼in (2–3cm) from the edge of the bottom of the nori sheet.

5 Drizzle a little of the dressing over the vegetables and scatter some of the remaining toasted sesame seeds over the top.

6 Lift the bottom edge of the sushi mat (or paper) and roll up the nori with the ingredients inside. To seal the nori roll, wet your fingers in the small bowl of water, dampen the top edge of the nori sheet, and finish rolling the nori. Repeat with the remaining nori sheets, vegetables, and dressing.

7 When ready to serve, slice the nori rolls into three sections, and stand each one upright on a serving plate. Sprinkle each nori roll with toasted sesame seeds, and use any remaining dressing as a dip.

MINT AND CUCUMBER SIDE SALAD WITH CASHEW NUT CREAM

INGREDIENTS

1 medium cucumber, peeled
a few fresh mint leaves,
   finely chopped, to garnish

FOR THE CASHEW
NUT CREAM

½ cup (75g) raw cashew
   nuts, pre-soaked
2 garlic cloves, crushed
2 tsp white miso
2 tbsp freshly squeezed
   lemon juice
1 tbsp fresh mint leaves,
   finely chopped
1 tbsp fresh cilantro, finely
   chopped

MAKES 4 SERVINGS

You can happily share this fresh-tasting, minty raita with friends who do not eat milk or milk-related products. Cucumbers are cooling, so this dish is ideal for summer dining; if you serve it in winter, add some finely chopped fresh chile. Use young cucumbers, which have small, compact seeds, or scoop out the larger seeds from a mature cucumber with a spoon.

METHOD

1 Cut the cucumber in half lengthwise and scoop out any large seeds with a spoon. Dice the cucumber finely and place in a serving bowl.
2 Put all the ingredients for the cashew nut cream in a blender or food processor, and blend thoroughly. Add ½ cup of water or more to adjust the consistency to that of heavy cream.
3 Pour the cashew nut cream over the cucumber and stir together well. Sprinkle with finely chopped mint leaves.

CAYENNE-TOASTED ALMONDS AND KALE SALAD

INGREDIENTS

2 tbsp chopped almonds
pinch of cayenne pepper
½ tsp sweet paprika
pinch of salt
a little lemon juice
9oz (250g) kale, washed,
   and cut into thin strips
1 tbsp olive oil

MAKES 3–4 SERVINGS

Kale is the perfect winter green for this warming salad. It is touted as a "superfood" because it contains vitamins B, C, E, and K, as well as most of the minerals we need every day, in particular selenium, which supports the immune system. This recipe also contains cayenne pepper to add warmth on cold winter days.

METHOD

1 Toast the almonds first: heat a heavy-bottomed frying pan over medium heat, add the almonds, and toast for a couple of minutes. Then add the cayenne pepper, paprika, and salt, and toss the almonds in the spices. Add the lemon juice, remove the pan from the heat before the juice begins to burn, and set aside.

2 Heat a saucepan over medium heat, add 2 tablespoons of water, let the water heat up, add the kale, and close the lid tightly. Lower the heat and allow the kale to sweat for 2–3 minutes so that it wilts, rather than cooks.

3 Place the kale in a serving dish, toss with the olive oil and another dash of lemon, and garnish with the spicy almonds.

Note: Do not include cayenne pepper if you have stomach or duodenal ulcers.

MAKING FRUIT BARS

These recipes will help you incorporate more wild fruits, nuts, and grains into your diet. The variations on these basic ingredients are endless, and depend mainly on the way the grains are prepared, as well as your choice of dried fruits, nuts, and seeds.

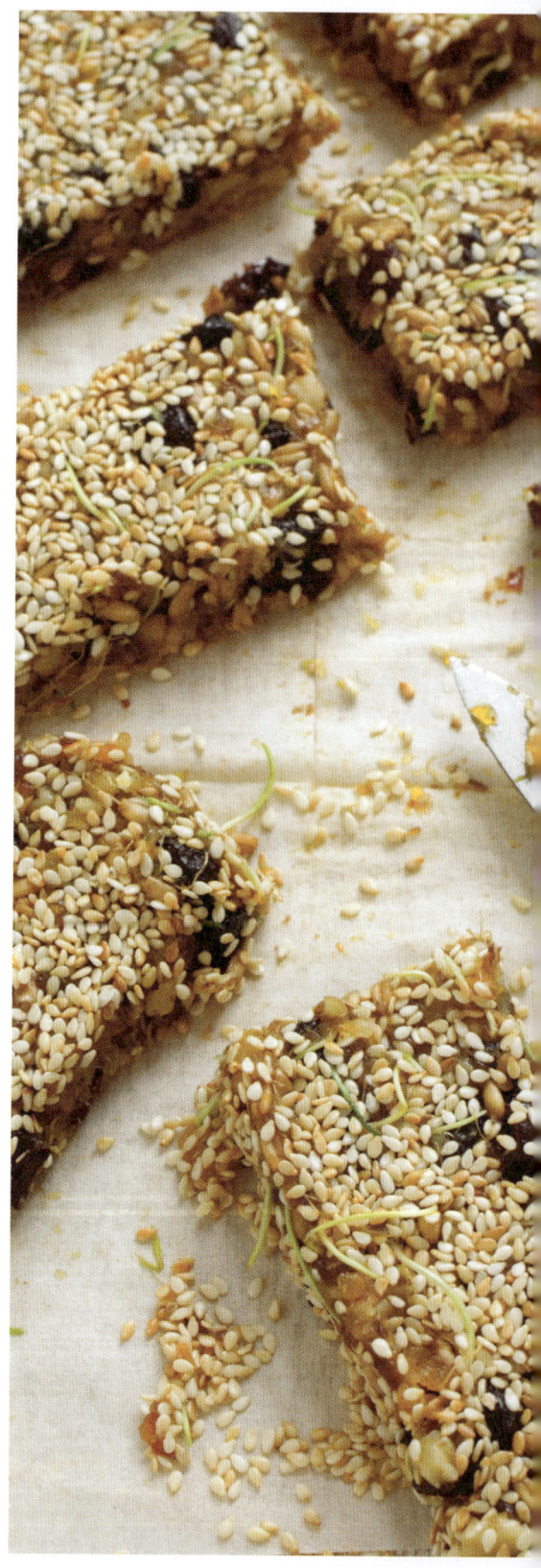

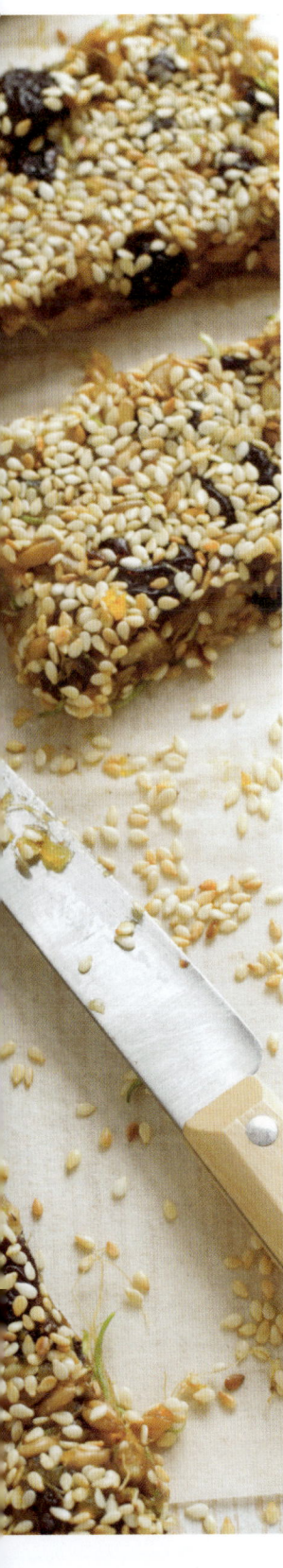

FOUR FRUITS POWER BAR

INGREDIENTS

1⅓ cup (150g) wheat grains
1 cup (150g) dry apricots
⅓ cup (50g) raisins
⅓ cup (50g) black currants
⅓ cup (50g) sour cherries
½ cup (50g) walnuts, soaked
   for 4 hours, dried, and
   lightly pan-toasted
⅓ cup (50g) sesame seeds,
   pan-toasted

MAKES 16 BARS

Sour cherries bring a sharp, lively flavor to these power bars. Add a combination of other dried berries, fruits, or nuts if you like, to complement the flavor of the sour cherries. These bars are best eaten the day you make them, not only to keep them from spoiling, but to get the maximum goodness from the freshly sprouted grains.

METHOD

1 To sprout the wheat grains, soak for 12 hours or overnight. Rinse the grains thoroughly and put in a large glass jar (grains expand to two to three times their initial volume). Cover the opening and neck of the jar with muslin cloth and attach it with string or a strong rubber band. Place at a 45-degree angle in a well-lit spot but not in direct sunlight. Rinse the grains each morning and evening by pouring water through the muslin and emptying it out.

2 The sprouts are ready when seedlings approximately ¼in (0.5–1 cm) in length appear. Rinse the seedlings thoroughly in clean water, strain, and spread on a clean cloth to dry. The sprouted grains are ready to use when they are dry to the touch. Place the apricots and raisins in a blender and blend to a paste. Add half of the sprouted grains and black currants and blend until crushed (but not blended to a puree).

Transfer to a mixing bowl and add the rest of the grains, berries, and the cherries. Mix well with a wooden spoon. Chop the walnuts into small chunks and add them to the mix. Sprinkle the sesame seeds on a flat surface. Roll out the mixture, or press it with clean hands, over the seeds into a rectangle ½in (1cm) thick. Use a sharp knife to cut the mixture into small rectangular bars. Place the bars on a rack and leave to dry out for a few hours.

CRANBERRY AND APRICOT POWER BARS

INGREDIENTS

¾ cup (100g) dried cranberries (presoaked and dried on a dish towel or paper towels)

1½ cups (200g) dried apricots (washed and dried on a dish towel or paper towels)

½ cup (60g) pistachios, coarsely chopped

5½oz (150g) lightly toasted barley, ground to a powder (see note)

⅓ cup (40g) pistachios, finely ground

MAKES 12–16 BARS

Barley has long had a reputation as a highly nutritious cereal; it was eaten by Ancient Greek athletes and Roman gladiators, who were known as hordearii ("barley eaters"). Cranberries are packed with antioxidants and apricots are an excellent source of iron, so these power bars make a highly nutritious and sustaining snack to keep your energy levels up.

METHOD

1 Put the fruit and coarsely chopped pistachios in a blender or food processor and blend into a thick puree. Then add just enough of the toasted barley powder to make a pliable dough.

2 Sprinkle half the finely ground pistachios onto a flat surface, place the fruit dough on top, and roll it out into a rectangular shape about ¼–½in (6–8mm) thick. Sprinkle the top of the dough with the remaining finely ground pistachios and press them by hand into the mixture.

3 Cut into 1¼ × 4in (3 × 10cm) rectangles and place on a baking sheet. Bake in a preheated 125°F (50°C) oven for 2–3 hours until the bars have dried out.

4 Carefully lift the bars off the sheet, allow to cool on a wire rack, then wrap them individually in plastic wrap or parchment paper. If wrapped and stored in a can in a cool place, the bars can last for more than a week.

Note: To roast barley, soak it overnight in lukewarm water, drain, and leave to dry on a baking sheet covered with a clean dish towel. When the barley is still damp, heat a large frying pan over high heat. Turn the heat down to medium and add a quarter of the barley, stirring constantly. When the grain is golden brown and makes a gravely noise as you stir it, transfer it out of the pan and allow to cool completely on a plate. Repeat with the remaining 3 batches. Allow the grain to cool completely and store in an airtight container. Grind the toasted grains in a pestle and mortar to make a barley powder.

FLAXSEED AND CHILE CRACKERS

INGREDIENTS

9oz (250g) flaxseeds

juice of 5 medium-sized
   carrots

juice of 2 celery ribs

1 small or medium chile
   (according to taste),
   chopped

4 tbsp fresh parsley, finely
   chopped

4 tbsp dulse or wakame
   flakes

a large pinch of salt

a sprinkle of chili powder
   (optional)

MAKES APPROX 12

These healthy crackers can be enjoyed by everyone.
Flaxseed is a valuable food in a balanced diet owing
to its high levels of omega-3 fatty acids, which play
an essential role in strengthening immunity and
maintaining good blood vessel health. The addition of
seaweeds, chile, and fresh parsley make these crackers
taste very addictive.

METHOD

1 Add the flaxseeds to the freshly made carrot and celery juices,
then stir in the chile, parsley, seaweed flakes, salt to taste, and chili
powder (if using). Leave for up to 2 hours to allow the flaxseeds
to soak up the juices.

2 Spread the soaked flaxseeds in a thin layer on a piece of
parchment paper on a baking sheet. Bake in a preheated 125°F
(50°C) oven for 3–4 hours.

3 Use a knife to cut the crackers into squares. Thicker pieces can
be served instead of bread with soup.

BLACK CURRANT AND WALNUT BARS

INGREDIENTS
1¼ cups (250g) barley grains
½ cup (50g) walnut pieces
4 dates, pitted
¾ cup (100g) dried black
    currants (or blueberries)

MAKES 8 OR MORE BARS

If barley grain is soaked in warm water, it cooks very slowly, allowing for little loss of nutrients. Toasted grain is very crunchy and can be partially cracked or milled by laying it in a thin layer on a wooden cutting board and rolling over it with a rolling pin before rolling out the bars. Eat the bars within 1–2 days while still fresh.

METHOD
1 Wash the barley grains, then soak them in warm water overnight. In the morning, drain the grains and allow them to dry out for a few minutes in a strainer. Set aside ⅔ cup (150g) of the grain and spread the rest in a thin layer over a clean, dry dish towel to dry until the next day.
2 The ⅔ cup (150g) of grain you set aside should still be damp, but no longer wet, and will be ready to toast. Heat a large frying pan over high heat, then turn the heat down and add the barley in small batches to toast. Make sure that the pan is not too crowded, and that the size of the pan allows for an equal toasting of all the barley grains. Stir constantly until the grain is a golden tan color and makes gravely noises as you stir it.
3 Allow the grain to cool completely, then move it in batches into a pestle and mortar and grind until lightly milled.
4 Toast the walnuts in the same way as the barley, toasting it lightly until golden with a nutty scent.
5 Once the barley grain and walnuts are ready to use, place the untoasted batch of barley grains in a blender or food processor with the dates and process to a paste. Transfer to a mixing bowl and stir in the black currants and walnuts. Spread the toasted barley grains over a work surface and place the paste mixture on top, rolling it out into a rectangle or pressing it into shape with clean hands. Cut into bars and place them on a rack to dry.

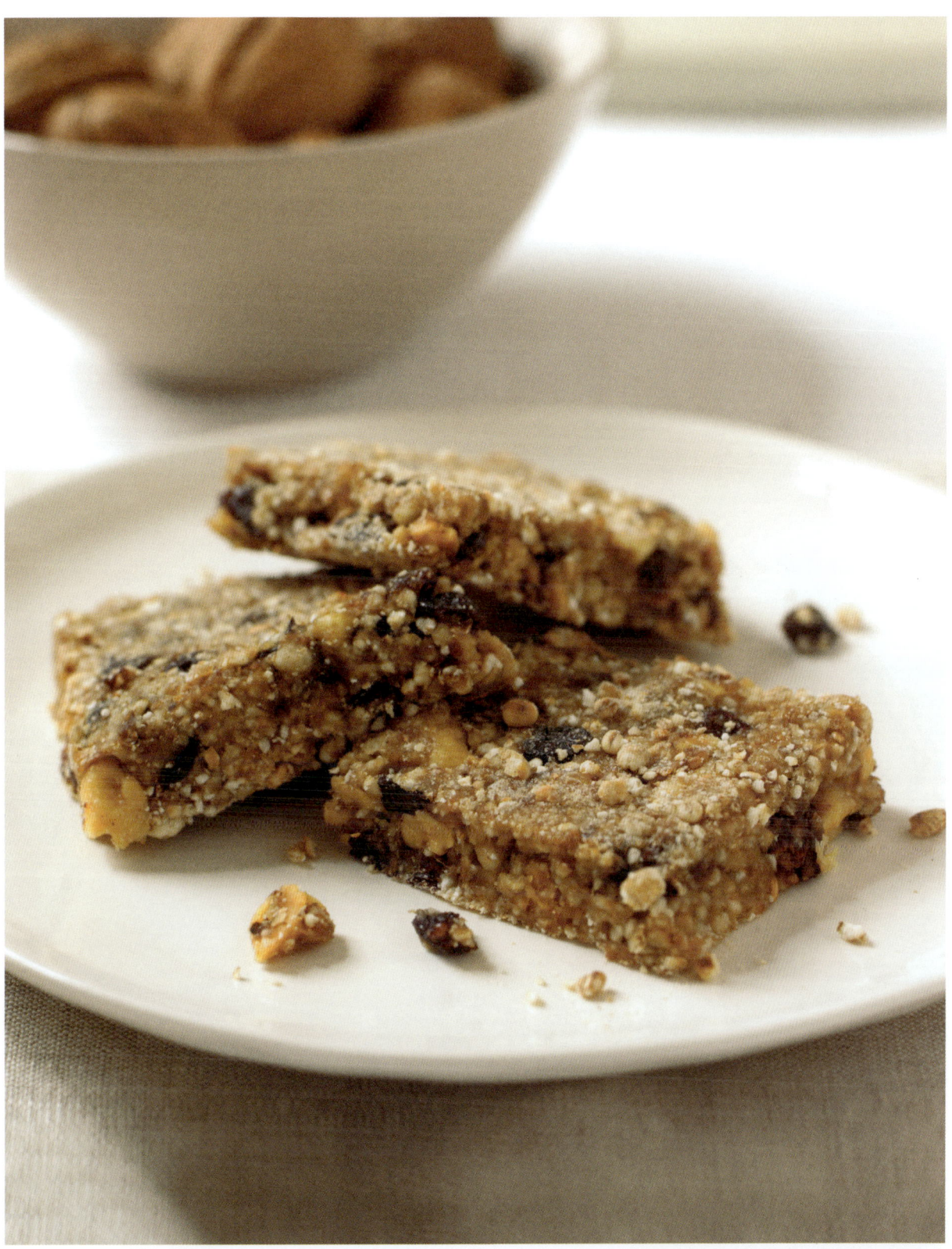

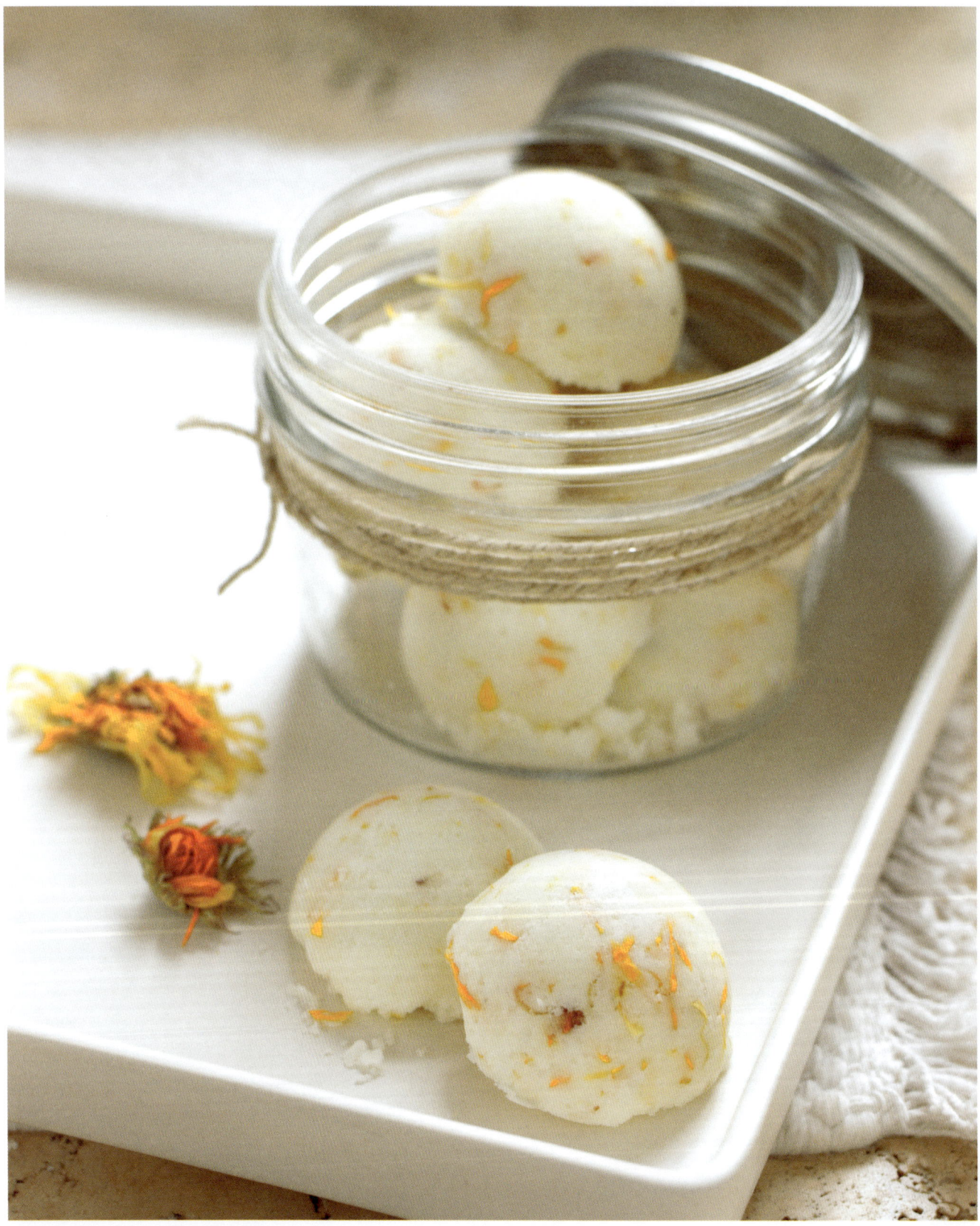

HEAL FROM THE OUTSIDE

MAKING FACE AND BODY CREAMS

Most of us use a moisturizer every day; you can perfect yours by choosing plant oils and extracts that are exactly suited to your skin type. If you have very sensitive skin, test any skin product on a small area of skin first to check that it does not provoke a reaction.

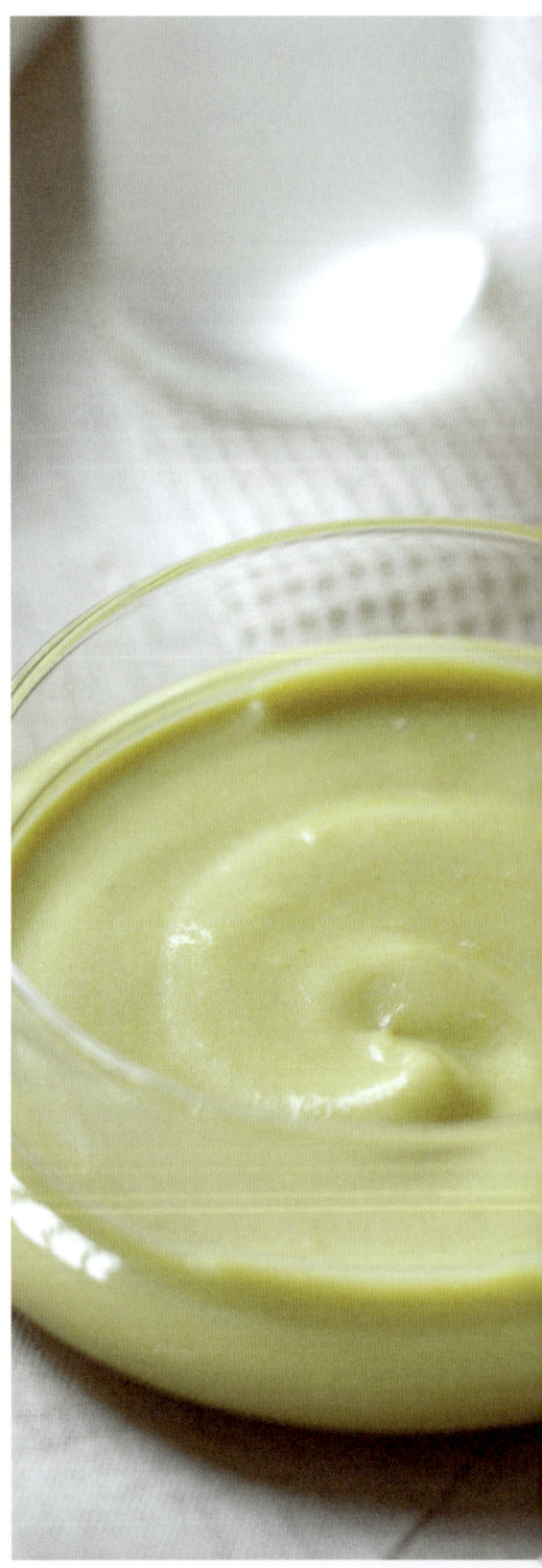

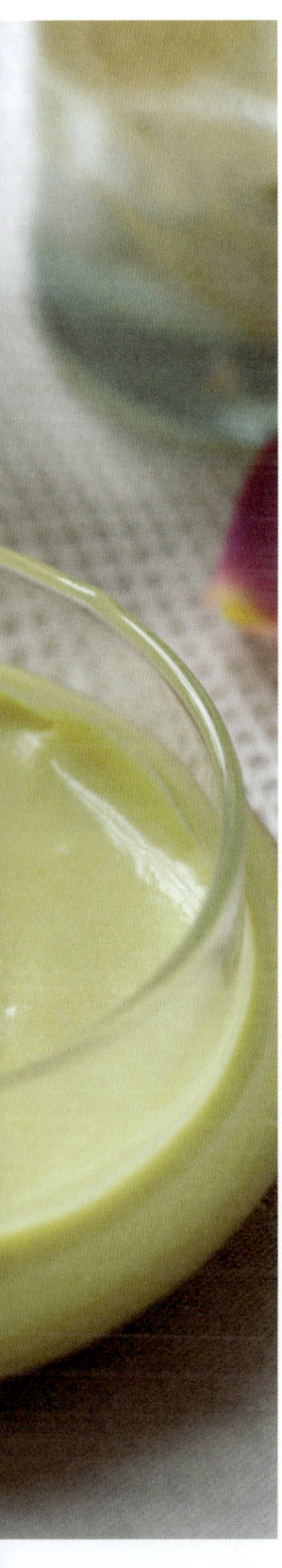

ROSE AND AVOCADO BODY MOISTURIZER

MAKES 1¼OZ (40G)

Moisturizing cocoa butter and shea nut butters are combined here with vitamin-rich avocado oil to give skin a nourishing, enriching treat to boost suppleness, banish dry patches, and leave a feeling of velvety smoothness. The beautiful rose fragrance adds a touch of luxury to delight the senses.

MOISTURIZES SKIN

INGREDIENTS
½ tsp cocoa butter and shea nut butter mix
1 tsp avocado oil
2 tbsp rose petal infusion
2 tbsp emulsifying wax
2 drops rose otto
3 drops geranium essential oil

METHOD

1 Melt the cocoa butter and shea nut butter with the avocado oil in a bowl set over a saucepan of boiling water (bain-marie).

2 Gently heat the rose petal infusion (p.176) and emulsifying wax in a small saucepan until the wax has completely dissolved in the infusion. Slowly add the infusion to the oil mixture, whisking it together for about 10 seconds.

3 When the mixture has cooled down, add the oils. Store in a sterilized glass jar (p.210) with a tight-fitting lid, and use within three months.

GOTU KOLA AND GINGER BODY TONING CREAM

MOISTURIZES SKIN

INGREDIENTS
1 tbsp apricot oil
2 tbsp gotu kola infusion
2 tsp emulsifying wax
2 drops black pepper
essential oil
3 drops ginger essential oil
2 drops lemon essential oil

MAKES 1½OZ (40G)

This is a nourishing cream with stimulating herbal extracts to restore suppleness and tone. Gotu kola has anti-inflammatory properties and encourages the formation of collagen, which firms and boosts the suppleness of the skin, while ginger, black pepper, and lemon essential oils encourage circulation and help tone the skin.

METHOD
1 Heat the apricot oil in a bowl set over a saucepan of boiling water (bain-marie).
2 Heat the gotu kola infusion and emulsifying wax gently in a saucepan until the emulsifier has dissolved in the infusion.
3 Slowly add the infusion to the apricot oil, stirring constantly. When the mixture has cooled, stir in the essential oils.
4 Store in a sterilized dark glass jar (p.210) with a tight-fitting lid in the refrigerator, and use within 2 months.

VIOLA AND EVENING PRIMROSE SKIN CREAM

MOISTURIZES SENSITIVE SKIN

INGREDIENTS
1 tsp lanolin
1 tsp avocado oil
1 tsp evening primrose oil
2 tbsp viola and chamomile
infusion (50:50 mix)
¼oz (10g) emulsifying wax

MAKES 1½OZ (40G)

This gently soothing and moisturizing skin cream is ideal for sensitive skin. Viola (heartsease) calms and soothes irritated skin and is traditionally used to ease conditions such as eczema. Here it is combined with essential fatty acid–rich avocado and evening primrose oils and gentle chamomile to soothe and nurture delicate skin.

METHOD
1 Melt the lanolin, avocado oil, and evening primrose oil in a bowl set over a saucepan of boiling water (bain-marie).
2 Put the viola and chamomile infusion and emulsifying wax into a saucepan and heat gently until the emulsifier has dissolved.
3 Slowly add the infusion to the lanolin and oil mixture, whisking it together for about 10 seconds.
4 Pour into a sterilized dark glass jar (p.210) with a tight-fitting lid, store in the refrigerator, and use within 2 months.

FRANKINCENSE AND WILD ROSE SKIN CREAM

INGREDIENTS
½ tsp cocoa butter
1 tsp calendula oil
1 tsp rose hip seed oil
¼oz (10g) emulsifying wax
2 tbsp (30ml) water
2 drops frankincense essential oil
1 drop neroli essential oil

MAKES 1½OZ (40G)

Frankincense is renowned for its toning, restorative, and anti-aging properties while rose hip oil helps improve skin elasticity and prevent moisture loss. Neroli oil, the precious essential oil from the blossom of the bitter orange tree, helps treat fine lines and encourages a bright, radiant complexion.

METHOD

1 Heat the cocoa butter, calendula oil, and rose hip oil in a bowl set over a saucepan of boiling water (bain-marie).
2 Gently heat the emulsifying wax and water in a saucepan until the emulsifier has dissolved. Slowly add this to the cocoa butter and oil mixture, whisking it together for about 10 seconds.
3 When the mixture has cooled, stir in the essential oils.
4 Store in a sterilized dark glass jar (p.210) with a tight-fitting lid in the refrigerator, and use within 2 months.

COCOA BUTTER AND ROSE BODY LOTION

INGREDIENTS
½oz (15g) cocoa butter
1 tsp lanolin
5 tbsp wheat germ oil
3 tbsp rose infusion (p.176)
1 tsp honey
scant 1oz (25g) emulsifying wax
5 drops benzoin tincture
5 drops vanilla extract
2 drops rose absolute
5 drops ylang-ylang essential oil
2 drops geranium essential oil
1 drop vetiver essential oil

MAKES 3½ (FL OZ) 100ML

This enriching lotion includes soothing honey and nourishing, cooling rose blended with vitamin E–rich wheat germ oil to smooth and soften skin. It has a subtle fragrance created by the blend of ylang-ylang, benzoin, geranium, and vetiver essential oils.

METHOD

1 Melt the cocoa butter, lanolin, and wheat germ oil in a bowl set over a pan of boiling water (bain-marie).
2 Make the rose infusion and while it is still hot, dissolve the honey and emulsifying wax in it.
3 Add this infusion mixture to the cocoa butter and oil mixture 1 tablespoon at a time, whisking all the while. Then add the benzoin tincture, vanilla extract, rose absolute, and essential oils.
4 Store in a sterilized glass bottle (p.210) with a tight-fitting lid in the refrigerator for up to 3 weeks. Shake before use.

GERANIUM AND ORANGE BODY BUTTER

MOISTURIZES SKIN

HARMONIZES EMOTIONS

INGREDIENTS
1 tbsp beeswax
3 tbsp calendula
 macerated oil
4 tsp grape-seed oil
4 tsp almond oil
20 drops geranium
 essential oil
20 drops orange essential oil

MAKES 3½OZ (100G)

A rich and deeply nourishing body butter like this is ideal for dry skin. The essential fatty acid combination of grape-seed and almond oils act to enrich and nourish the skin by strengthening and improving its suppleness. Geranium and orange essential oils also help tone the skin and impart a bright, sunny scent.

METHOD

1 Heat the beeswax, calendula, grape-seed and almond oils in a bowl set over a saucepan of boiling water (bain-marie). As the mixture cools, stir in the essential oils.
2 Pour into a sterilized dark glass jar (p.210) with a tight-fitting lid, and leave to set. Use within 3 months.

ROSE BODY BUTTER

MOISTURIZES SKIN

REVITALIZES

INGREDIENTS
1 tbsp beeswax
3 tbsp rose macerated oil
2 tbsp almond oil
2 tsp rose hip oil
10 drops rose absolute
10 drops geranium
 essential oil
5 drops patchouli
 essential oil

MAKES 3½OZ (100G)

If you want a luxurious and gorgeously scented body butter for nurturing the skin, this is the best choice. This aromatic balm features a triple dose of roses—macerated petal oil, rose absolute, and wild rose hip seed oil—to create a nurturing blend that softens, smooths, and scents the skin. Geranium and patchouli give depth to the fragrance, making it truly special.

METHOD

1 Heat the beeswax, rose, almond, and rose hip oils in a bowl set over a saucepan of boiling water (bain-marie). As the mixture cools, stir in the rose absolute and essential oils.
2 Pour into a sterilized dark glass jar (p.210) with a tight-fitting lid, and leave to set. Use within 3 months.

LAVENDER BODY BALM

MAKES 3½OZ (100G)

In this creamy and rich body balm with a deeply relaxing fragrance, skin-softening coconut oil is blended with gently moisturizing and soothing almond oil to nourish and nurture the skin. Lavender and its richly scented cousin, lavandin, are both healing and soothing on the skin and are combined here to give a relaxing fragrance.

METHOD

1 Heat the coconut and almond oils with the beeswax in a bowl set over a saucepan of boiling water (bain-marie). As the mixture cools, stir in the essential oils.
2 Pour into a sterilized dark glass jar (p.210) with a tight-fitting lid, and leave to set. Use within 3 months.

MOISTURIZES SKIN

RELAXES

INGREDIENTS
2oz (55g) coconut oil
2 tbsp almond oil
1 tbsp beeswax
30 drops lavender essential oil
10 drops lavandin essential oil

SOOTHING HERBAL BALM

MAKES 1½OZ (40G)

An all-purpose emergency salve for bumps, bruises, bites, and scrapes, this is an essential first aid remedy to keep at home. The therapeutic blend of herbal extracts, including St. John's wort, calendula, and gotu kola, are combined with antiseptic myrrh and niaouli oils to help ease all types of skin irritations and soothe scrapes.

METHOD

1 Heat the calendula oil and St. John's wort oil with the beeswax in a bowl set over a saucepan of boiling water (bain-marie). As the mixture cools, stir in the essential oils and tinctures.
2 Pour into a sterilized dark glass jar (p.210) with a tight-fitting lid, and leave to set. Use within 3 months.

TREATS BRUISES, SCRAPES, AND STINGS

INGREDIENTS
4½ tsp calendula macerated oil
2 tsp St. John's wort (Hypericum perforatum) macerated oil
1½ tsp (8g) beeswax
12 drops myrrh essential oil
12 drops lavender essential oil
4 drops niaouli essential oil
4 drops echinacea tincture
4 drops gotu kola tincture

BALANCING LEMON MOISTURIZER

MOISTURIZES OILY AND PROBLEM SKIN

INGREDIENTS

1 tsp beeswax
1 tsp cocoa butter
3 tbsp grape-seed oil
2 tsp emulsifying wax
2 tbsp lavender and nettle (50:50 mix) infusion (p.176)
10 drops lemon essential oil

MAKES 1½OZ (40G)

Mineral-rich, anti-inflammatory nettle and cleansing lavender infusions make this light cream an ideal moisturizer for oily or problem skin. The addition of lemon essential oil, which is machine-pressed from the peel of the ripe fruit then distilled, has a tightening effect on the pores and helps regulate the oils in the skin.

METHOD

1 Heat the beeswax, cocoa butter, and grape-seed oil in a bowl set over a saucepan of boiling water (bain-marie).
2 Dissolve the emulsifying wax in the freshly made, and still warm, lavender and nettle infusion.
3 Slowly add the infusion to the oil mixture, using a fast whisking action for about 10 seconds. When the mixture has cooled, stir in the lemon essential oil.
4 Store in a sterilized dark glass jar (p.210) with a tight-fitting lid in the refrigerator, and use within 2 months.

MARSHMALLOW MOISTURIZER

MOISTURIZES DRY SKIN

INGREDIENTS

1 tsp beeswax
1 tsp cocoa butter
1 tbsp avocado oil
2 tbsp almond oil
2 tsp emulsifying wax
2 tbsp marshmallow infusion (p.176)
4 drops geranium essential oil
5 drops bergamot essential oil

MAKES 1½OZ (40G)

A deeply enriching, nourishing moisturizer suitable for dry skin, this rich blend of cocoa butter and avocado and almond oils ensures that skin will remain supple and well protected from any moisture loss. Marshmallow has a soothing, softening effect, and geranium and bergamot essential oils are toning and refreshing.

METHOD

1 Heat the beeswax, cocoa butter, avocado oil, and almond oil in a bowl set over a saucepan of boiling water (bain-marie).
2 Dissolve the emulsifying wax in the freshly made, and still warm, marshmallow infusion.
3 Slowly add the infusion to the oil mixture, using a fast whisking action for about 10 seconds. When the mixture has cooled, stir in the essential oils.
4 Store in a sterilized dark glass jar (p.210) with a tight-fitting lid in the refrigerator, and use within 2 months.

ROSE AND GERANIUM MOISTURIZER

INGREDIENTS

1 tsp beeswax
1 tsp cocoa butter
1 tbsp apricot kernel oil
2 tbsp grape-seed oil
2 tsp emulsifying wax
2 tbsp rose petal infusion
    (p.176)
10 drops geranium
    essential oil

MAKES 1½OZ (40G)

This is a light moisturizer for normal skin, with a fresh, floral scent. Apricot is a wonderful skin-conditioning oil, and here it is combined with light, easily absorbed grape-seed oil and nourishing cocoa butter to enrich and smooth. Soothing rose and balancing geranium are also included to regulate moisture levels for soft, dewy skin.

METHOD

1 Heat the beeswax, cocoa butter, apricot oil, and grape-seed oil in a bowl set over a saucepan of boiling water (bain-marie).
2 Dissolve the emulsifying wax in the freshly made, and still warm, rose petal infusion.
3 Slowly add the infusion to the oil mixture, using a fast whisking action for about 10 seconds. When the mixture has cooled, stir in the geranium essential oil.
4 Store in a sterilized dark glass jar (p.210) with a tight-fitting lid in the refrigerator, and use within 2 months.

CHAMOMILE AND EVENING PRIMROSE MOISTURIZER

INGREDIENTS

1 tsp beeswax
1 tsp cocoa butter
2 tbsp almond oil
1 tsp borage seed oil
2 tsp evening primrose oil
2 tsp emulsifying wax
2 tbsp chamomile infusion
    (p.176)

MAKES 3½FL OZ (100ML)

A soothing, unscented cream to nurture delicate skin. Starflower and evening primrose seed oils are nature's best sources of gamma-linolenic acid (GLA) and are renowned for helping to soothe dry, itchy, or inflamed skin. Almond and cocoa butter gently moisturize, and chamomile soothes.

METHOD

1 Heat the beeswax and cocoa butter with the almond, borage, and evening primrose oils in a bowl set over a saucepan of boiling water (bain-marie).
2 Dissolve the emulsifying wax in the freshly made, and still warm, chamomile infusion.
3 Slowly add the infusion to the oil mixture, using a fast whisking action for about 10 seconds. Allow to cool.
4 Store in a sterilized dark glass jar (p.210) with a tight-fitting lid in the refrigerator, and use within 2 months.

MINTY FRESH FOOT CREAM

MOISTURIZES SKIN

ENERGIZES

INGREDIENTS
2 tsp cocoa butter
2 tsp beeswax
2 tbsp almond oil
1 tbsp wheat germ oil
2 tbsp spearmint
    infusion (p.176)
2 tsp emulsifying wax
10 drops peppermint
    essential oil

MAKES 3½OZ (100G)

Tired, aching feet will benefit from this cooling, refreshing foot cream, which includes both peppermint and spearmint (also known as garden mint) for maximum effect. Its soothing effects will alleviate any discomfort after a long day on the move, and also help keep skin smooth and in good condition.

METHOD

1 Heat the cocoa butter, beeswax, almond oil, and wheat germ oil together in a bowl set over a saucepan of boiling water (bain-marie) until the ingredients have melted.

2 Warm the spearmint infusion gently in a saucepan, but do not allow to boil. Dissolve the emulsifying wax in it. Take the oil mixture off the heat, slowly add the infusion, and stir until cool.

3 Add the peppermint essential oil, decant into a sterilized (p.210) glass jar (such as a screw-cap jar) with a tight-fitting lid and store in the refrigerator. It will keep for at least 2 months.

"THIS COOLING, SOOTHING CREAM WILL BRING RELIEF TO HOT, ACHING FEET AFTER A LONG DAY ON THE MOVE"

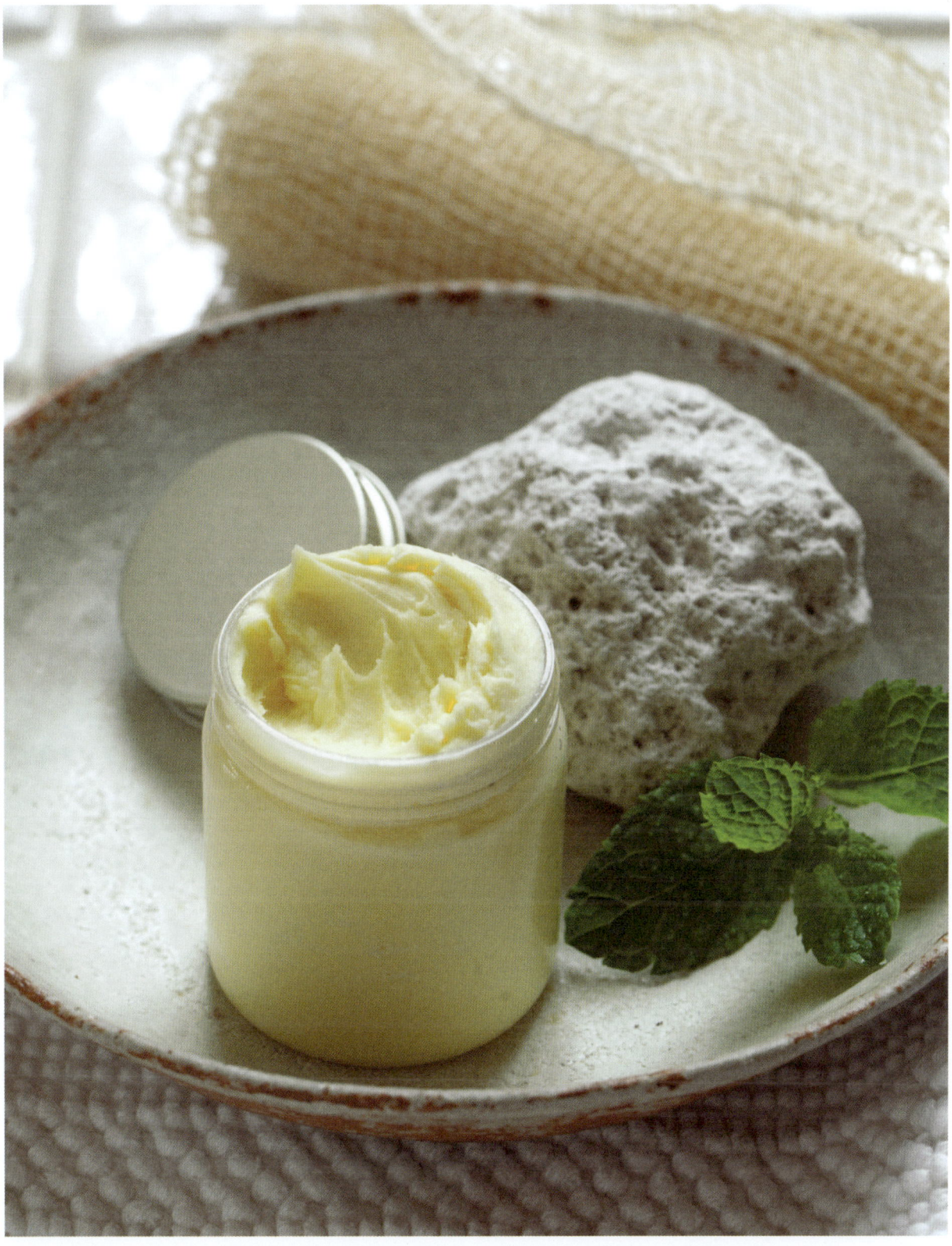

ROSE HAND CREAM

INGREDIENTS
1½ tsp cocoa butter
1 tsp beeswax
1 tbsp almond oil
1 tbsp rose hip oil
3 tbsp rosewater
2 tsp emulsifying wax
10 drops rose absolute

MAKES 3OZ (85G)

Fragrant, smoothing, and nourishing, this hand cream is a perfect treat for hard-working hands. It combines restorative cold-pressed seed oil from wild roses (*Rosa canina*) with soothing flower extracts from damask roses (*Rosa* x *damascena*) to revive dry, irritated, or weather-worn skin. It also includes almond oil and cocoa butter for added moisturizing.

METHOD
1 Melt the cocoa butter, beeswax, and almond oil in a bowl set over a saucepan of boiling water (bain-marie).
2 Warm the rosewater gently in a saucepan and dissolve the emulsifying wax into it.
3 Stir the rosewater and emulsifying wax into the oil mixture very slowly and continue stirring until the cream cools.
4 Add the rose absolute and stir.
5 Store in a sterilized glass jar (p.210) with a tight-fitting lid in the refrigerator, and use within 2 months.

FRANKINCENSE AND ORANGE FLOWER HAND CREAM

INGREDIENTS

1½ tsp cocoa butter

1 tsp beeswax

2 tsp calendula
   macerated oil

3 tbsp orange flower water

2 tsp emulsifying wax

10 drops orange essential oil

5 drops frankincense
   essential oil

MAKES 3OZ (85G)

Nurturing calendula oil is combined with moisturizing cocoa butter and a toning aromatherapy blend of frankincense and orange essential oils in this smoothing, revitalizing cream. A little orange flower water added to the blend imparts a beautiful scent and helps make a wonderfully restorative treatment for dry skin.

METHOD

1 Melt the cocoa butter, beeswax, and calendula oil in a bowl set over a saucepan of boiling water (bain-marie).

2 Warm the orange flower water gently and dissolve the emulsifying wax into it.

3 Stir the orange flower water and emulsifying wax into the oil mixture very slowly and continue to stir until the cream cools.

4 Add the orange and frankincense essential oils and stir.

5 Store in a sterilized glass jar (p.210) with a tight-fitting lid in the refrigerator, and use within 2 months.

MAKING BODY SCRUBS

Scrubs boost circulation and smooth the skin, leaving it feeling radiant with a healthy glow. If you have sensitive skin or eczema, this may be exacerbated by scrubbing; the best treatment is a moisturizer or anti-inflammatory cream such as Chamomile and Evening Primrose Moisturizer (p.269).

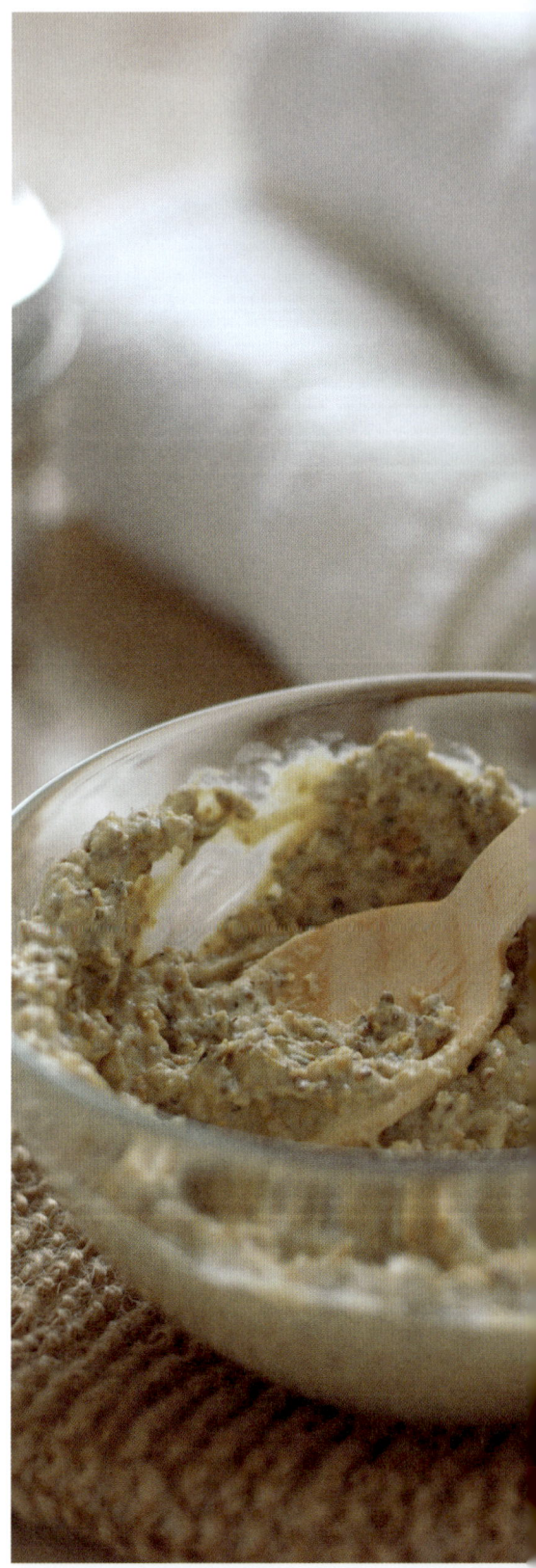

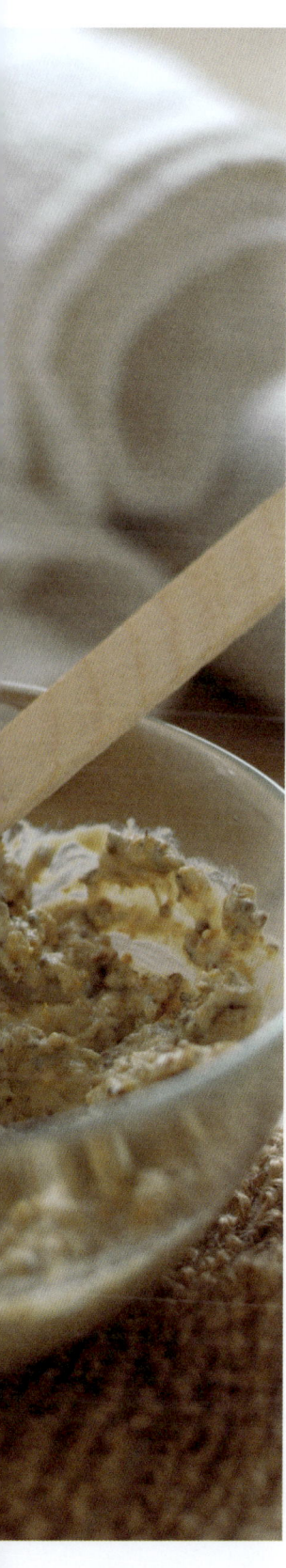

ALOE AND ELDERFLOWER BODY SCRUB

EXFOLIATES

INGREDIENTS
¾oz (20g) dried elderflowers
2 tbsp aloe vera juice
scant 1oz (25g) ground rice
3 drops benzoin tincture
4 tsp organic plain yogurt
4 drops lavender
  essential oil

MAKES ENOUGH FOR 1 APPLICATION

Aloe vera is an extremely soothing and cooling plant extract, and is rich in nourishing vitamins, amino acids, enzymes, and proteins. This body scrub combines fresh, thick, mucilaginous aloe vera juice with elderflowers, which have anti-inflammatory qualities, and ground rice to create an exfoliating paste that refreshes and smooths the skin.

METHOD

1 Cover the elderflowers with the aloe vera juice and leave for 15 minutes.
2 Add the ground rice and mix thoroughly.
3 Add the benzoin, yogurt, and lavender essential oil.
4 Apply to the skin using firm, circular hand movements.

HONEY AND AVOCADO BODY SCRUB

EXFOLIATES

INGREDIENTS

scant 1oz (25g) crushed
  pumice stone
1 ripe avocado
1 tbsp honey
1 tbsp olive oil
2 drops lemon balm
  essential oil (optional)

MAKES ENOUGH FOR 1 TREATMENT

Excellent for softening areas of dry, rough skin (but not eczema patches), this exfoliating paste can be quickly whipped up for skin-smoothing emergencies. Honey is a natural treat for the skin, with cleansing, soothing properties; when combined with avocado, olive oil, and exfoliating pumice powder, this simple recipe transforms dull, dry skin.

METHOD

1 Grind the pumice stone to a fine powder with a pestle and mortar.
2 Mash the avocado in a bowl with a fork.
3 Slightly warm the honey, then add it to the bowl followed by the olive oil (and lemon balm essential oil if using).
4 Stir the mixture well before gradually adding the pumice.
5 Blend carefully, adding enough pumice to enable the mixture to stick together. Use immediately.

LAVENDER SALT SCRUB

EXFOLIATES

INGREDIENTS

2 tbsp sea salt
1 tsp dried lavender flowers
2 tbsp almond oil
2 drops lavender
  essential oil

MAKES ENOUGH FOR 1 TREATMENT

For the simplest of scrubs, mix salt and oil into a paste for immediate use. By adjusting the texture and amount of salt, you can tailor the texture to suit your preference. Including powdered herbs and essential oils can add a fragrance that suits your mood; this scrub contains lavender, which is both refreshing and relaxing.

METHOD

1 Use a pestle and mortar to grind the sea salt if you want a finer scrub.
2 Grind the lavender flowers to a rough powder with the pestle and mortar.
3 Mix all the ingredients into a paste and use immediately.

CALENDULA AND OAT BODY SCRUB

INGREDIENTS
1½oz (45g) oats
¾oz (20g) bran
½oz (15g) calendula flowers

MAKES ENOUGH FOR 1 TREATMENT

A simple recipe like this gently cleanses, soothes, and enriches the skin. Oats have long been used for their skin soothing properties, and they create a nurturing wash for dry skin; they are rich in natural polysaccharides, which become gelatinous in water. Here they are combined with calendula and exfoliating bran to cleanse and smooth the skin.

METHOD

1 Place the oats, bran, and flowers in a muslin or cheesecloth bag, tie firmly at the top with string, and use the ends of the string to hang it from the tap so the bath water runs through it.
2 When you are in the bath, rub your skin with the bag, especially on any patches of dry skin.

HONEY AND ORANGE BODY SCRUB

INGREDIENTS
¼oz (10g) kaolin powder
1oz (30g) ground rice
1 tsp orange flower water
1 tbsp honey
5 drops calendula tincture
2 drops orange essential oil
1 drop geranium
   essential oil

MAKES APPROX 1¾OZ (50G)

Suitable for all skin types, this is an enriching scrub to effectively exfoliate and cleanse the skin. Ground rice provides the exfoliating action, clay is included to draw impurities from the skin, and honey moisturizes and smooths. Geranium and orange essential oils have a toning effect and also impart a bright, sunny fragrance.

METHOD

1 Grind the kaolin and ground rice together using a pestle and mortar to create a fine powder.
2 Add the orange flower water and slightly warmed honey (warming makes the honey easier to blend) to the powder mixture and mix thoroughly with the calendula tincture and essential oils. Decant into a sterilized glass jar (p.210) with a tight-fitting lid.
3 To use, mix the scrub with a little warm water to form a paste and apply to damp skin with a circular motion. Rinse with warm water. Use within 2 months.

CLEANSING CHAMOMILE HAND SCRUB

EXFOLIATES

INGREDIENTS
2 tbsp vegetable glycerin
1¾ tbsp cornstarch
1 tsp chamomile flower
  water (or infusion)
2 tsp ground rice
2 tsp finely ground oats

MAKES 1½OZ (40G)

Use this gentle hand cleanser as an alternative to soap. With its gently exfoliating action, enriching oats to soften and smooth, and glycerin to reduce moisture loss from the skin, it both cleans and cares for hard-working hands. Chamomile flower water, which is naturally nurturing, has also been included to bring extra relief and soothe the skin.

METHOD
1 Warm the vegetable glycerin in a bowl set over a saucepan of hot or boiling water (bain-marie).
2 Slowly add the cornstarch, stirring constantly to make a paste.
3 Take off the heat and gradually add the chamomile water, still stirring. Mix in the ground rice and oats.
4 Store in a sterilized glass jar (p.210) with a tight-fitting lid and use in the same way as liquid soap. Use within 2 months.

MANDARIN AND MYRRH FOOT SCRUB

EXFOLIATES

INGREDIENTS
½oz (15g) crushed pumice
  stone
¼oz (10g) cocoa butter
¼oz (10g) beeswax
3 tbsp apricot kernel oil
¼oz (10g) emulsifying wax
2 tbsp marshmallow
  infusion (p.176)
12 drops myrrh essential oil
8 drops mandarin
  essential oil

MAKES 1½OZ (40G)

Foot scrubs effectively smooth away hard skin and cleanse and nourish feet to leave them feeling soft and fresh. In this scrub, pumice powder removes rough skin and boosts circulation, while a blend of skin-softening marshmallow herb, deeply moisturizing cocoa butter, enriching apricot kernel oil, and cleansing mandarin and myrrh essential oils nourish the skin.

METHOD
1 Grind the pumice stone with a pestle and mortar to a fine powder.
2 Warm the cocoa butter, beeswax, and apricot kernel oil together in a bowl set over a saucepan of boiling water (bain-marie) until all the ingredients have melted. Then remove from the heat.
3 Dissolve the emulsifying wax in the freshly made, and still warm, marshmallow infusion. Slowly add the infusion to the oil mixture and stir until cool.
4 Add the pumice stone and essential oils and mix thoroughly.
5 Store in a sterilized dark glass jar (p.210) with a tight-fitting lid in the refrigerator, and use within 3 months.

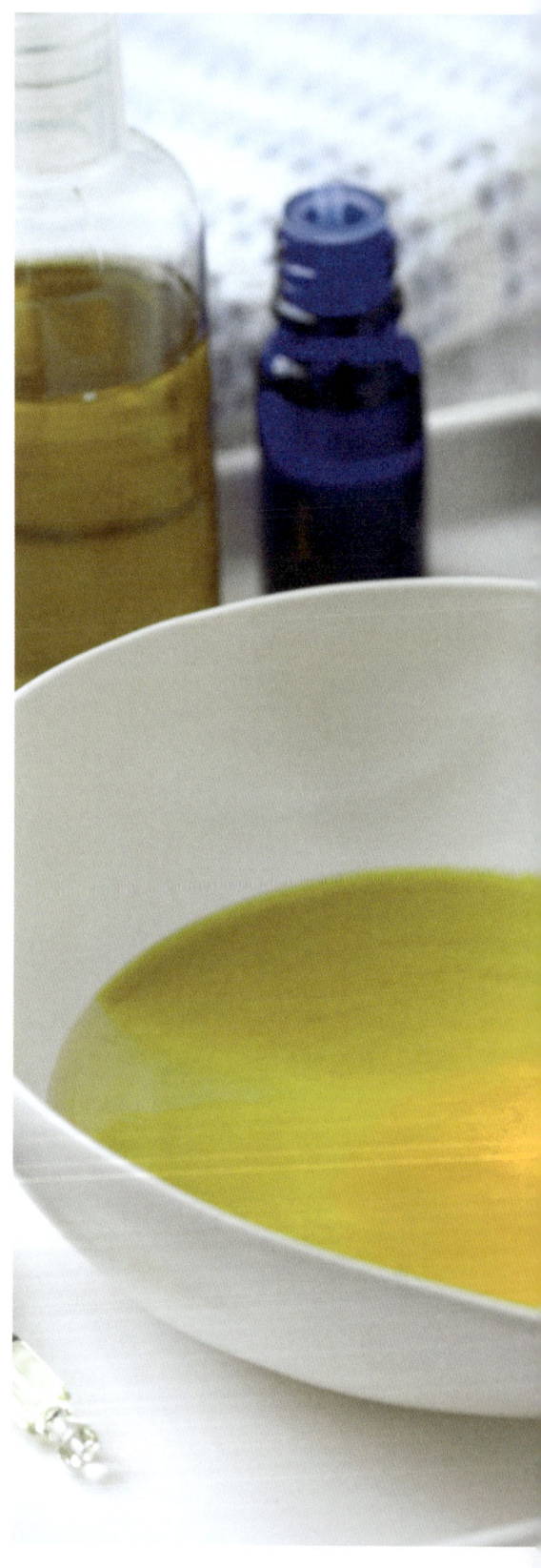

MAKING BODY OILS

Whether used for massages or to condition the skin, enriching, nourishing, and moisturizing body oils are a real treat. If you have very sensitive skin, test any skin care product on a small area of skin first to check that it does not provoke a reaction.

LAVENDER AND BERGAMOT SOOTHING SKIN OIL

MAKES 3½FL OZ (100ML)

A relaxing aromatherapy mix of floral geranium; soothing lavender; calming cypress; and fresh, uplifting bergamot is blended into a nourishing base of different vegetable oils to help restore your skin's suppleness and give it maximum protection from moisture loss.

METHOD

1 Blend all the ingredients together.
2 Store in a sterilized dark glass bottle (p.210) with a tight-fitting lid away from sunlight. This skin oil will keep for up to 6 months.

MOISTURIZES SKIN

RELAXES

INGREDIENTS
4 tsp almond oil
4 tsp sunflower oil
4 tsp coconut oil
4 tsp grape-seed oil
2 tsp avocado oil
2 tsp wheat germ oil
10 drops geranium
   essential oil
10 drops bergamot
   essential oil
10 drops lavender
   essential oil
10 drops cypress
   essential oil

STIMULATING BODY OIL

INGREDIENTS
4 tsp almond oil
4 tsp sunflower oil
4 tsp coconut oil
4 tsp grape-seed oil
2 tsp avocado oil
2 tsp wheat germ oil
10 drops lavender
  essential oil
10 drops peppermint
  essential oil
10 drops juniper
  essential oil
10 drops rosemary
  essential oil

MAKES APPROX 3½FL OZ (100ML)

The wonderfully enriching base of plant oils in this body oil is rich in natural essential fatty acids, minerals, and vitamins to restore suppleness and elasticity to the skin. A stimulating aromatherapy blend of peppermint, juniper, lavender, and rosemary also boosts the circulation and invigorates the senses.

METHOD

1 Blend all the ingredients together.
2 Store in a sterilized dark glass bottle (p.210) with a tight-fitting lid and use within 3 months.

GERANIUM AND ORANGE BODY OIL

INGREDIENTS
2½ tbsp almond oil
2½ tbsp sunflower oil
4 tsp calendula
  macerated oil
20 drops geranium
  essential oil
20 drops orange essential oil

MAKES APPROX 3½FL OZ (100ML)

This enriching body oil treats both body and mind to bring a deep sense of well-being. It is an excellent all-purpose skin-conditioning or massage oil, with a bright, sunny scent. Geranium essential oil has a balancing effect on the skin and is used by aromatherapists to help treat anxiety and tension, while orange essential oil is toning and refreshing.

METHOD

1 Blend all the ingredients together.
2 Store in a sterilized dark glass bottle (p.210) with a tight-fitting lid and use within 3 months.

DETOX BODY OIL

MAKES APPROX 3½FL OZ (100ML)

A stimulating and detoxifying blend of oils like this can help boost the circulation and strengthen and tone the skin for a smoother appearance. For the best results, try dry-skin brushing your body with a natural bristle brush before having a warm bath or shower, then massage the body oil into your skin.

METHOD

1 Blend all the ingredients together.
2 Store in a sterilized dark glass bottle (p.210) with a tight-fitting lid and use within 3 months.

MOISTURIZES SKIN

STIMULATES CIRCULATION

INGREDIENTS
2½ tbsp soy oil
2½ tbsp almond oil
4 tsp wheat germ oil
5 drops lemon essential oil
5 drops frankincense
   essential oil
5 drops orange essential oil
2 drops juniper essential oil
2 drops black pepper
   essential oil
2 drops vetiver essential oil
2 drops eucalyptus
   essential oil

CALENDULA AND ST. JOHN'S WORT SOOTHING OIL

MAKES ENOUGH FOR 1 TREATMENT

Always try to protect your skin from overexposure to the sun, but if you do accidentally get sunburned, use this soothing oil to ease the discomfort. Do not apply before any exposure to the sun, as St. John's wort is known to be photosensitizing. This oil blend can also be applied to relieve the pain of shingles.

METHOD

Blend the ingredients together and gently apply to the skin.

SOOTHES SUNBURN
AND SHINGLES

INGREDIENTS
1 tsp calendula oil
1 tsp St. John's wort oil
2 drops lavender
   essential oil

SESAME AND SOY SKIN OIL

NOURISHES SKIN

INGREDIENTS
2½ tbsp soy oil
2½ tbsp sesame oil
2½ tbsp coconut oil
4 tsp grape-seed oil
40 drops petitgrain
    essential oil
5 drops lavender
    essential oil

MAKES APPROX 3½FL OZ (100ML)

If you are going on vacation, take this deeply nourishing skin oil to restore suppleness to your skin if it becomes dehydrated by the sun and ocean. Sesame is rich in antioxidant vitamin E, coconut replenishes moisture, and grape-seed and soy feed the skin with nourishing essential fatty acids. Toning petitgrain essential oil has a clean, refreshing scent.

METHOD
1 Blend all the ingredients together.
2 Store in a sterilized dark glass bottle (p.210) with a tight-fitting lid and use within 3 months.

COCONUT AND LIME
SKIN OIL

NOURISHES SKIN

INGREDIENTS
2 tsp wheat germ oil
¾oz (20g) cocoa butter
3½ tbsp coconut oil
10 drops lime essential oil
5 drops benzoin tincture

MAKES APPROX 2FL OZ (60ML)

Easily absorbed, skin-softening coconut oil is combined with deeply moisturizing cocoa butter and nourishing vitamin E–rich wheat germ oil in this blend to restore radiance to dull, dry skin. A few drops of lime essential oil give the oil a refreshing, uplifting aroma. Apply in the evening to nourish the skin overnight.

METHOD
1 Blend all the ingredients together in a bowl (if necessary, gently warm the cocoa butter and coconut oil over a bain-marie first to liquefy and aid blending).
2 Store in a sterilized dark glass bottle (p.210) with a tight-fitting lid and use within 3 months.

BABY MASSAGE OIL

INGREDIENTS

5½ tbsp sunflower oil

4 tsp calendula
  macerated oil

8 drops lavender
  essential oil

6 drops Roman chamomile
  essential oil

6 drops rose absolute

MAKES APPROX 3½FL OZ (100ML)

Suitable for use from 3 months, this is a gentle, soothing oil for delicate skin. Rose absolute and lavender and Roman chamomile essential oils, which are renowned for their soothing and skin-conditioning properties, are combined with a base of gentle sunflower and calendula oils to give a mild and soothing skin oil that is excellent for babies or anyone with sensitive skin.

METHOD

1 Blend all the ingredients together.

2 Store in a sterilized dark glass bottle (p.210) with a tight-fitting lid and use within 3 months.

BABY BATH OIL

INGREDIENTS

5½ tbsp sunflower oil

4 tsp calendula
  macerated oil

10 drops mandarin
  essential oil

MAKES APPROX 3½FL OZ (100ML)

Gently nourishing sunflower and calendula oils form a soothing base for this simple bath oil that moisturizes dry or delicate skin with a calming, comforting scent. Mandarin oil, which is expressed from the peel of the fruit, is excellent for children, as its sweet, citrus fragrance is calming and has a soothing effect. Suitable for use from 3 months.

METHOD

1 Blend all the ingredients together.

2 Store in a sterilized dark glass bottle (p.210) with a tight-fitting lid and use within 3 months. Use 2 teaspoons of blend per bath.

MAKING BODY SPRITZES

Creating your own fragrant body splashes with essential oils and herbal blends is a simple way of keeping your skin fresh and enhancing your sense of well-being. If you have very sensitive skin, test any skin product on a small area of skin first to check that it does not provoke a reaction.

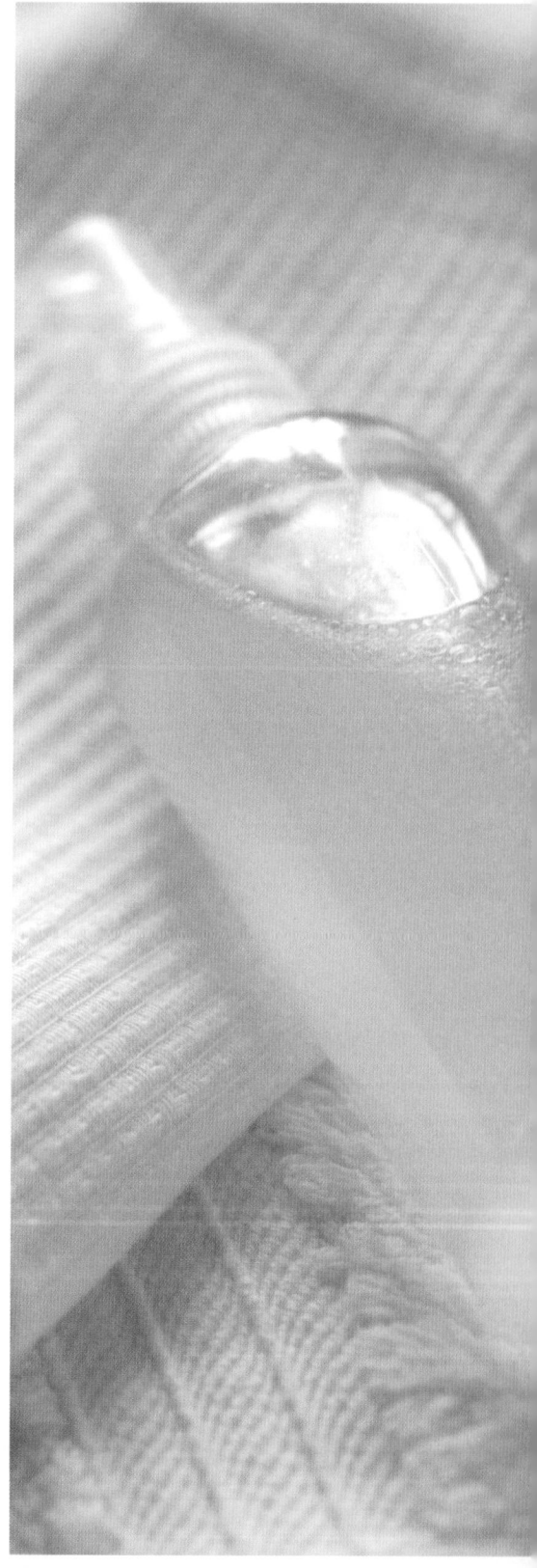

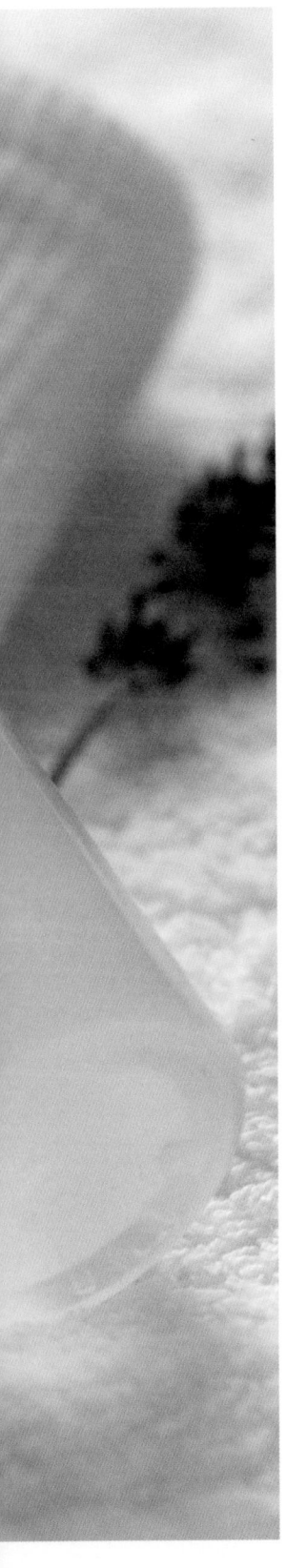

SPICY WITCH HAZEL DEODORANT

DEODORIZES

INGREDIENTS
3fl oz (90ml) witch hazel
2 tsp vegetable glycerin
2 drops clove essential oil
2 drops coriander
  essential oil
5 drops grapefruit
  essential oil
2 drops lavender
  essential oil
10 drops lemon essential oil
5 drops lime essential oil
5 drops palmarosa
  essential oil

MAKES 3½FL OZ (100ML)

This fresh, fragrant-smelling underarm spray is ideal if you wish to avoid products containing aluminum derivatives. Witch hazel is gently astringent and acts as a perfect base for an antibacterial blend of essential oils. Spray the deodorant onto clean, dry skin after bathing and reapply as often as required. It can also be used to freshen feet.

METHOD
1 Mix the witch hazel and vegetable glycerin together.
2 Add the essential oils, and mix well.
3 Store in a sterilized dark glass bottle (p.210) with a fine mist atomizer. Shake well before use to ensure the ingredients are well blended. Use within 6 months.

BERGAMOT AND MINT DEODORANT

INGREDIENTS
1 tsp vegetable glycerin
2½ tbsp witch hazel
2½ tbsp lavender water
10 drops bergamot
  essential oil
8 drops grapefruit
  essential oil
7 drops lemon essential oil
4 drops peppermint
  essential oil
1 drop cypress essential oil

MAKES APPROX 2¾FL OZ (85ML)

A refreshing combination of witch hazel and lavender water are the main ingredients for this fragrant underarm body spray, which keeps skin fresh. It also contains a cleansing, antibacterial blend of essential oils that includes citrusy bergamot, grapefruit, and lemon; invigorating peppermint; and woody cypress. Spray on clean, dry skin. May also be used on the feet.

METHOD
1 Combine the vegetable glycerin with the witch hazel and lavender water.
2 Stir in the essential oils.
3 Store in a sterilized dark glass bottle (p.210) with a fine mist atomizer. Shake well before use to ensure the ingredients are well blended. Use within 6 months.

GERANIUM AND ORANGE BODY SPLASH

INGREDIENTS
⅓ cup distilled water
2 tsp aloe vera juice
1 tsp orange flower water
2 drops patchouli
   essential oil
1 drop geranium
   essential oil

MAKES APPROX 3¼FL OZ (95ML)

With its bright, sunny fragrance, this body spray refreshes the skin, lifts the spirits, and leaves the skin lightly scented. Aloe vera, which makes a cooling, soothing base, is combined with earthy vetiver, brightly scented geranium oil, and delicately scented orange flower water, made from the blossom of the bitter orange tree.

METHOD
1 Combine all the ingredients.
2 Store in a sterilized dark glass bottle (p.210) with a fine mist atomizer. Shake well before use to ensure the ingredients are well blended. Use within 2 months.

CITRONELLA SPRAY

MAKES APPROX 5 TSP

The two essential oils in this insect-repellent spray are distilled from citronella grass and the leaves of *Eucalyptus citriodora*, the Australian lemon-scented gum tree. Both oils have a sharp, citrus scent and are traditionally used to keep mosquitoes at bay. Apply this fragrant mist every two hours on exposed skin.

METHOD

1 Combine the lavender water and essential oils.
2 Store in a sterilized dark glass bottle (p.210) with a fine mist atomizer. Shake before use to ensure the ingredients are well blended. Use within 6 months.

PROTECTS AGAINST INSECT BITES

INGREDIENTS

5 tsp lavender flower water

3 drops *Eucalyptus citriodora* essential oil

2 drops citronella essential oil

AFTER-BITE SOOTHER

MAKES APPROX 2 TBSP

Witch hazel, yarrow, and plantain all have styptic and anti-inflammatory properties; when combined with soothing calendula, cooling aloe vera, and a cleansing blend of lavender and tea tree essential oils, they become a handy herbal extract spray that will bring immediate relief from the irritation and pain of bites and stings.

METHOD

1 Combine all the ingredients.
2 Store in a sterilized dark glass bottle (p.210) with a fine mist atomizer. Shake before use to ensure the ingredients are well blended. Use within 6 months.

SOOTHES

INGREDIENTS

4 tsp witch hazel

1 tsp aloe vera juice

30 drops (1.5ml) plantain tincture

30 drops (1.5ml) calendula tincture

30 drops (1.5ml) yarrow tincture

24 drops lavender essential oil

6 drops tea tree essential oil

ROSE BODY SPLASH

INGREDIENTS

¼ cup distilled water

2 tsp aloe vera juice

2 tsp rosewater

3 drops rose absolute

3 drops geranium
   essential oil

1 drop patchouli essential oil

MAKES APPROX 3¼FL OZ (95ML)

This subtle, floral body splash features a luxurious blend of damask rose flower water, earthy patchouli, and bright geranium essential oils. Aloe vera and rosewater are both gentle, soothing, and cooling—a perfect combination to pep up tired skin. For extra refreshment in hot weather, store the bottle in the refrigerator in between each use.

METHOD

1 Combine all the ingredients.

2 Store in a sterilized dark glass bottle (p.210) with a fine mist atomizer. Shake before use to ensure the ingredients are well blended. Use within 2 months.

FRANKINCENSE BODY SPLASH

INGREDIENTS

5½ tbsp distilled water

2 tsp aloe vera juice

1 tsp lavender flower water

4 drops frankincense
   essential oil

2 drops mandarin
   essential oil

2 drops bergamot
   essential oil

MAKES APPROX 3¼FL OZ (95ML)

Frankincense essential oil, which is distilled from the resin of the tree, is gently astringent and has a toning effect on the skin. Combined with fresh citrus oils of mandarin and bergamot, it creates a subtly scented blend that has cleansing and revitalizing properties and will refresh all skin types.

METHOD

1 Combine all the ingredients.

2 Store in a sterilized dark glass bottle (p.210) with a fine mist atomizer. Shake before use to ensure the ingredients are well blended. Use within 2 months.

MAKING BODY POWDERS

Body powders help keep the skin soft, smooth, and silky. Essential oils can be added to the powder base to give a subtle fragrance to the skin. If you have very sensitive skin, test any skin product on a small area of skin first to check that it does not provoke a reaction.

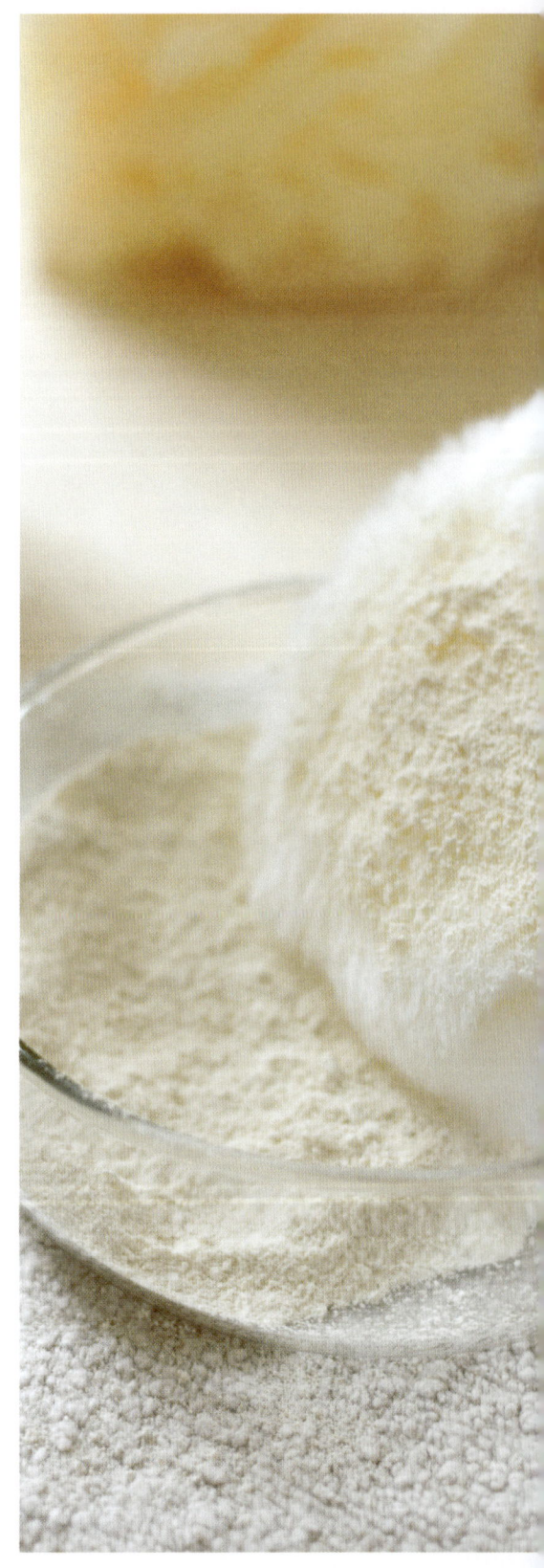

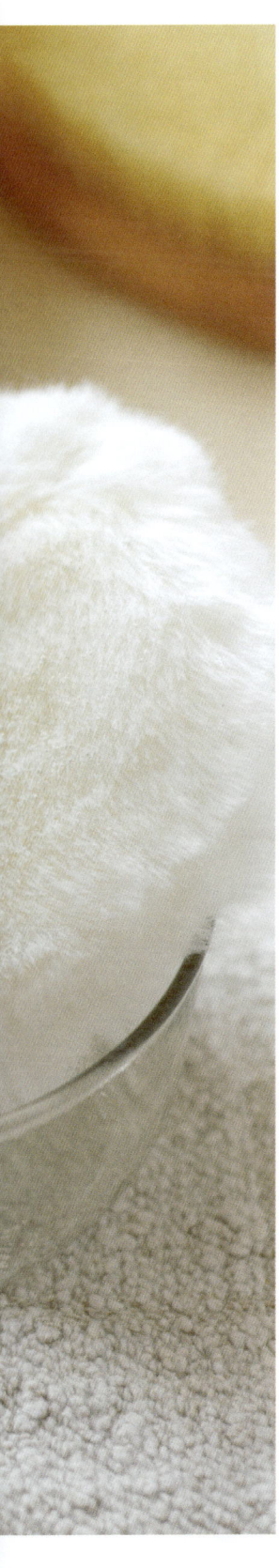

CALENDULA BODY POWDER

SOOTHES SKIN

INGREDIENTS
¾oz (20g) kaolin powder
5 drops calendula tincture
5 drops lemon essential oil

MAKES ¾OZ (20G)

A talc-free body powder such as this is perfect for delicate or sensitive skin, for keeping skin dry in hot or humid weather, or for soothing and protecting areas of skin that are prone to chafing or rubbing. Apply to clean, dry skin after bathing using cotton balls, or just sprinkle the powder on your body and lightly smooth it over the skin.

METHOD
1 Sift the kaolin evenly onto a wide, flat plate.
2 Mix the tincture and essential oil together and decant into a clean container with a fine mist atomizer.
3 Spray this mix onto the kaolin, taking care to spray evenly and not to saturate the powder, which may cause lumps. Allow the powder to dry.
4 Store the dry powder in an old, clean body powder dispenser or clean pepper shaker. Use within 6 months.

"TRY ONE OF THESE FRAGRANT HOMEMADE BODY POWDER RECIPES AS A TREAT AFTER A RELAXING AROMATHERAPY BATH"

LAVENDER AND TEA TREE POWDER

INGREDIENTS

2¾ tbsp cornstarch

20 drops (1ml) propolis tincture

5 drops lavender essential oil

5 drops tea tree essential oil

MAKES APPROX ¾OZ (20G)

A cleansing, talc-free, lightly scented body powder such as this is ideal for use before and after sports or strenuous activity to keep skin fresh and to protect against chafing. Apply after bathing to freshly dried skin. Use cotton balls to apply the powder, or just sprinkle it on your body and lightly smooth it over the skin.

METHOD

1 Sift the cornstarch evenly onto a wide, flat plate.

2 Mix the propolis tincture and essential oils together and decant into a clean container with a fine mist atomizer.

3 Spray this mix onto the cornstarch, being sure to spray evenly and not to saturate the powder, which may cause lumps. Allow the powder to dry.

4 Store the dry powder in a used, clean body powder dispenser or clean pepper shaker. Use within 6 months.

ROSE BODY POWDER

INGREDIENTS

2¾ tbsp cornstarch

5 drops rose absolute
  essential oil

4 drops geranium
  essential oil

1 drop patchouli essential oil

MAKES APPROX ¾OZ (20G)

This fragrant, talc-free, floral body powder includes soothing, cooling rose to smooth the skin. Geranium complements and strengthens the scent of rose, while earthy patchouli gives lasting depth. Apply after bathing to freshly dried skin. Use cotton balls to apply the powder, or just sprinkle it on your body and lightly smooth it over the skin.

METHOD

1 Sift the cornstarch evenly onto a wide, flat plate.

2 Mix the essential oils together and decant into a clean container with a fine mist atomizer.

3 Spray this mix onto the cornstarch, being sure to spray evenly and not to saturate the powder, which may cause lumps. Allow the powder to dry.

4 Store the dry powder in a used, clean body powder dispenser or clean pepper shaker. Use within 6 months.

BLACK CURRANT AND SAGE FOOT POWDER

INGREDIENTS

1 tbsp dried sage

2 tbsp dried black currant leaves

¼oz (10g) kaolin powder

5 drops lemon essential oil

MAKES APPROX ½OZ (15G)

This is a cleansing powder to help keep feet dry and fresh. Sage is known for its cool, drying character and black currant for its astringent properties. Lightly dust the powder over the feet after cleaning and drying them, then rub the powder gently into the skin. It can also be sprinkled into your footwear for added protection.

METHOD

1 Grind the dried herbs together with a pestle and mortar to a fine powder.

2 Add the kaolin and mix thoroughly, then add the lemon essential oil and mix again. Allow the powder to dry.

3 Store the dry powder in an old, clean body powder dispenser or clean pepper shaker. Use within 2 months.

BABY POWDER

INGREDIENTS

3 tsp cornstarch
5 drops propolis tincture
2 drops Roman chamomile
  essential oil

MAKES APPROX ¾OZ (20G)

A light, fine powder such as this is designed to soothe and dry a baby's delicate skin. It is so mild and gentle that it is suitable even for newborn babies: Roman chamomile, which has soothing and anti-inflammatory properties, and propolis, a natural antiseptic, are mixed into a base of smoothing cornstarch. Always keep powder away from a baby's mouth and nose.

METHOD

1 Sift the cornstarch evenly onto a wide, flat plate.
2 Mix the propolis tincture and Roman chamomile essential oil together and decant into a clean container with a fine mist atomizer.
3 Spray this mix onto the cornstarch, taking care to spray evenly and not to saturate the powder, which may cause lumps. Allow the powder to dry.
4 Store the dry powder in an old, clean body powder dispenser or clean pepper shaker. Use within 6 months.

MAKING SOAPS

Soap-making is fun, and soaps make lovely gifts. With careful preparation you can make your own, but read the safety information on page 177 first and follow the instructions closely. It is worth noting that the cheapest olive oil makes better soap. Store the soaps in an airtight container.

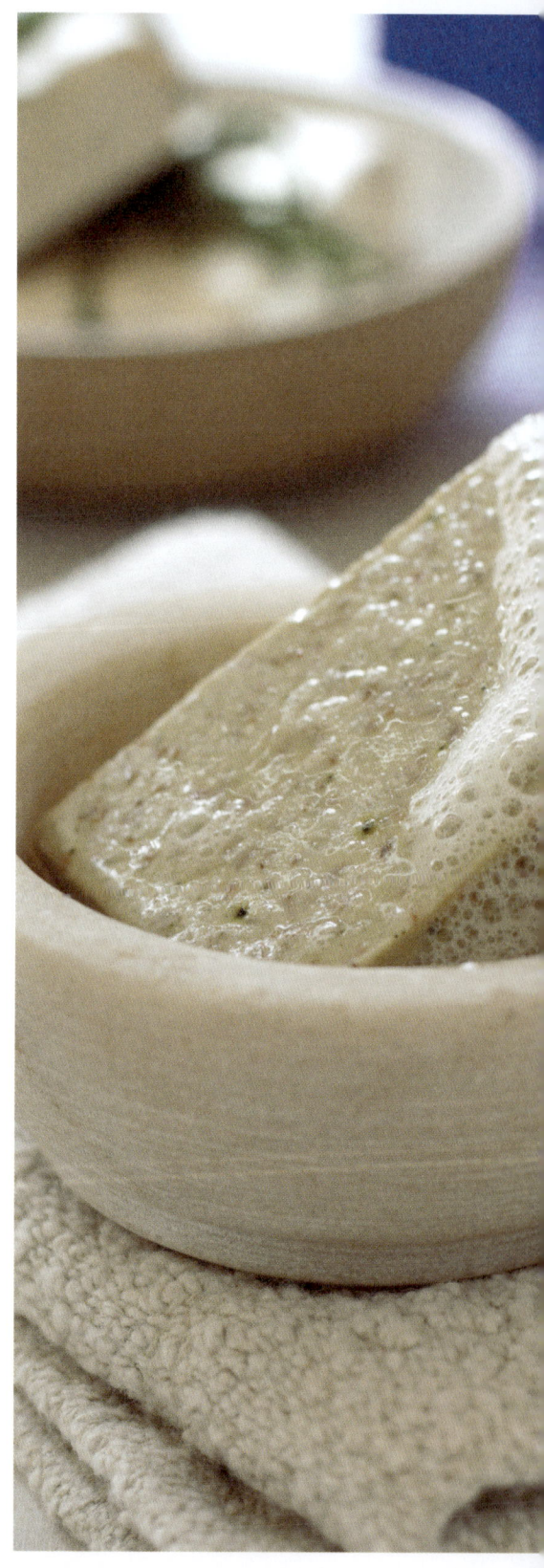

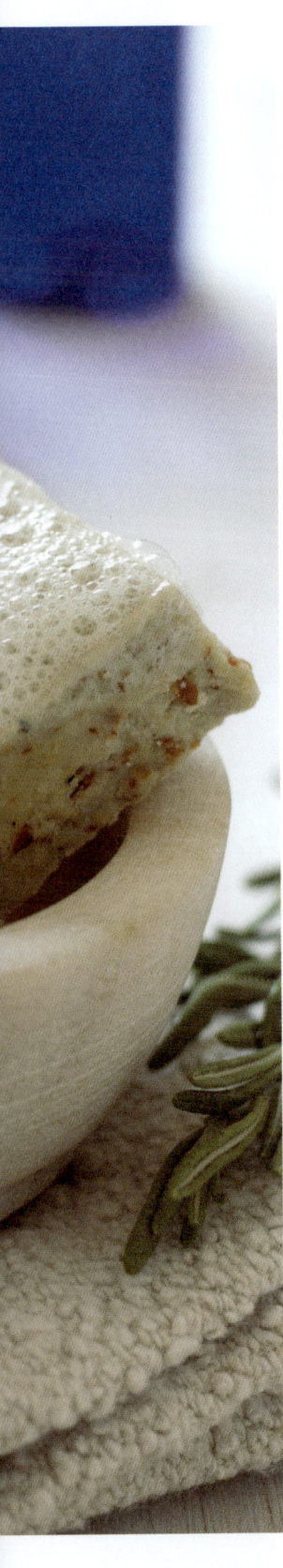

ROSEMARY GARDENER'S SOAP

INGREDIENTS

1¼ cups olive oil
¾ cup coconut oil
½ cup cooled boiled or
    distilled water
2oz (60g) caustic soda
    (lye crystals)
1 tbsp green clay
4 crushed spirulina tablets
1 tbsp bran or oatmeal
30 drops rosemary
    essential oil

MAKES 16 BARS

Rosemary adds to the cleansing properties of this soap, which also contains gently exfoliating oatmeal to smooth roughened hands. Spirulina and green clay lend color. Sprinkle a few dried rosemary flowers on top of the soap when it is semi-set as a decoration, if you wish.

METHOD

1 Whisk together the olive and coconut oils in a saucepan over low heat until the temperature reaches 140°F (60°C).
2 To make the lye mix, pour the water into a stainless steel or glass bowl, then place the bowl in a sink in case the contents froth over when the caustic soda is added. Wearing protective goggles, gloves, and an apron, add the caustic soda to the water and mix with a wooden spoon until the crystals have dissolved (always add the caustic soda to the water rather than the other way around). Leave to cool.
3 Add the cooled lye mixture to the hot oils in the saucepan and stir with a wooden spoon until well mixed. Then beat with a metal whisk for about 20 seconds. The consistency should now be similar to that of thick custard so that a line is visible if drawn on its surface. Stir in the green clay, crushed spirulina tablets, bran or oatmeal, and rosemary essential oil. Pour the mix into a 6 in (15 cm) square stainless steel dish 2 in (5 cm) deep and greased with olive oil. Cover with a cloth and leave for 24 hours.
4 While still soft enough to cut, remove the soap wearing plastic gloves, and cut into bars using a cheese slicer or knife. Arrange on trays and leave to dry out fully and harden; this will take several weeks. During this time the pH value of the soap will drop, becoming more neutral and therefore milder. You may find that a whitish residue appears on the surface; this can be scraped off if you prefer. The soap will continue to dry out for several months depending on the weather, but the reduction of the pH value will slow and remain stable after a few weeks. Check the pH of the finished soap before using (it should be around 10–10.5).

CALENDULA AND CHAMOMILE SOAP

INGREDIENTS
1¼ cups olive oil
¾ cup coconut oil
½ cup cooled boiled or distilled water
2oz (60g) caustic soda (lye crystals)
2 tsp calendula macerated oil
1 tsp evening primrose oil
25 drops chamomile essential oil
10 drops lavender essential oil

MAKES 16 BARS

Soothing calendula (marigold) and chamomile are combined with gentle evening primrose oil in this mild soap bar for delicate skin. Try adding a few flowers to the top of the soap when it is semi-set, if you wish, for a decorative touch. Read the safety information on p.177 carefully before you start, and follow the instructions closely.

METHOD

1 Mix the olive and coconut oils in a saucepan with a whisk over low heat until the temperature reaches 140°F (60°C).

2 To make the lye mixture, pour the water into a glass or stainless steel bowl, then place the bowl in a sink in case the contents froth over when the caustic soda is added. Wearing protective goggles, gloves, and an apron, add the caustic soda to the water and mix with a wooden spoon until the crystals have dissolved (always add the caustic soda to the water rather than the other way around). Leave to cool.

3 Add the cooled lye mixture to the hot oils in the saucepan and stir with a wooden spoon until well mixed. Then beat with a metal whisk for about 20 seconds. The consistency should now be similar to that of thick custard so that a line is visible if drawn on its surface. Stir in the remaining oils to fragrance the soap. Pour the mixture into a 6in (15cm) square stainless steel dish that is at least 2in (5cm) deep and greased with olive oil, cover with a cloth, and leave to set for 24 hours.

4 While still soft enough to cut, remove the soap wearing plastic gloves and cut into bars using a cheese slicer or knife. Arrange the bars on trays and leave to dry out fully and harden; this will take several weeks. During this time the pH value of the soap will drop, becoming more neutral and therefore milder. You may find that a whitish residue appears on the surface; this can be scraped off if you prefer. The soap will continue to dry out for several months depending on the weather, but the reduction of the pH value will slow and remain stable after a few weeks. Check the pH of the finished soap before using (it should be around 10–10.5).

NEEM CLEANSING SOAP

INGREDIENTS

1¼ cups olive oil

¾ cup coconut oil

½ cup cooled boiled or distilled water

2oz (60g) caustic soda (lye crystals)

1 tsp neem oil

5 drops propolis tincture

40 drops lavender essential oil

30 drops tea tree essential oil

MAKES 16 BARS

Neem has a long history of use in India and Africa for its cleansing properties. Here, antiseptic propolis, which is used by bees to protect their hives, has been added, as well as cleansing lavender and tea tree essential oils. Try adding a few lavender flowers to the soap when it is semi-set, if you wish. Read the safety information on p.177 carefully before you start.

METHOD

1 Mix the olive and coconut oils in a saucepan with a whisk over low heat until the temperature reaches 140°F (60°C).

2 To make the lye mixture, pour the water into a glass or stainless steel bowl, then place the bowl in a sink in case the contents froth over when the caustic soda is added. Wearing protective goggles, gloves, and an apron, add the caustic soda to the water and mix with a wooden spoon until the crystals have dissolved (always add the caustic soda to the water rather than the other way around). Leave to cool.

3 Add the cooled lye mixture to the hot oils in the saucepan and stir with a wooden spoon until well mixed. Then whisk for about 20 seconds. The consistency should now be similar to that of thick custard so that a line is visible if drawn on its surface. Stir in the neem oil, propolis tincture, and essential oils to fragrance the soap. Pour the mixture into a 6in (15cm) square stainless steel dish that is at least 2in (5cm) deep and greased with olive oil, cover with a cloth, and leave to set for 24 hours.

4 While still soft enough to cut, remove the soap wearing plastic gloves and cut into bars using a cheese slicer or knife. Arrange the bars on trays and leave to dry out fully and harden; this will take several weeks. During this time the pH value of the soap will drop, becoming more neutral and therefore milder. You may find that a whitish residue appears on the surface; this can be scraped off if you prefer. The soap will continue to dry out for several months depending on the weather, but the reduction of the pH value will slow and remain stable after a few weeks. Check the pH of the finished soap before using (it should be around 10–10.5).

RELAXATION SOAP

CLEANSES SKIN

RELAXES

INGREDIENTS

1¼ cups olive oil

¾ cup coconut oil

½ cup cooled boiled or distilled water

2oz (60g) caustic soda (lye crystals)

2 tsp almond oil

10 drops lavender essential oil

10 drops rose absolute

5 drops marjoram essential oil

MAKES 16 BARS

This delightful soap has a fragrant, aromatherapeutic combination of essential oils to help ease the cares of the day. Rose creates a relaxed sense of well-being, marjoram is warming and comforting, and lavender helps the mind unwind and restores a sense of balance. Read the safety information on p.177 carefully before you start.

METHOD

1 Mix the olive and coconut oils in a saucepan with a whisk over low heat until the temperature reaches 140°F (60°C).

2 To make the lye mixture, pour the water into a glass or stainless steel bowl, then place the bowl in a sink in case the contents froth over when the caustic soda is added. Wearing protective goggles, gloves, and an apron, add the caustic soda to the water and mix with a wooden spoon until the crystals have dissolved (always add the caustic soda to the water rather than the other way around). Leave to cool.

3 Add the cooled lye mixture to the hot oils in the saucepan and stir with a wooden spoon until well mixed. Then beat with a metal whisk for about 20 seconds. The consistency should now be similar to that of thick custard so that a line is visible if drawn on its surface. Stir in the remaining oils to fragrance the soap. Pour the mixture into a 6in (15 cm) square stainless steel dish that is at least 2 in (5 cm) deep and greased with olive oil, cover with a cloth, and leave to set for 24 hours.

4 While still soft enough to cut, remove the soap wearing plastic gloves and cut into bars using a cheese slicer or knife. Arrange the bars on trays and leave to dry out fully and harden; this will take several weeks. During this time the pH value of the soap will drop, becoming more neutral and therefore milder. You may find that a whitish residue appears on the surface; this can be scraped off if you prefer. The soap will continue to dry out for several months depending on the weather, but the reduction of the pH value will slow and remain stable after a few weeks. Check the pH of the finished soap before using (it should be around 10–10.5).

SKIN-SMOOTHING SOAP

INGREDIENTS
1¼ cups olive oil

¾ cup coconut oil

½ cup cooled boiled or
distilled water

2oz (60g) caustic soda
(lye crystals)

2 tsp avocado oil

12 drops ylang-ylang
essential oil

12 drops geranium
essential oil

12 drops clary sage
essential oil

5 drops rose absolute

1 tsp vanilla extract

MAKES 16 BARS

Ylang-ylang essential oil is distilled from the flowers of the cananga tree (*Cananga odorata*), a member of the custard apple family native to the Philippines and Indonesia. The fragrant oil is combined here with rose, geranium, and clary sage to make a delicately aromatic and skin-smoothing soap. Read the safety information on p.177 carefully before you start.

METHOD
1 Mix the olive and coconut oils in a saucepan with a whisk over low heat until the temperature reaches 140°F (60°C).

2 To make the lye mixture, pour the water into a glass or stainless steel bowl, then place the bowl in a sink in case the contents froth over when the caustic soda is added. Wearing protective goggles, gloves, and an apron, add the caustic soda to the water and mix with a wooden spoon until the crystals have dissolved (always add the caustic soda to the water rather than the other way around). Leave to cool.

3 Add the cooled lye mixture to the hot oils in the saucepan and stir with a wooden spoon until well mixed. Then beat with a metal whisk for about 20 seconds. The consistency should now be similar to that of thick custard so that a line is visible if drawn on its surface. Stir in the remaining oils to fragrance the soap. Pour the mixture into a 6in (15cm) square stainless steel dish that is at least 2in (5cm) deep and greased with olive oil, cover with a cloth, and leave to set for 24 hours.

4 While still soft enough to cut, remove the soap wearing plastic gloves and cut into bars using a cheese wire or knife. Arrange the bars on trays and leave to dry out fully and harden; this will take several weeks. During this time the pH value of the soap will drop, becoming more neutral and therefore milder. You may find that a whitish residue appears on the surface; this can be scraped off if you prefer. The soap will continue to dry out for several months depending on the weather, but the reduction of the pH value will slow and remain stable after a few weeks. Check the pH of the finished soap before using (it should be around 10–10.5).

MAKING CLEANSERS

A cleansing routine is essential to support and maintain healthy skin, especially if you live or work in an urban environment with higher levels of pollution. Test any product on a small area of skin first to check that it does not provoke a reaction.

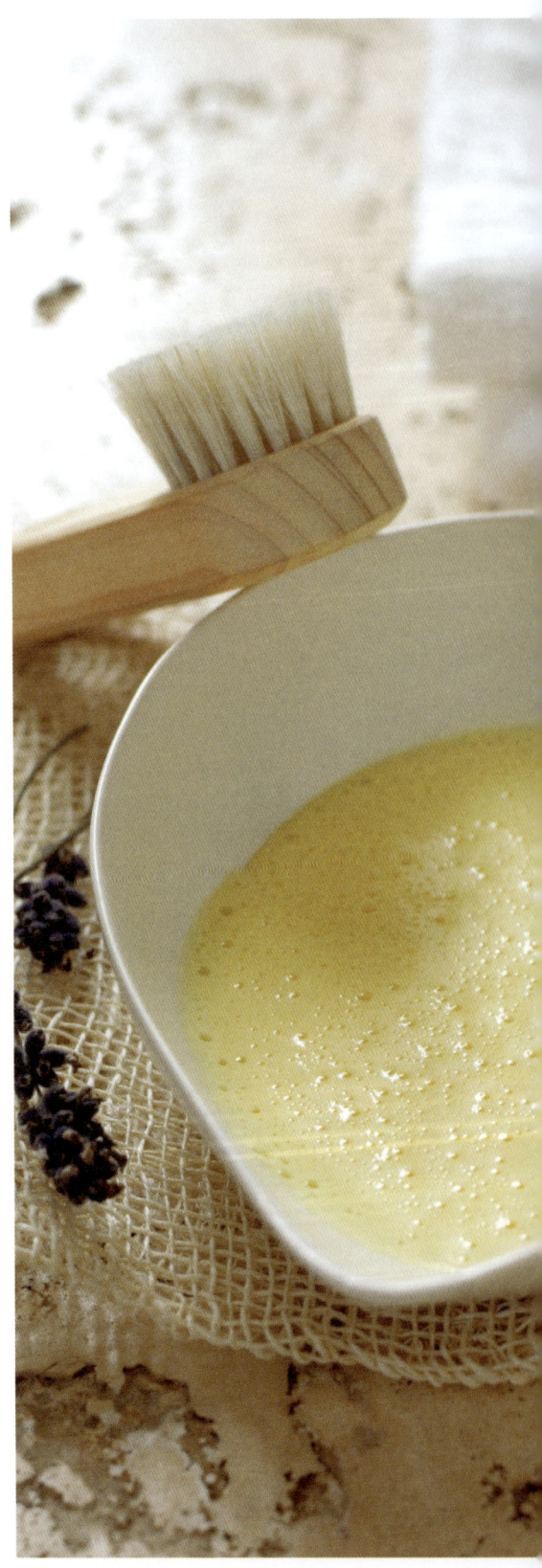

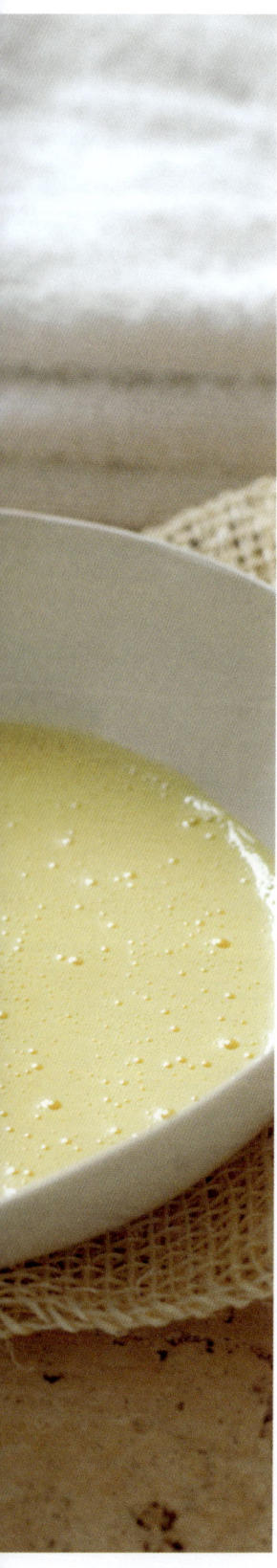

SOOTHING LAVENDER CLEANSER

CLEANSES SKIN

INGREDIENTS
scant 1oz (25g) organic oats
a little mineral water
1 egg yolk
3½ tbsp almond oil
5 drops lavender
   essential oil

MAKES 2FL OZ (60ML)

This is a simple cleanser for sensitive or dry skin. Oats have long been used for their skin-soothing properties, as they are rich in natural polysaccharides that become glutinous in water to create a nurturing wash for delicate skin. Almond oil also soothes and enriches skin, helping prevent moisture loss, while lavender soothes the skin and adds a gentle fragrance.

METHOD

1 Put the oats in a bowl, pour over enough mineral water to cover, and leave to soak for at least 1 hour.
2 Whisk the egg yolk in a blender or food processor, adding a drop of almond oil at a time. The mixture should be a thick emulsion when all the oil has been added. Add the lavender essential oil, adding a drop at a time so it blends in well.
3 Strain the oats, squeezing all the liquid (oat milk) into a bowl. Reserve the oat milk (but discard the oats). Add the oat milk slowly to the egg mixture, stirring or blending it in gently so that it thins to the consistency of a lotion.
4 Store in a sterilized glass bottle (p.210) with a tightly fitting lid. Refrigerate and use within 3 days.

HONEY AND ROSE PETAL FACE SCRUB

INGREDIENTS
scant 1oz (25g) dried
  rose petals
1 cup boiling water
2 tbsp dried lavender
  flowers
1 drop lavender essential oil
1 drop rose otto
2 tsp honey

MAKES ENOUGH FOR 1 APPLICATION

Honey is one of nature's best skin treatments. It softens, soothes, and protects the skin from moisture loss, as well as acting as a lubricant. Rose oil, with its cooling and toning properties, and lavender oil, which freshens, and purifies, are also added to this gently exfoliating scrub to help condition and balance the skin and give you a feeling of relaxed well-being.

METHOD
1 Make an infusion (p.176) using half the rose petals and the boiling water. Cover and leave to one side.
2 Using a pestle and mortar, grind the remaining rose petals and the lavender flowers until they are of a powdery consistency. Combine the powdered herbs with the essential oils and honey, and add enough rose infusion for the mixture to form a soft paste.
3 To use, apply to the face and gently rub in a circular motion to cleanse the skin.

ELDERFLOWER AND ALOE VERA FACIAL POLISH

INGREDIENTS

scant 1oz (25g) elderflower
or 10 elderflower tea bags

scant 1oz (25g) chamomile
or 10 chamomile tea bags

2 cups boiling water

2 tsp aloe vera juice

2 tbsp plain yogurt

MAKES ENOUGH FOR 1 TREATMENT

Elderflower is mildly astringent and its emollient and anti-inflammatory properties mean that it has long been beneficial for skin. Combined with cooling aloe vera and soothing chamomile, this gentle, refreshing facial polish is suitable for all skin types. As it contains fresh dairy ingredients, this polish is for immediate use.

METHOD

1 Make an infusion (p.176) using half the herbs and the boiling water. Cover and set aside.

2 Grind the rest of the herbs to a fine powder using a pestle and mortar. If using tea bags, the herbs will already be chopped to a fine powder so they are ready to use.

3 Mix the herbs, aloe vera, and yogurt, then add the infusion a teaspoon at a time, stirring as you go, until it makes a thin paste (but thick enough not to run off your skin).

4 Apply to the face after cleansing (be sure to avoid the area directly around the eyes and mouth). To exfoliate, gently massage the paste onto your skin with your fingertips in small circular movements.

5 Use the remaining infusion (with extra water as necessary) to rinse off the paste and tone the skin.

MAKING TONERS

Toners are used after cleansing to help refine the skin and maintain its pH balance; they also remove any last traces of cleanser before moisturizing. Test any product on a small area of skin first to check that it does not provoke a reaction.

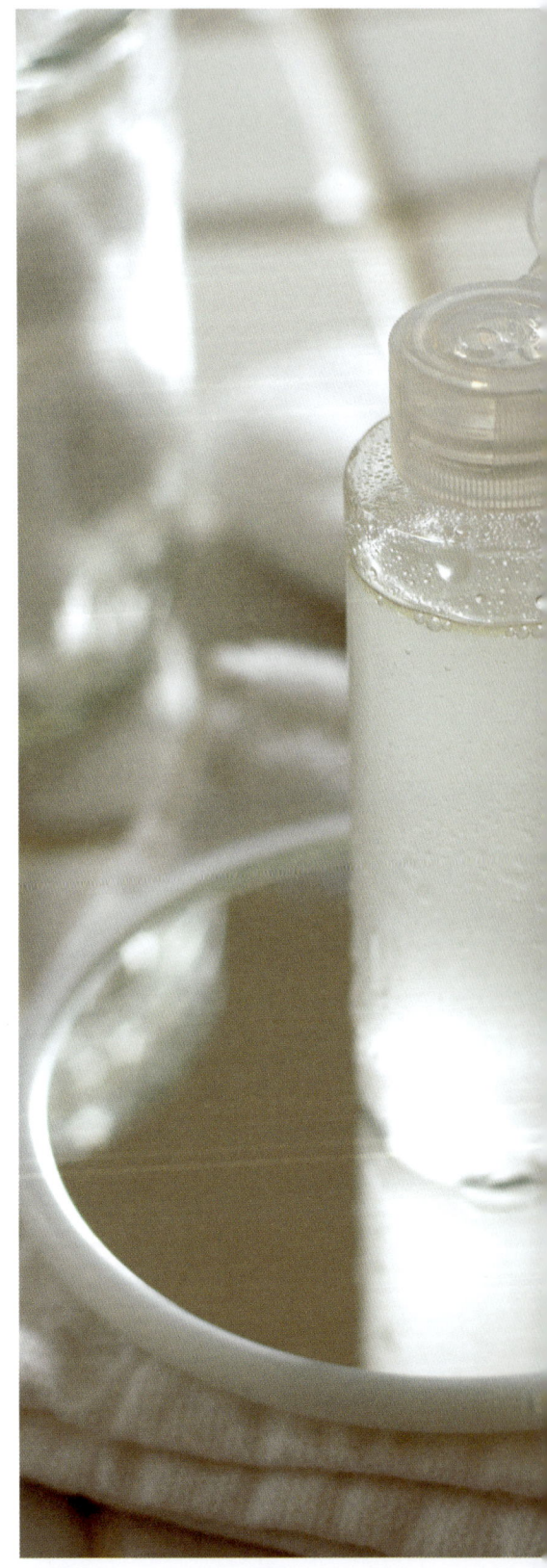

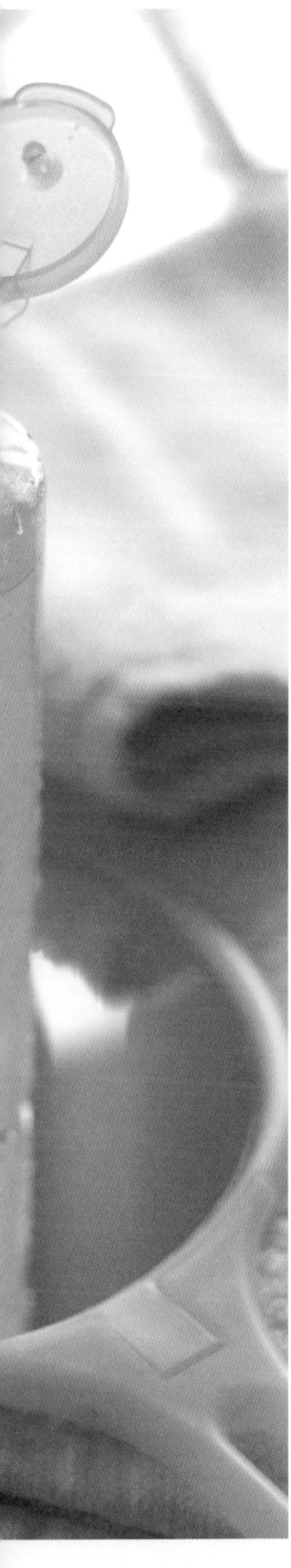

LAVENDER AND ALOE VERA TONER

INGREDIENTS
2¾fl oz (80ml) lavender
  flower water
2 tsp witch hazel
1 tsp aloe vera juice
14 drops bergamot
  essential oil
4 drops lemon essential oil
4 drops petitgrain
  essential oil
4 drops lavender
  essential oil
2 drops rosemary
  essential oil
2 drops black pepper
  essential oil

MAKES 3½FL OZ (100ML)

This refreshing toner is suitable for all skin types, especially problem skin, and contains a stimulating aromatherapy blend to cleanse the skin and regulate oiliness: witch hazel and lavender waters create a purifying and gently astringent base to tone the pores of the skin and promote a clear complexion.

METHOD
1 Combine all the ingredients thoroughly.
2 Store in a sterilized glass bottle (p.210), preferably with an atomizer spray, out of direct sunlight, and shake well before use. Use within 6 months.

ROSE TONER

INGREDIENTS

¼ cup mineral water

2 heaping tsp dried
or 4 heaping tsp fresh
rose petals

1 tsp dried or 2 tsp
fresh elderflower

1 tbsp apple cider vinegar

MAKES 3½FL OZ (100ML)

This simple toner refreshes and balances the skin. Rose soothes while vinegar, which has a tonic action, stimulates circulation and helps regulate the skin's natural pH. Apple cider vinegar—produced by a simple fermentation process that retains all the apples' nutritional goodness—is fortified with extra enzymes produced during fermentation.

METHOD

1 Make an infusion (p.176) with the water, rose petals, and elderflower. Once cooled, add the cider vinegar and pour into a sterilized glass bottle (p.210) with a tight-fitting lid.
2 Shake well before each use to blend. Apply after cleansing with cotton balls or a muslin cloth. Gently wipe over the skin. Refrigerate and use within 3 months.

HERBAL TONER

INGREDIENTS

¼ cup distilled water

1 tbsp witch hazel

2 tsp aloe vera

3 drops chamomile
essential oil

3 drops rosemary
essential oil

3 drops rose absolute

MAKES 3½FL OZ (100ML)

Witch hazel extract is a useful remedy that helps calm and refresh tired skin. Its astringent properties also help regulate the production of sebum and minimize pores for a more even skin tone. Combined with anti-inflammatory chamomile, balancing rose, and stimulating rosemary, this gentle toner is suitable for all skin types

METHOD

1 Combine all the ingredients and decant into a sterilized glass bottle (p.210) with a tight-fitting lid.
2 Shake well before each use to blend. Apply after cleansing with cotton balls or a muslin cloth. Gently wipe over the skin. Refrigerate and use within 3 months.

HERBAL FACE AND BODY SPRITZ

INGREDIENTS
3 heaping tsp fresh mint
1 heaping tsp fresh dill
1 heaping tsp fresh parsley
¼ cup mineral water

MAKES 3½FL OZ (100ML)

Revitalizing fresh mint is the essential ingredient of this refreshing, fragrant herbal spritz, which is ideal for hot summer days and nights to help cool your skin. Spray it in a fine mist over exposed skin on the face and body as often as required.

METHOD
Make an infusion (p.176) with the herbs (using just enough boiling water to cover the herbs). Once brewed, add the mineral water and pour into a sterilized glass bottle (p.210) with an atomizer spray. Refrigerate and use within 2 days.

REFRESHING FACIAL SPRITZ

INGREDIENTS
¼ cup distilled water
2 tsp aloe vera juice
1 tsp orange flower water
1 drop propolis tincture
1 drop lemon essential oil
1 drop rosemary essential oil

MAKES 3½FL OZ (100ML)

Orange flower water is a wonderfully restorative remedy for the skin, and aromatherapists use its delicate scent to help treat stress. This refreshing spritz is ideal to use when traveling to refresh the skin and ease the mind.

METHOD
Combine all the ingredients and decant into a sterilized glass bottle (p.210) with an atomizer spray. Shake well before each use. Refrigerate and use within 2 days.

MAKING FACE MASKS

Taking some quiet time to relax with a soothing face mask can be one of life's indulgent pleasures. For extra purification, try a clay mask for a real home spa treat. Test any product on a small area of skin first to check that it does not provoke a reaction.

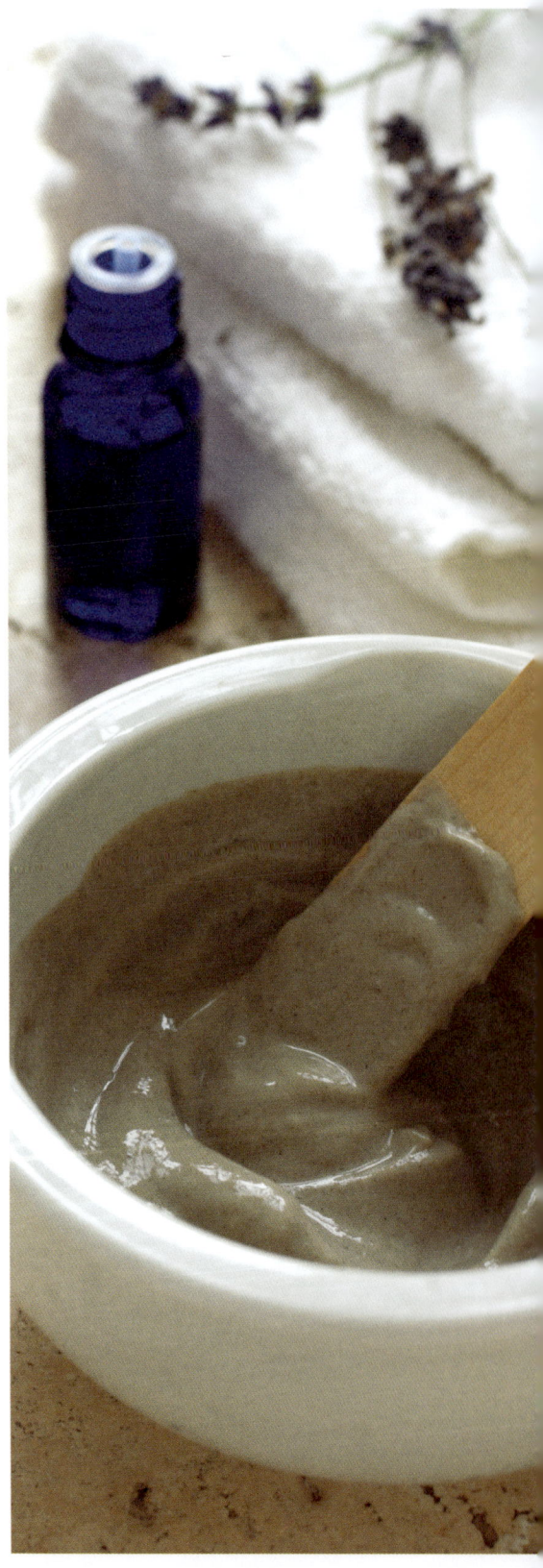

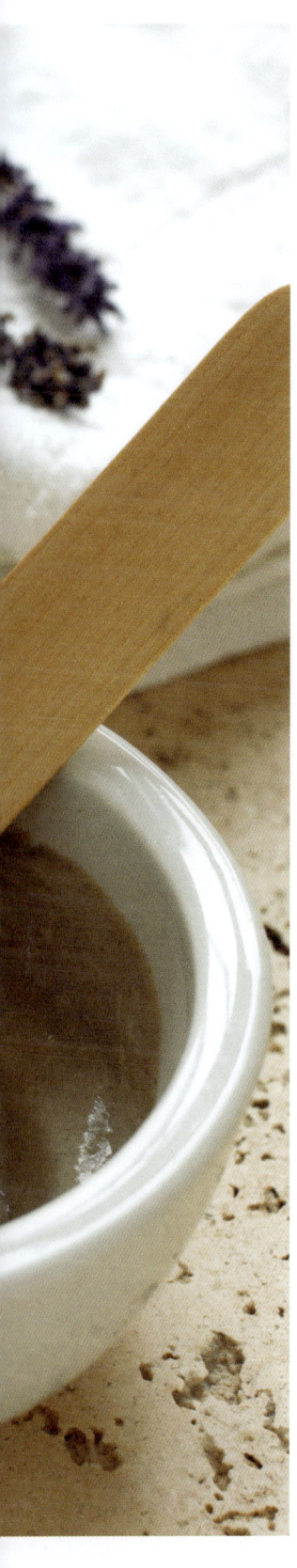

WITCH HAZEL AND LAVENDER FACE MASK

CONDITIONS SKIN

INGREDIENTS
2 tsp green clay powder
2 tsp witch hazel
1 egg, lightly beaten
2 drops lavender
   essential oil

MAKES ENOUGH FOR 1 TREATMENT

Green clay is the common name for *montmorillonite*, a naturally occurring mineral-rich clay with highly absorbent properties. As it dries, it draws impurities from the skin and cleanses pores. At the same time, gently astringent witch hazel and soothing lavender tighten the pores and help promote a clear complexion.

METHOD
1 Mix the green clay with the witch hazel to make a paste. Add the beaten egg and mix in the lavender essential oil.
2 Apply the mask to your face and leave on for 10 minutes. Gently remove with cool water, then pat dry with a clean towel.

"SPEND 10 MINUTES RELAXING WITH A NATURAL HOMEMADE FACE MASK AS AN INDULGENT, FRAGRANT TREAT FOR YOUR SKIN AND YOUR MIND"

STRAWBERRIES AND CREAM EXFOLIATING FACIAL MASK

INGREDIENTS
2 tbsp ground oats
3 large ripe strawberries
1 tsp half-and-half

MAKES ENOUGH FOR 1 TREATMENT

This fruity mask refreshes and brightens the skin. Strawberries, which are rich in natural fruit acids that help exfoliate the skin, are combined with ground oats to give texture and extra polish, unclog pores, and smooth the skin. As it uses fresh fruit and dairy ingredients, this recipe is for immediate use.

METHOD

1 Using a pestle and mortar, grind the oats to a fine powder. Mash the strawberries with a fork and combine with the oats. Add the half-and-half and mix to a thick paste (add a little more cream if needed to create the right consistency).

2 Apply the paste to freshly cleansed skin (avoiding the area directly around the eyes and mouth) and leave for 10 minutes.

3 Remove the paste by applying a little water in the palms of your hands to loosen it, then rub it away in gentle circular movements. Rinse with cool water and pat dry with a towel.

LAVENDER CLAY MASK

CONDITIONS SKIN

INGREDIENTS
2 tbsp aloe vera juice
1 tsp lavender water
1 tsp honey
½ tbsp kaolin powder
1 tbsp bentonite powder
1 drop lavender essential oil

MAKES ENOUGH FOR 1–2 TREATMENTS

Natural clay minerals draw impurities from the skin and deeply cleanse it. With moisturizing honey and antioxidant-rich aloe vera, and reviving, balancing lavender water and essential oil, this soothing, purifying mask leaves skin feeling fresh and smooth.

METHOD

1 Combine the aloe vera, lavender water, and honey. Add the clay powders by sprinkling them gradually over the mixed liquids while stirring continually. Press the mixture through a sieve. Add the essential oil and stir again to mix well.

2 Apply to freshly cleansed skin (avoiding the area directly around the eyes and mouth). Leave for 10 minutes. Rinse with warm water and pat dry with a towel.

3 Store in a sterilized dark glass jar (p.210) with a tight-fitting lid. Use within 2 months.

GRAPEFRUIT CLAY MASK

CONDITIONS SKIN

INGREDIENTS
2 tbsp aloe vera juice
1 tsp witch hazel
1 tsp fresh grapefruit juice
1½ tsp kaolin powder
½ tbsp bentonite powder
1 drop lemon essential oil

MAKES APPROX 1¾FL OZ (50ML)

This variation on a clay mask is more suited to oilier skin types. Grapefruit is naturally rich in fruit acids, and combined with cleansing clay minerals; mildly astringent and toning witch hazel; and soothing, nutrient-rich aloe vera, it leaves skin cleansed, refreshed, and revitalized.

METHOD

1 Combine the aloe vera juice, witch hazel, and grapefruit juice. Add the clay powders by sprinkling them gradually over the mixed liquids while stirring continually. Press the mixture through a sieve. Add the essential oil and stir again to mix well.

2 Apply to freshly cleansed skin (avoiding the area directly around the eyes and mouth). Leave for 10 minutes. Rinse with warm water and pat dry with a towel.

3 Store in a sterilized dark glass jar (p.210) with a tight-fitting lid. Use within 2 months.

ROSE CLAY MASK

INGREDIENTS

2 tbsp aloe vera juice
1 tsp rosewater
1 tsp honey
½ tbsp kaolin powder
1 tbsp bentonite powder
1 drop rose absolute

MAKES ENOUGH FOR 1–2 TREATMENTS

This nourishing mask purifies and smooths the skin. Rose, used for its cooling and balancing properties, is combined with aloe vera—an extremely soothing plant extract that is rich in vitamins, amino acids, enzymes, and proteins, and has excellent moisturizing properties.

METHOD

1 Combine the aloe vera, rosewater, and honey. Add the clay powders by sprinkling them gradually over the mixed liquids while stirring continually. Press the mixture through a sieve. Add the rose absolute and stir again to mix well.
2 Apply to freshly cleansed skin (avoiding the area directly around the eyes and mouth). Leave for 10 minutes. Rinse with warm water and pat dry with a towel.
3 Store in a sterilized dark glass jar (p.210) with a tight-fitting lid. Use within 2 months.

GOLDEN BANANA FACIAL MASK

INGREDIENTS

1 ripe banana
1 egg yolk
2 tsp calendula
   macerated oil

MAKES ENOUGH FOR 1 TREATMENT

This rich, nourishing treatment revitalizes dry skin. Fresh banana is richly moisturizing and smoothing, while golden calendula oil contains carotenoids, a precursor to skin-nurturing vitamin A. The oil also has excellent healing and anti-inflammatory properties. As it uses fresh fruit ingredients, this recipe is for immediate use.

METHOD

1 Peel the banana, place in a bowl, and mash with a fork. Add the egg yolk and calendula oil and mix all the ingredients together.
2 Apply to freshly cleansed skin (avoiding the area directly around the eyes and mouth). Leave for 10 minutes. Rinse with cool water and pat dry with a towel.

AVOCADO AND ALOE VERA FACIAL MASK

INGREDIENTS
1 ripe avocado
1 tsp honey
1 tsp lemon juice
1 tsp yogurt
1 tsp aloe vera juice

MAKES ENOUGH FOR 1 TREATMENT

A deeply nourishing and soothing facial mask suitable for all skin types. Avocado is vitamin- and mineral-rich, as well as being high in fatty acids, phytosterols, and lecithin, which makes it an excellent moisturizer for dry skin. As it uses fresh fruit and dairy ingredients, this recipe is for immediate use.

METHOD
1 Split the avocado in two and scoop out the flesh into a bowl. Mash with a fork to make a paste, then add the other ingredients and mix.
2 Apply to freshly cleansed skin (avoiding the area directly around the eyes and mouth). Leave for 10 minutes. Rinse with cool water and pat dry with a towel.

APPLE AND CINNAMON FACIAL MASK

INGREDIENTS
1 ripe apple, peeled and grated
½ tsp half-and-half
1 tsp honey
1 tbsp ground oats
½ tsp ground cinnamon

MAKES ENOUGH FOR 1 TREATMENT

This cleansing mask is ideally suited to oily or problem skin, as it gently regulates and cleanses the skin. Apples contain natural fruit acids, which help gently exfoliate the skin, while moisturizing honey and ground oats help smooth and polish it. As it uses fresh fruit and dairy ingredients, this recipe is for immediate use.

METHOD
1 Mix all the ingredients together in a bowl with a fork to form a paste.
2 Apply to freshly cleansed skin (avoiding the area directly around the eyes and mouth). Leave for 10 minutes. Rinse with cool water and pat dry with a towel.

MAKING BALMS

Balms are a simple way to nourish skin and protect it from moisture loss. Make sure that the containers you use to store your homemade balms are sterilized (p.210). Test any product on a small area of skin first to check that it does not provoke a reaction.

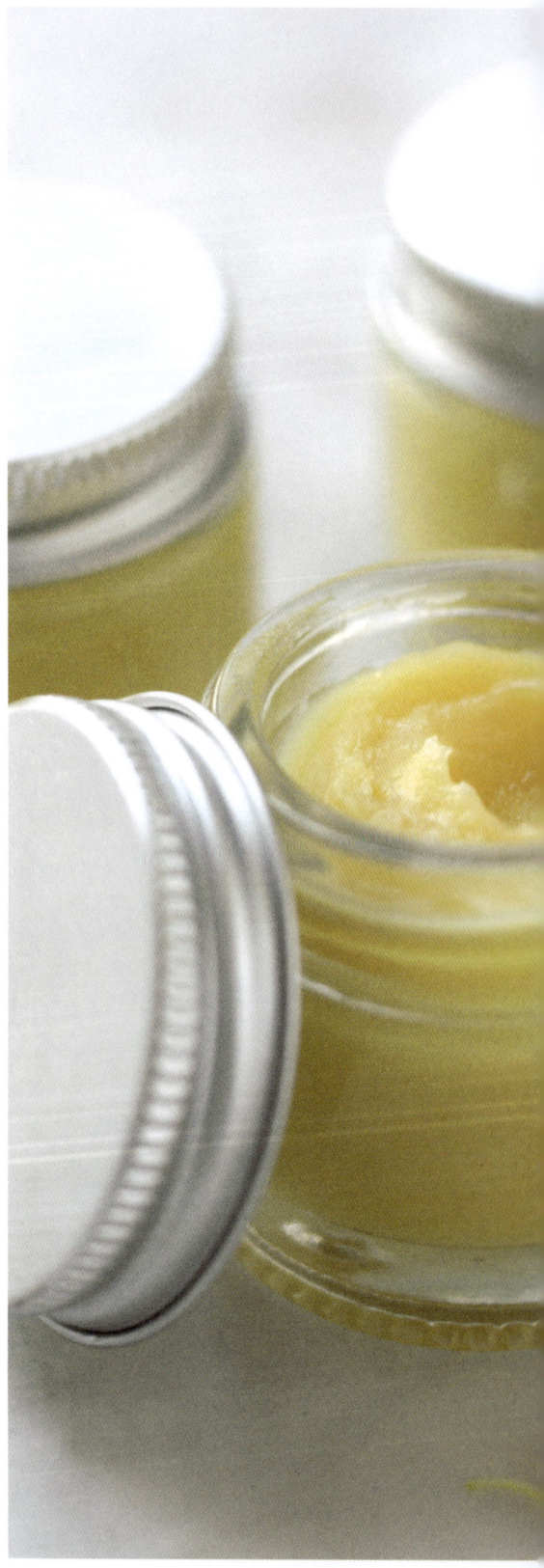

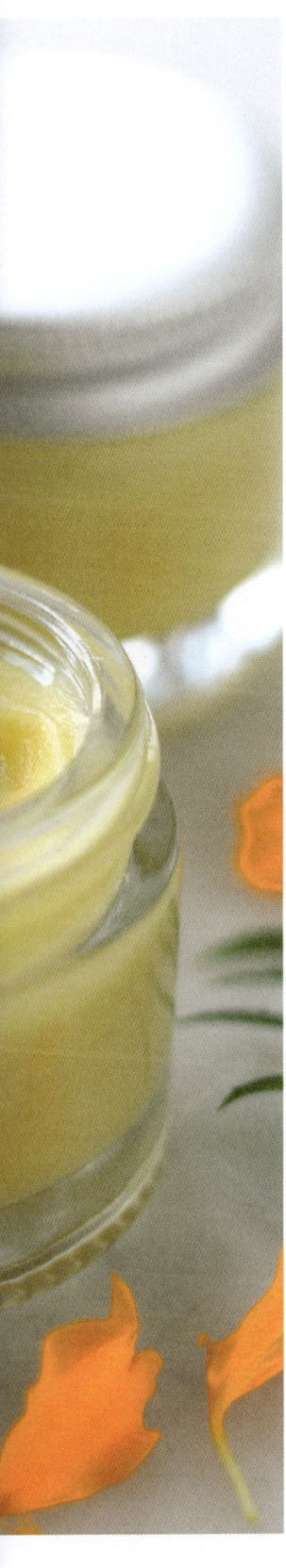

CALENDULA AND MANDARIN LIP BALM

MAKES 2¾OZ (80G)

Mandarin essential oil, expressed from the fresh peel of the fruit, is gently antiseptic and cleansing. Lemon balm is active against the herpes virus, so this balm will also help prevent or treat cold sores. Cocoa butter helps condition, soothe, and protect lips.

METHOD

1 Melt the beeswax, cocoa butter, and coconut oil in a bowl set over a saucepan of hot water (bain-marie). Add the tinctures and essential oil to the mixture, then stir.
2 Divide between two small sterilized jars (p.210) and allow to set. This may take up to 12 hours (depending on the room temperature). Use within 3 months.

MOISTURIZES SKIN

HELPS PREVENT COLD SORES

INGREDIENTS
1 tsp beeswax
2¼oz (70g) cocoa butter
1 tsp coconut oil
5 drops lemon balm tincture
5 drops calendula tincture
10 drops mandarin
  essential oil

LAVENDER AND MYRRH SOOTHING LIP BALM

INGREDIENTS
2 tsp cocoa butter and shea butter, combined
2 drops lavender essential oil
1 drop myrrh essential oil

MAKES ¼OZ (10G)

This very simple blend of ingredients is quick to make, but provides long-lasting relief by effectively smoothing, moisturizing, and protecting lips from drying out. The nourishing combination of therapeutic lavender and myrrh essential oils also helps condition the lips and soothe any chapped or cracked skin.

METHOD

1 Melt the cocoa butter and shea butter in a bowl set over a saucepan of boiling water (bain-marie). Add the essential oils and stir.
2 Pour into a small sterilized jar (p.210) with a tight-fitting lid. Allow to cool and set. This may take up to 12 hours (depending on the room temperature). Use within 6 months.

MOTHER-TO-BE BALM

INGREDIENTS
1 tsp beeswax
5 tsp coconut oil
1 tsp apricot oil
1 tsp calendula macerated oil

MAKES 1½OZ (40G)

This nourishing, fragrance-free balm will help soothe the discomfort of expanding skin and improve resistance to stretch marks. Deeply moisturizing coconut and apricot kernel oils help increase the skin's strength and suppleness, while beeswax locks in moisture and has protective properties. Antioxidant-rich calendula has a soothing action.

METHOD

1 Heat the beeswax with the coconut, apricot, and calendula oils in a bowl set over a saucepan of boiling water (bain-marie) until the beeswax has melted.
2 Pour into a sterilized dark glass jar (p.210) with a tight-fitting lid and leave to cool and set. This may take up to 12 hours (depending on the room temperature). Use within 3 months.

TEA TREE AND THYME FOOT BALM

INGREDIENTS
2 tsp beeswax
3 tbsp almond oil
1 tbsp wheat germ oil
1 tsp marshmallow tincture
1 tsp comfrey tincture
5 drops thyme essential oil
5 drops tea tree essential oil

MAKES APPROX 2¾OZ (80G)

A cleansing and soothing balm to help in the treatment of ailments such as athlete's foot or fungal infections. Research on tea tree and thyme essential oils has shown their potent antifungal and antibacterial properties. Combined here with marshmallow and comfrey extracts to soothe, they also promote the regeneration of healthy skin.

METHOD
1 Combine the beeswax and almond and wheat germ oils in a bowl set over a saucepan of boiling water (bain-marie). Heat until the beeswax has melted.
2 Take off the heat and, when cooled slightly, add the tinctures and essential oils.
3 Decant into a sterilized jar (p.210) with a tight-fitting lid and allow to cool and set. This may take up to 12 hours (depending on the room temperature). Use within 6 months.

MAKING BATH BOMBS

Fizzing bath bombs, which are easy to make and require only simple ingredients, are a delight to the senses. They make great gifts, too—once you have pressed the mixture into a ball and wrapped it in aluminum foil, simply cover it in colorful tissue paper and decorate it with ribbons.

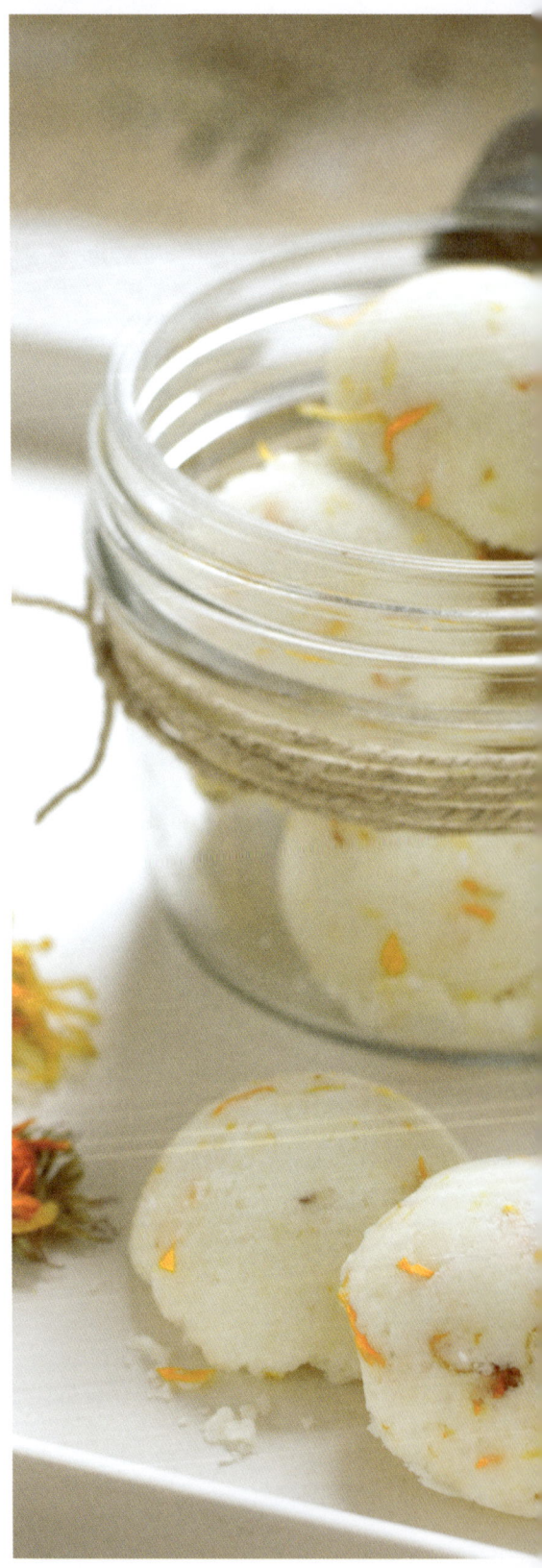

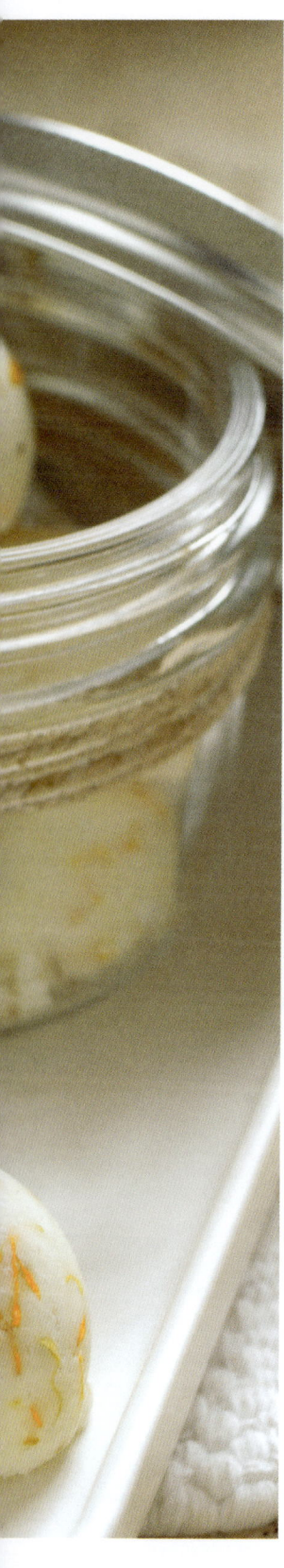

CITRUS BATH BOMB

MAKES 4 SMALL BATH BOMBS

This citrus bath bomb will always liven up bath time. Grapefruit, lemon, and lime essential oils are combined with fresh-scented rosemary essential oil to release a vibrant fragrance as the ingredients fizz and dissolve in the water. You can add some color by replacing the almond oil with green avocado oil or orange carrot oil.

METHOD

1 Mix the baking soda and citric acid together on a plate. Sprinkle the essential oils onto the baking soda mixture and add the calendula petals.
2 If you want to add some color to your bath bomb, add a dash of carrot oil to give an orange color, or avocado oil for a green tint. You might also like to add finely chopped herbs, such as mint, or flowers, such as lavender.
3 Use this mixture as a powder sprinkled directly into the bath; or press firmly into shaped molds, such as ice-cube trays and pastry cutters; or simply hand-mold the ingredients into balls. Store in a dry place, and use within 2 months.

SOOTHES TIRED MUSCLES

REVITALIZES

INGREDIENTS
2¾oz (80g) baking soda
1 tbsp citric acid
4 drops grapefruit essential oil
4 drops lemon essential oil
1 drop lime essential oil
1 drop rosemary essential oil
a pinch of dried calendula petals, chopped
a dash of carrot oil (optional)
a dash of avocado oil (optional)
finely chopped herbs or flowers (optional)

SENSUAL BATH BOMBS

INGREDIENTS

3 tbsp baking soda

1 tbsp citric acid

4 drops mandarin essential oil

3 drops vetiver essential oil

2 drops ylang-ylang essential oil

1 petitgrain essential oil

2 tsp St. John's wort macerated oil

a pinch of rose petals, finely chopped

MAKES 4 SMALL BATH BOMBS

Just add this sensually scented fizzing bath bomb to running bath water to make bath time a special occasion. The powdery mix softens the water, while the aromatherapeutic blend of earthy vetiver; Madagascan ylang-ylang flowers; and warm, relaxing citrus brings peace of mind and a deep sense of well-being.

METHOD

1 Mix the baking soda and citric acid together on a flat plate. Add the essential oils by sprinkling them over the powder.

2 Use a spoon to heap the powder into the center of the plate. Make a small well in the center of the powder and add the deep red St. John's wort oil and the rose petals.

3 Gradually mix the powder, oil, and rose petals together. The St. John's wort oil helps the ingredients bind together, as well as adding color.

4 Press the mixture firmly into shaped molds such as ice-cube trays or pastry cutters, or simply hand-mold the ingredients into balls. Store in a dry place and use within 2 months.

SUNSHINE BATH BOMB

SOOTHES TIRED MUSCLES

REVITALIZES

INGREDIENTS
3 tbsp baking soda
1 tbsp citric acid
7 drops mandarin
    essential oil
2 drops orange essential oil
1 drop lavender essential oil
2 tsp calendula oil
a pinch of orange, mandarin,
    or lemon peel, finely grated

MAKES 4 SMALL BATH BOMBS

This gentle yet warmly scented fizzing bath bomb is ideal for children, lifting the spirits but also calming the emotions with its warm, citrus scents of mandarin and orange combined with soothing, relaxing lavender. Golden calendula oil and grated citrus zest give the bomb added color and texture.

METHOD

1 Mix the baking soda and citric acid on a flat plate. Add the essential oils by sprinkling them over the powder.

2 Use a spoon to heap the powder into the center of the plate. Make a small well in the center, add the calendula oil, and gradually mix it into the powder to bind the bath bomb together. It will also add a little color. Add the citrus peel zest while mixing.

3 Press the mixture firmly into shaped molds such as ice-cube trays or pastry cutters, or simply hand-mold the ingredients into balls. Store in a dry place, and use within 2 months.

MAKING BATH INFUSIONS

Adding herbs to your bath is one of the easiest and most enjoyable ways to benefit from their amazing natural properties. Simply lie back and let the fragrant essences in the infusions lift your spirits, ease any tension headaches, and help you relax. There's no better way to get a good night's sleep.

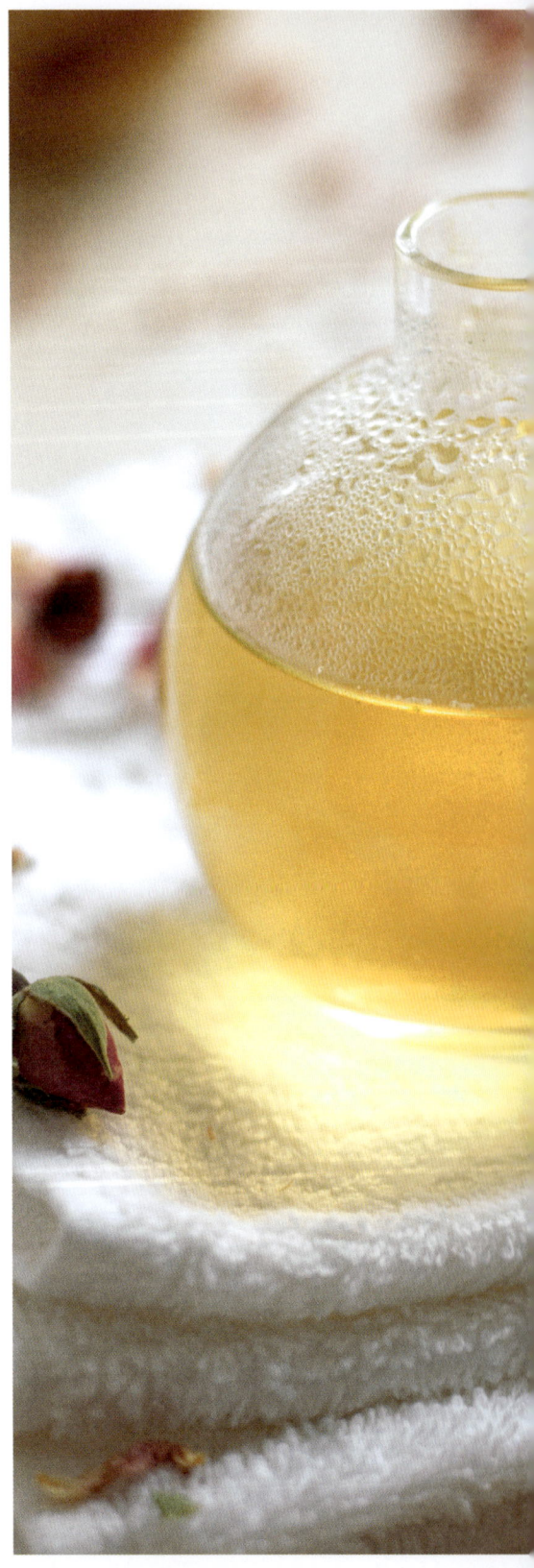

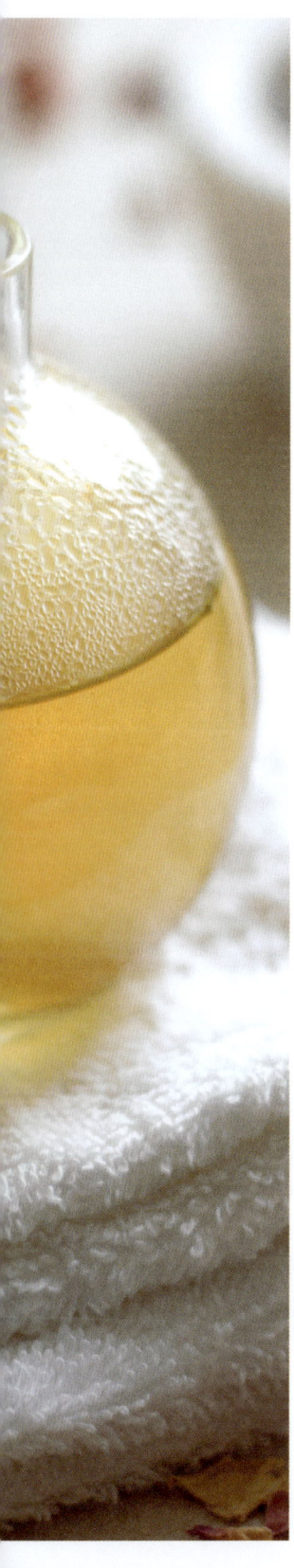

ROSE AND CALENDULA BATH INFUSION

SOOTHES TIRED MUSCLES

RELAXES

INGREDIENTS
2 tsp dried rose
    petals/buds
1 tsp dried rose hips
2 cups hot water
1 tsp salt
1 tsp cider vinegar
5 drops calendula tincture
8 drops rose otto
2 drops geranium
    essential oil

MAKES ENOUGH FOR 1 BATH

This gentle bath infusion nurtures and refreshes, making it a wonderful tonic for dry and sensitive skin. The cooling and balancing properties of roses are renowned; this recipe uses extracts from both the flowers and the vitamin- and flavonoid-rich hips. It also includes cider vinegar to soften the skin and calendula to soothe it.

METHOD
1 Make an infusion (p.176) using the rose petals, rose hips, and hot water.
2 Strain the infusion and add the rest of the ingredients. Use immediately by adding to a freshly run bath.

LEMONGRASS AND ROSEMARY BATH INFUSION

RELAXES

SOOTHES TIRED MUSCLES

INGREDIENTS
2 cups hot water
2 tsp dried bay leaves, chopped
1 tsp dried rosemary
5 drops lemongrass essential oil

MAKES ENOUGH FOR 1 BATH

Lemongrass, bay, and rosemary are all herbs that are well known for their fragrant, culinary use, but they can be just as useful in body care. This stimulating and warming aromatic bath blend eases tired muscles and is ideal for restoring the body after physical activity, sports, or periods of over-exertion.

METHOD
1 Make an infusion (p.176) with the hot water, bay leaves, and rosemary.
2 When cooled, add the lemongrass essential oil. Use immediately by adding to a freshly run bath.

LAVENDER AND ALOE VERA BATH INFUSION

RELAXES

SOOTHES TIRED MUSCLES

INGREDIENTS
2 cups hot water
2 tsp lavender
2 tsp chamomile
2 tbsp aloe vera juice
10 drops lavender essential oil

MAKES ENOUGH FOR 1 BATH

This bath infusion will soothe sensitive skin and encourage a sense of well-being and relaxation. Lavender, which initially has a reviving, restorative effect, has been long used to ease both body and mind. This makes it a perfect remedy in this gentle bath blend, along with soothing aloe vera and nurturing chamomile.

METHOD
1 Make an infusion (p.176) with the water and the lavender and chamomile flowers.
2 When cooled, add the aloe vera juice and lavender essential oil. Use immediately by adding to a freshly run bath. Be sure that your bath is not too hot if you have dry or sensitive skin.

SEAWEED AND ARNICA BATH INFUSION

MAKES ENOUGH FOR 1 BATH

This revitalizing blend restores the body after a long day. Nutrient-rich bladder wrack seaweed is traditionally used to soothe irritated and inflamed tissues in the body, and here it is partnered with arnica—a famous remedy for bumps, bruises, and strains—and a stimulating blend of essential oils. Add to your bath water, lie back, and relax.

METHOD

1 Make an infusion (p.176) with the water, herbs, and berries.
2 Add the salt and stir until well dissolved. Mix in the arnica tincture and the essential oils. Use immediately by adding to a freshly run bath.

RELAXES

SOOTHES TIRED MUSCLES

INGREDIENTS
2 cups hot water
½ tsp dried bladder wrack
1 tsp dried comfrey
2 tsp juniper berries
2 heaping tsp sea salt
5 drops arnica tincture
2 drops pine essential oil
2 drops lavender
  essential oil
2 drops lemon essential oil
2 drops juniper essential oil

DETOX BATH INFUSION

MAKES ENOUGH FOR 1 BATH

To encourage the elimination of toxins from the body, nutrient-rich bladder wrack is combined with cleansing sea salt, circulation-boosting juniper, black pepper, and lemon essential oils. For the best results, try dry body brushing with a natural bristle brush or body mitt before your bath to exfoliate the skin and energize the body.

METHOD

1 Make an infusion (p.176) with the water, bladder wrack, and celery and fennel seeds.
2 Add the essential oils to the salt, then add the salt to the infusion and stir until well dissolved. Use immediately by adding to a freshly run bath.

STIMULATES
CIRCULATION

SOOTHES TIRED MUSCLES

INGREDIENTS
2 cups hot water
½ tsp dried bladder wrack
1 tsp celery seeds
2 tsp fennel seeds
2 heaping tsp sea salt
2 drops juniper essential oil
2 drops black pepper
  essential oil
2 drops lemon essential oil
2 drops eucalyptus
  essential oil

GINGER AND JUNIPER WARMING FOOT SOAK

WARMS UP THE BODY

STIMULATES CIRCULATION

INGREDIENTS
1 tbsp dried rose hips
2 tbsp dried hibiscus
1 tsp cloves
1 tsp juniper berries
3 bay leaves, crushed
1 tbsp orange peel, fresh or dried
3 drops ginger essential oil

MAKES ENOUGH FOR 1 TREATMENT

This aromatic soak boosts the circulation and eliminates the chill from cold feet. Ginger has long been used for its warming action, while juniper is stimulating and cloves have mild pain-relieving properties. The aromatic bay leaves and orange peel in this therapeutic blend also delight the senses as the foot soak takes effect.

METHOD
1 Place all the ingredients in a muslin (cheesecloth) bag and gently stir the bag in a large bowl of boiling water.
2 After 10 minutes, add enough cold water to make the soak a comfortable temperature, but still hot. Immerse your feet in the liquid for as long as is comfortable, or until the water has cooled.

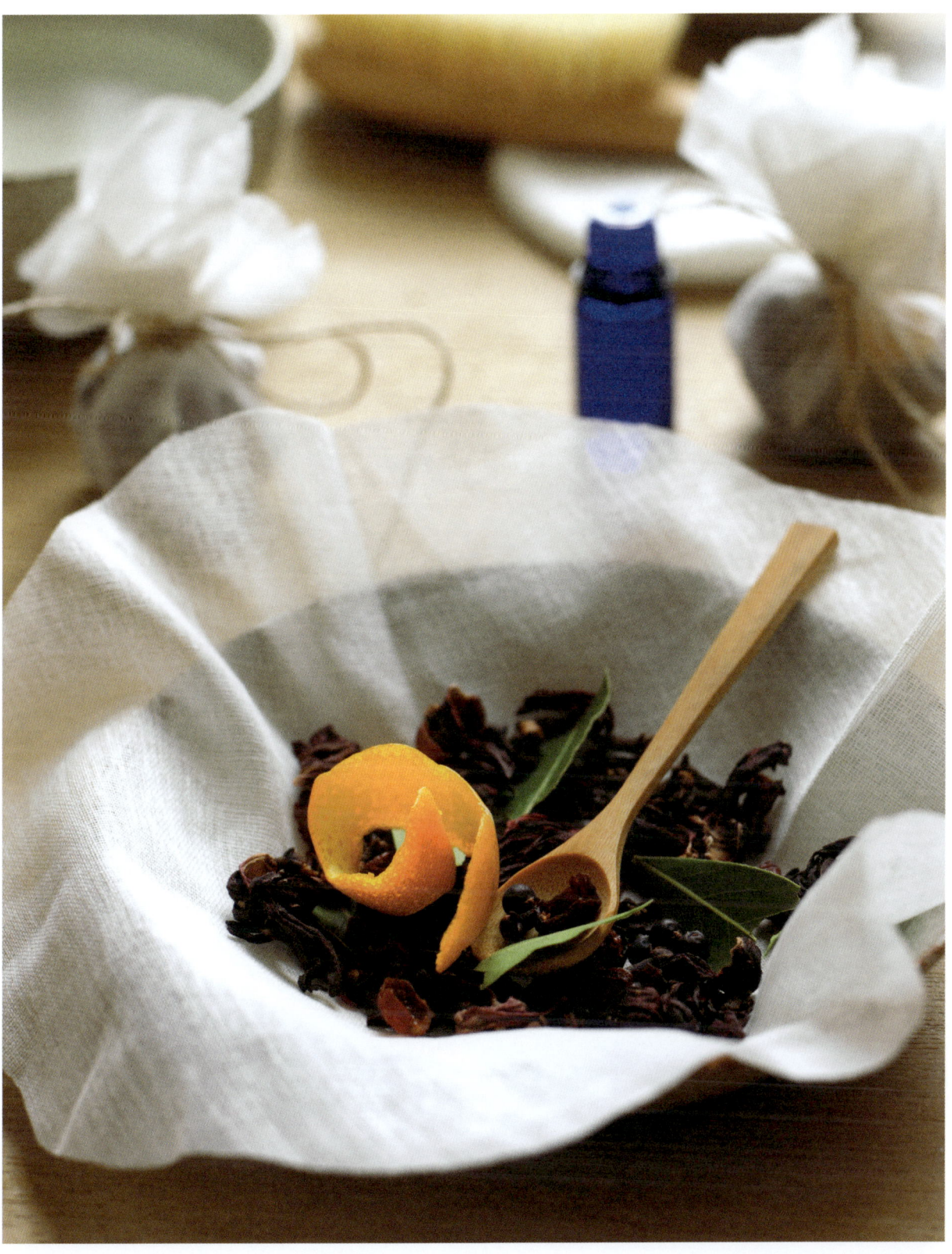

RELAX AND RESTORE BATH HERBS

RELAXES

SOOTHES TIRED MUSCLES

INGREDIENTS
2 tbsp raspberry leaves
2 tbsp violet leaves
2 tbsp lavender
2 tbsp oatmeal, powdered

MAKES ENOUGH FOR 1 BATH TREATMENT

Mildly astringent, tannin-rich raspberry leaves blend well with skin-soothing violet and relaxing lavender to create this fragrant, skin-friendly wash that eases the mind and body. Oatmeal has also been included, as it is known to be an excellent remedy for dry skin: it gently softens and nurtures the skin to leave it feeling smooth and moisturized.

METHOD

1 Combine the herbs and oatmeal and grind using a pestle and mortar (or a coffee grinder or blender) to make a coarse powder.
2 Place the powder in a muslin (cheesecloth) bag. Hang the bag under the faucet while running your bath so that the warm water flows through the herbs, then add the bag to your bath water. Lie back and relax.

POSTNATAL SITZ BATH

INGREDIENTS
2 tbsp calendula
2 tbsp chamomile
2 tbsp lavender
1 tbsp yarrow
1 tbsp shepherd's purse
   (*Capsella bursa-pastoris*)

MAKES ENOUGH FOR 1 BATH TREATMENT

A soothing herbal blend to encourage postnatal recovery. Calendula helps encourage natural cellular regeneration, while chamomile is gentle and soothing. Yarrow and shepherd's purse have anti-inflammatory properties. Cleansing lavender nurtures the skin and also provides a calming fragrance to aid relaxation.

METHOD
1 Boil enough water to make an infusion with the herbs (p.176).
2 When the infusion is cool, add to a warm, shallow bath (the water should only come up to the level of your hips). Allow yourself 10 minutes to soak in the bath. If you have had stitches, limit yourself to one sitz bath per day.

MAKING HAIR AND SCALP TREATMENTS

Beautiful hair depends on a healthy scalp.
Keep your scalp in good condition by washing
your hair in warm, not hot, water, and using
homemade herbal treatments to add extra
nutrition. Then rinse through for shiny,
revitalized hair with bounce.

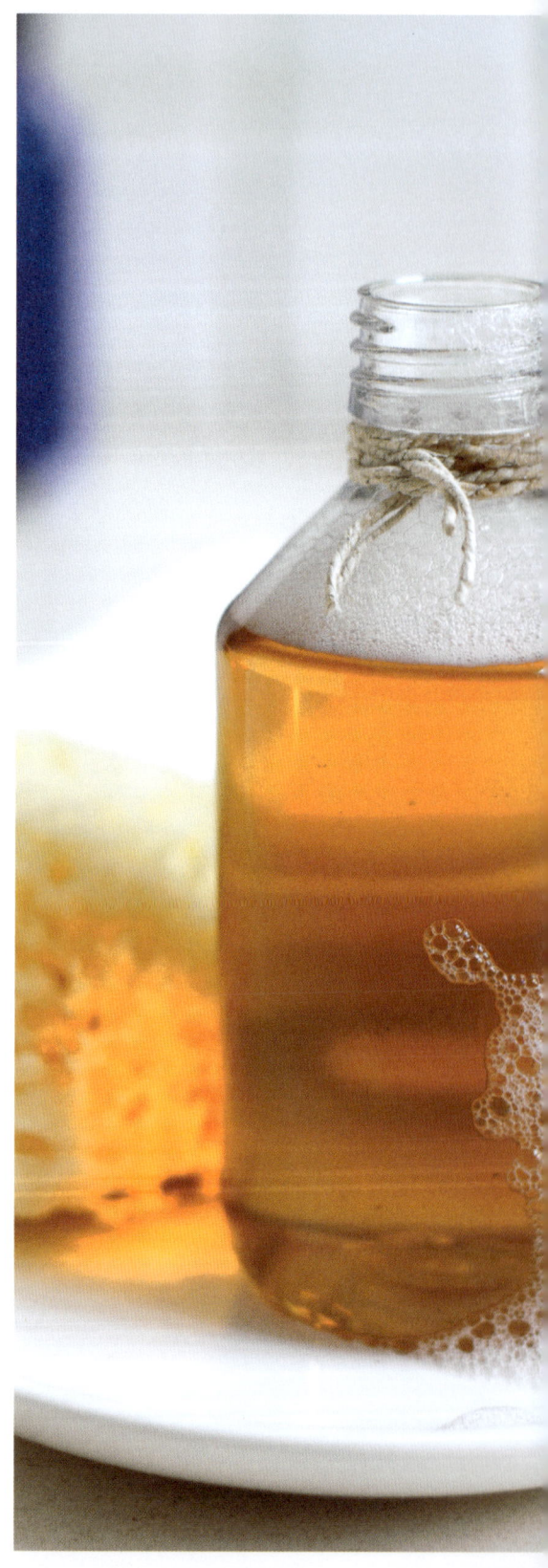

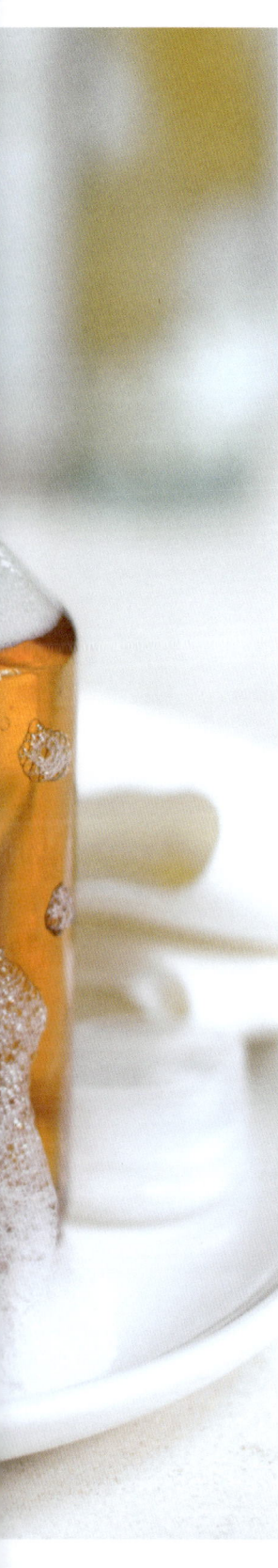

TREATS ALL HAIR TYPES

INGREDIENTS
3 tsp dried calendula
3 tsp dried comfrey
1 tsp dried horsetail

COMFREY HAIR TONIC

MAKES 1 TREATMENT

Comfrey has a conditioning effect on the hair and scalp, as it is rich in allantoin, which helps encourage natural cellular regeneration. Calendula soothes the scalp and is an excellent rinse for hair alongside shine-enhancing horsetail. This simple tonic nourishes both the hair and scalp to restore your hair's natural vitality.

METHOD
1 Infuse the dried herbs with ⅓ cup boiling water in a bowl.
2 Allow to stand and cool for 20 minutes, then strain through a sieve into a bowl. Discard the herbs.
3 Add the strained liquid to your shampoo up to a maximum ratio of 50 percent (the more you add, the thinner the shampoo will be). Use any excess infusion as a final rinse for the hair. Use within 1 week, or keep refrigerated and use within 2 weeks.

HORSETAIL SHAMPOO FOR DULL HAIR

INGREDIENTS
3 tbsp shampoo
3 tbsp infusion of equal
   parts horsetail, rosemary,
   and sage
scant 1 tsp almond oil
6 drops rosemary
   essential oil

MAKES 3½FL OZ (100ML)

Silica-rich horsetail is a traditional remedy used to restore vitality to lackluster hair. Combined with classic, shine-boosting, growth-encouraging rosemary; cooling, oil-balancing sage; and rich almond oil, it moisturizes and nourishes hair to make it stronger and healthier. It also enhances natural shine and bounce.

METHOD
Blend all the ingredients together well. Use within 1 week, or keep refrigerated and use within 2 weeks.

NETTLE SHAMPOO FOR DANDRUFF

INGREDIENTS
3 tbsp shampoo
3 tbsp infusion of equal
   parts lavender, nettle,
   and sage
scant 1 tsp borage
   (starflower) oil
6 drops cedarwood
   essential oil
2 drops lemon essential oil

MAKES 3½FL OZ (100ML)

Borage, also known as starflower oil, is rich in essential fatty acids, including gamma-linolenic acid, and is especially nourishing to dry, irritated skin. Combined with mineral-rich nettle, calming lavender, and cooling sage, this rinse helps soothe irritated scalps prone to dandruff. Cedarwood and lemon essential oils add to the restorative properties of the herbs.

METHOD
Blend all the ingredients together well. Use within 1 week, or keep refrigerated and use within 2 weeks.

NOURISHING CONDITIONER FOR DRY AND DAMAGED HAIR

TREATS DRY AND DAMAGED HAIR

INGREDIENTS
3 tbsp conditioner

3 tbsp infusion of equal
parts comfrey,
marshmallow,
and calendula

scant 1 tsp calendula oil

8 drops frankincense
essential oil

2 drops chamomile Roman
essential oil

MAKES 3½FL OZ (100ML)

Softening marshmallow and nourishing comfrey are combined here with a double calendula boost—both the soothing herbal infusion and the nutrient-rich oil—to bring first aid to brittle, fragile hair. Frankincense and Roman chamomile essential oils also lend their soothing, toning properties to this herbal conditioner.

METHOD

Blend all the ingredients together well. Use within 1 week, or keep refrigerated and use within 2 weeks.

ROSEMARY CONDITIONER FOR ALL HAIR TYPES

TREATS ALL HAIR TYPES

INGREDIENTS
3 tbsp conditioner

3 tbsp infusion of equal
parts rose, rosemary,
thyme

scant 1 tsp avocado oil

5 drops cedarwood
essential oil

3 drops orange essential oil

3 drops rosemary
essential oil

MAKES 3½FL OZ (100ML)

Stimulating rosemary is probably the most well-known herb included in treatments to encourage thick, healthy hair. It is sometimes used to darken the hair, so blondes may want to halve the quantity of the rosemary and add a chamomile infusion to make up the correct quantity. Avocado is a rich, nourishing oil that enriches the scalp and deeply moisturizes the hair.

METHOD

Blend all the ingredients together well. Use within 1 week, or keep refrigerated and use within 2 weeks.

THYME AND CIDER RINSE

TREATS DANDRUFF

INGREDIENTS
3¹/₂fl oz (100ml) apple
   cider vinegar
10 drops thyme essential oil

MAKES 3½FL OZ (100ML)

Thyme essential oil is warming and stimulating, has strong antifungal and antibacterial properties, and is traditionally used to give hair added strength. Apple cider vinegar makes a wonderfully cleansing, shine-enhancing hair tonic. This simple combination makes an excellent pre-wash treatment for anyone prone to dandruff.

METHOD
Blend the ingredients together and massage into the scalp. Leave for up to 5 minutes. Rinse with warm water and shampoo as usual. Use within 6 months.

ENRICHING COCONUT CONDITIONER

INGREDIENTS
3½oz (100g) jar coconut oil
8 drops lavender
  essential oil
7 drops mandarin
  essential oil
5 drops petitgrain
  essential oil

MAKES 3½FL OZ (100ML)

Coconut makes a wonderful, nurturing treatment for all hair types. It is easily absorbed into the scalp, enriches and moisturizes the skin, and softens and smooths hair. A combination of lavender, mandarin, and petitgrain essential oils bring a cleansing, fresh fragrance to this deeply conditioning treatment.

METHOD
1 Melt the coconut oil by standing the jar in a bowl of hot water (the water only needs to come half way up the sides of the jar). When the coconut oil is has melted, remove the jar from the bowl. Add the essential oils to the coconut oil, and stir before it sets. Allow to cool.
2 To use, melt a little of the infused oil in the palms of your hands and massage into the hair and scalp. Leave on for at least 2 hours, then shampoo off. Applying your shampoo before wetting your hair makes it easier to remove the coconut treatment. Use within 6 months.

"COCONUT OIL IS ONE OF NATURE'S BEST TREATMENTS FOR MOISTURIZING THE SKIN AND HAIR. LOOK FOR ORGANIC OR VIRGIN COLD-PRESSED COCONUT OIL FOR MAXIMUM NUTRITIONAL BENEFIT"

LAVENDER AND ROSEMARY CONDITIONER

INGREDIENTS

3½oz (100g) jar coconut oil

10 drops lavender essential oil

8 drops rosemary essential oil

6 drops geranium essential oil

MAKES 3½OZ (100G)

Super-enriching coconut is one of the greatest treats for the hair and scalp. It moisturizes the skin while smoothing and softening the hair, and is perfect for conditioning unruly curls or taming flyaway ends. The addition of lavender, rosemary, and geranium essential oils will stimulate hair growth and restore vitality to dull hair.

METHOD

1 Melt the coconut oil by standing the sealed jar in a bowl of hot water so that the water reaches halfway up the side of the jar.

2 Remove the jar, add the essential oils to the melted coconut oil, and mix thoroughly. Allow to cool and set. (In hot weather you may want to keep this blend in the fridge to keep it solid.)

3 To use, warm some of the blend by rubbing it in the palm of your hand to melt it, then work it methodically through the hair, concentrating on massaging the scalp. Then wrap a warm towel around your head and leave for 30 minutes.

4 Remove the oil by applying shampoo and working it into the hair before adding water. Rinse the hair and repeat with shampoo if necessary.

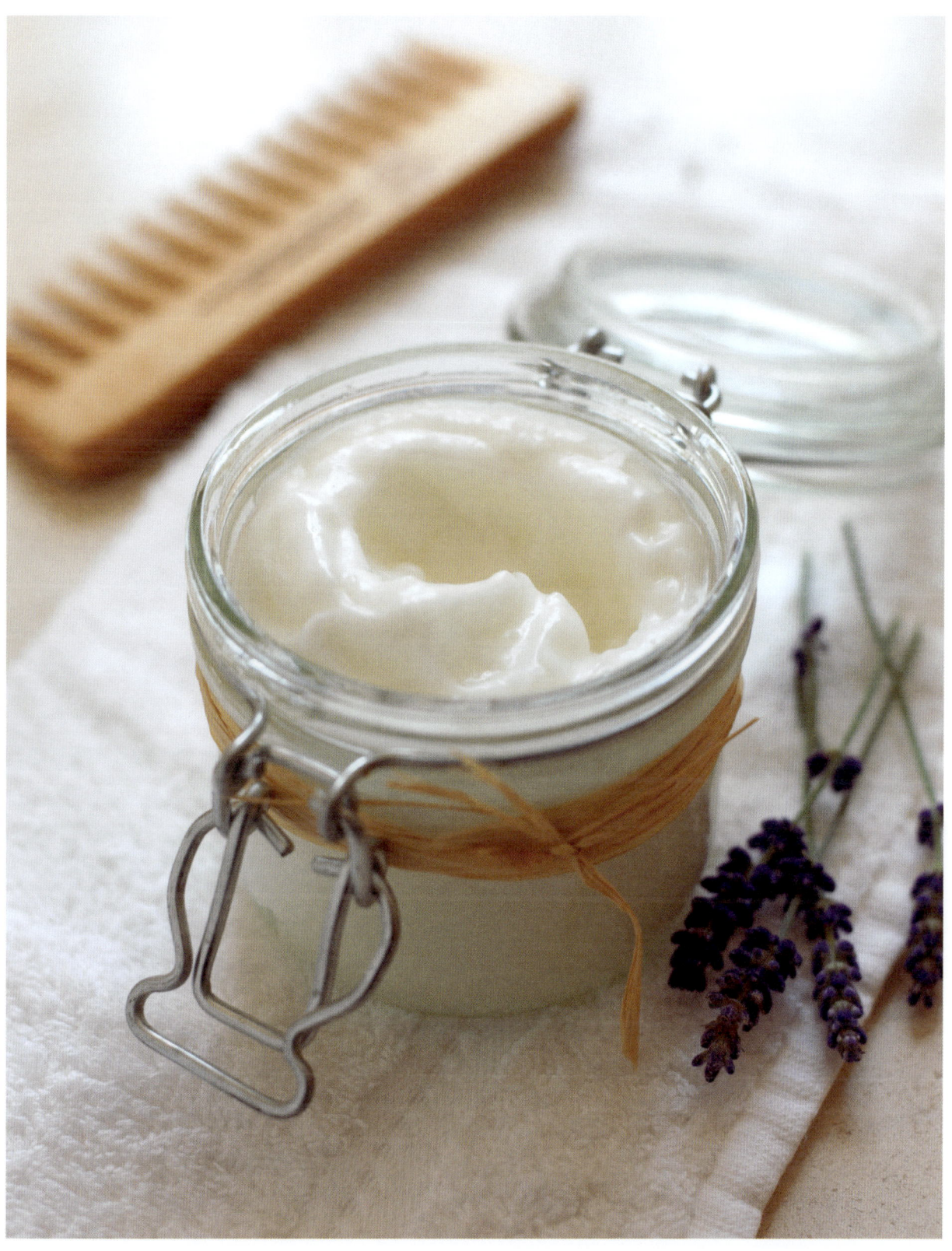

STIMULATING HAIR OIL

INGREDIENTS
2 tsp avocado oil
2 drops rosemary
  essential oil
2 drops basil essential oil

MAKES ENOUGH FOR 1 TREATMENT

Rich, green avocado oil is pressed from the flesh of the fruit rather than the seed. It is vitamin- and mineral-rich, as well as being high in essential fatty acids, and is extremely moisturizing. Toning rosemary and basil essential oils are also added to stimulate hair growth in this intensive conditioning treatment.

METHOD
1 Mix the avocado oil and essential oils together and decant into a bottle. Heat the oils by placing the bottle in a bowl of hot water.
2 Massage the oil into the scalp with firm circular movements with the pads of your fingers. Leave the mixture on the hair for 30 minutes, then shampoo. Applying your shampoo before wetting your hair makes it easier to remove the hair oil.
Use within 6 months.

CALENDULA AND BANANA HAIR TREATMENT

TREATS ALL HAIR TYPES

INGREDIENTS
1 ripe banana

2 tsp calendula
  macerated oil

3 drops ylang-ylang
  essential oil

a dash of lemon juice to add
  to shampoo

MAKES ENOUGH FOR 1 TREATMENT

Bananas are rich in potassium and amino acids, and make a great treatment for smoothing and nourishing dry or damaged hair. Combined with calendula macerated oil and ylang-ylang, this simple and moisturizing hair mask is particularly effective for taming unruly or frizzy curls.

METHOD

1 Use a blender to puree the banana to a smooth paste (this will make it easier to rinse from your hair), then combine with the calendula and ylang-ylang oils.

2 Wet your hair, squeeze out the excess water with a towel to leave hair damp, comb through, then apply the banana paste by massaging it into the hair.

3 Cover your hair with plastic wrap, an old shower cap, or a large plastic food bag (this will keep the mixture from drying out) and leave for 30 minutes. Wash out the mask using your normal shampoo with a dash of added lemon juice.

GLOSSARY

Adaptogenic
A restorative herb which helps increase the body's resistance to fatigue or stress

Alterative
Normalizes or reestablishes healthy nutritive processes

Analgesic
Relieves pain

Anaphrodisiac
Represses sexual desire

Anodyne
Allays pain

Antacid
Helps neutralize stomach acid

Anthelmintic
Treats infections by parasitic worms

Antiallergenic
Alleviates allergic reactions

Antiarrhythmic
Relieves an abnormal heart rate

Antibacterial
Kills bacteria or inhibits their growth or replication

Antibiotic
With properties that can destroy or inhibit the growth of microorganisms

Anticatarrhal
Efficacious against catarrh

Anticoagulant
Hinders blood clotting

Antidepressant
Helps alleviate depression

Antidiarrheal
Helps treat diarrhea

Antiemetic
Helps reduce vomiting

Antifungal
Destroying or inhibiting the growth of fungi

Antihidrotic
Reduces sweating

Antihistaminic
Counteracts the effect of histamine or inhibits its production in the body

Anti-inflammatory
Helps counteract inflammation

Antioxidant
A substance that reduces the damage caused by oxidation, such as the harm caused by free radicals

Antiparasitic
Kills or inhibits the growth or reproduction of parasites

Antiprostatic
Reduces symptoms relating to the prostate gland

Antirheumatic
Relief of symptoms of rheumatism

Antiscorbutic
Helps prevent scurvy (a condition caused by lack of vitamin C)

Antispasmodic
Reduces muscle spasm and tension

Antithrombotic
Preventing or interfering with the formation of a thrombus or blood clotting

Antitumorous
Reduces or inhibits the growth of tumors

Antitussive
Helps alleviate coughing

Antiviral
With properties that can destroy or inhibit the growth of viruses

Astringent
Causes contraction of tissues and inhibits the flow of blood or other secretions

Bitter
A digestive tonic, alterative, or appetizer

Bronchodilator
Opens up the bronchial tubes (air passages) of the lungs

Carminative
Reduces flatulence and gastric discomfort

Choleretic
Increases secretion of bile by the liver

Cholagogue
Stimulates the flow of bile

Demulcent
Softens and soothes inflamed surfaces

Diaphoretic
Promotes sweating

Diuretic
Encourages flow of urine

Emmenagogue
Stimulates blood flow to the pelvis and uterine area, may stimulate menstruation

Emollient
Softening and soothing, especially to the skin

Estrogenic
Promote or mimic the action of female hormones

Expectorant
Promotes the discharge of mucous or phlegm from the respiratory system

Febrifuge
Helps to reduce a fever

Galactagogue
Increases milk flow

Hemostatic
Capable of stopping hemorrhaging or bleeding

Hepatic restorative
Supports the liver

Hypoglycemic
Lowers the concentration of glucose in the blood

Hypolipidemic
Regulates cholesterol levels

Hypotensive
Helps lower blood pressure

Laxative
Encourages bowel movements

Nervine
Affects the nervous system (can be either stimulating or relaxing)

Nutritive
Beneficially nutritious

Oxytocic
Stimulates the smooth muscle of the uterus to contract, hastening or facilitating childbirth

Peripheral vasodilator
Improves blood flow, especially to hands and feet, used to treat conditions of poor circulation

Progesterogenic
Having or stimulating a progesterone-like activity

Purgative
Strong laxative

Relaxant
Tending to relax or to relieve tension

Rubefacient
Stimulates the flow of blood to the skin, causing localized reddening

Sedative
Soothing and calming

Soporific
Inducing or tending to induce sleep

Spasmolytic
Reduces muscle spasms

Stomachic
Beneficial to or stimulating digestion in the stomach

Styptic
Stops external bleeding

Vasodilator
Increases diameter of blood vessels

INDEX

ACKNOWLEDGMENTS

FIRST EDITION

Neal's Yard Remedies would like to thank the following for their valuable contribution to making this book happen: Julie Wood, Elly Phillips, Dr. Pauline Hili and the NYR technical team past and present, and Dr. Merlin Willcox.

Dorling Kindersley would like to thank the team at Neal's Yard Remedies, Peacemarsh, for the use of the organic physic garden in July and August 2010 for many of the herb photographs in this book. We would also like to thank Philip Robbshow at Sheepdrove Organic Farm for his help.

Thanks to the following for supplying plants for photography: Arne Herbs, Jekka's Herb Farm, Petersham Nurseries, Poyntzfield Herb Nursery, and South Devon Chilli Farm.

Thanks to the following for creating the first edition of the book: Susannah Steel, Peter Anderson, Peter Kindersley, William Reavell, Sarah Ruddick, Kathryn Wilding, Dawn Henderson, Marianne Markham, Nicola Powling, Caroline de Souza, Ben Marcus, Alice Sykes, Sonia Charbonnier, Alicia Ingty, Chitra Subramanyam, Tina Jindal, Ekta Sharma, Neha Ahuja, Devika Dwarkadas, Shruti Soharia Singh, Era Chawla, Glenda Fernandes, Navidita Thapa, Pankaj Sharma, Sunil Sharma, Dheeraj Arora, Jagtar Singh, Neeraj Bhatia, Tarun Sharma, Sourabh Challariyan, Debbie Maizels, Luis Peral, Nicky Collings, Jane Lawrie, Wei Tang, Jennifer Latham, Hilary Bird, Katy Greenwood, Roxanne Benson-Mackey, Kajal Mistry, Danaya Bunnag, Emma Forge, Lucy Claxton, and Romaine Werblow.

SECOND EDITION

Dorling Kindersley would like to thank Julia Behrens for her assistance in reviewing and updating content for the second edition. Thanks also to Toby Mann, Dawn Titmus, and Connor Kelly for editorial support.

Picture credit: 138 Steven Foster Group Inc.: (l).

ABOUT THE AUTHORS

Julia Behrens

Julia is a qualified medical herbalist with more than 20 years' experience. She has her own clinic in Brighton and also works with several doctors' offices. She has two children and is passionate about growing herbs, designing herb gardens, and teaching people how to take their health into their own hands.

Susan Curtis

Susan runs a busy practice as a homeopath and naturopath and is the Senior Brand Ambassador for Neal's Yard Remedies. She is the author of several books, including *Essential Oils*, and coauthor of *Natural Healing for Women*. Susan has two children and is passionate about helping people live a more natural and healthy lifestyle.

Louise Green

An avid supporter of the organic movement and eco-living, Louise has spent 25 years at Neal's Yard Remedies in a variety of roles ranging from buying to product development, and is currently the Head of Ethics & Sustainability. Louise lives in London with her artist husband and two children.

Penelope Ody MNIMH

Penelope qualified as a medical herbalist in the 1980s and practiced as a consultant herbalist for 12 years. Since then she has written more than 20 books on both Western and Chinese herbalism and runs workshops on traditional uses of culinary and medicinal herbs at her home in Hampshire.

Dragana Vilinac

A fourth-generation herbalist widely respected for her vast knowledge and expertise, Dragana's passion for herbal medicine has taken her around the world, and has led her to train in disciplines including Western Herbal Medicine and Traditional Chinese Medicine.

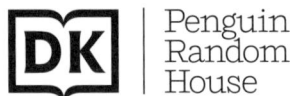

DK UK

Project editor Amy Slack
Senior designers Sara Robin, Glenda Fisher
Editor Helena Caldon
US editor Megan Douglass
US consultant Jane Wotton
Editorial assistant Millie Andrew
Production editors Heather Blagden, Jennifer Murray
Production controller Stephanie McConnell
Jacket designer Amy Cox
Jackets coordinator Lucy Philpott
Managing editors Stephanie Farrow, Ruth O'Rourke
Managing art editor Christine Keilty
Art director Maxine Pedliham
Publisher Mary-Clare Jerram

DK INDIA

Senior DTP designer Pushpak Tyagi
DTP designer Manish Upreti
Pre-production manager Sunil Sharma

This American Edition, 2020
First American Edition, 2011
Published in the United States by DK Publishing
1450 Broadway, Suite 801, New York, NY 10018

Copyright © 2011, 2020 Dorling Kindersley Limited
DK, a Division of Penguin Random House LLC
25 10 9 8 7 6
006 017024 Jul/2020

A catalog record for this book
is available from the Library of Congress.
ISBN: 978-1-4654-9430-6

DK books are available at special discounts when purchased in bulk for
sales promotions, premiums, fund-raising, or educational use.
For details, contact: DK Publishing Special Markets, 1450 Broadway,
Suite 801, New York, NY 10018
SpecialSales@dk.com

Printed and bound in China

www.dk.com

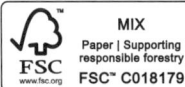

This book was made with Forest
Stewardship Council™ certified
paper – one small step in DK's
commitment to a sustainable future.
Learn more at **www.dk.com/uk/
information/sustainability**

DISCLAIMER: Herbs contain natural medicinal properties and should be treated with respect. This book is not intended as a medical reference book, but as a source of information. Do not take any herbal remedies if you are undergoing any other course of medical treatment without seeking professional advice. Before trying herbal remedies, the reader is advised to sample a small quantity first to establish whether there is any adverse or allergic reaction. The reader is advised not to attempt self-treatment for serious or long-term problems, during pregnancy, or for children without consulting a qualified medicinal herbalist. Neither the authors nor the publisher shall be liable or responsible for any loss or damage allegedly arising from any recipes, recommendations, and instructions contained herein, and the use of any herb or derivative is entirely at the reader's own risk.